Client-Centered Reasoning

Client-Centered Reasoning
Narratives of People with Mental Illness

Pat Precin, M.S., O.T.R./L.

*Director, P.R.I.D.E. 2000, Adult Rehabilitation Services,
Brooklyn Bureau of Community Services, Brooklyn, New York*

With a Contribution by

Marilyn Maxwell, Ph.D.

*Teacher, English Department, George W. Hewlett High School,
Hewlett, New York*

With a Foreword by

Anne Hiller Scott, Ph.D., O.T.R., F.A.O.T.A.

*Director, Division of Occupational Therapy,
School of Health Professions, Long Island University,
Brooklyn, New York*

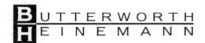

An imprint of Elsevier Science

Boston   Oxford   Auckland   Johannesburg   Melbourne   New Delhi

Butterworth–Heinemann is an imprint of Elsevier Science.

Every effort has been made to ensure that the drug dosage schedules within this text are accurate and conform to standards accepted at time of publication. However, as treatment recommendations vary in the light of continuing research and clinical experience, the reader is advised to verify drug dosage schedules herein with information found on product information sheets. This is especially true in cases of new or infrequently used drugs.

 Recognizing the importance of preserving what has been written, Elsevier Science prints its books on acid-free paper whenever possible.

Library of Congress Cataloging-in-Publication Data

Precin, Pat.
    Client-centered reasoning : narratives of people with mental illness / Pat Precin ; with a contribution by Marilyn Maxwell ; with a foreword by Anne Hiller Scott.
        p. cm.
    Includes bibliographical references and index.
    ISBN 0-7506-7374-5 (pbk. : alk. paper)
    1. Mental illness—Personal narratives. 2. Mentally ill—United States—Biography.
I. Maxwell, Marilyn. II. Title.

RC464.A1 P74 2002
616.89′0092′273—dc21
[B]   2001052928

British Library Cataloguing-in-Publication Data
A catalogue record for this book is available from the British Library.

The publisher offers special discounts on bulk orders of this book.
For information, please contact:

Manager of Special Sales
Elsevier Science
225 Wildwood Avenue
Woburn, MA 01801-2041
Tel: 781-904-2500
Fax: 781-904-2620

For information on all Butterworth–Heinemann publications available, contact our World Wide Web home page at: http://www.bh.com

10 9 8 7 6 5 4 3 2 1

Printed in the United States of America

To My Family:
Marilyn, Virginia, Paul, Bentley, and Devon

Contents

Foreword

The art and science of practice—in this time of evidence-based practice, we can surely teach the science, but how well do we convey the art of working with people who have psychosocial issues? Our own research in the health professions has documented that students have prejudices toward this population similar to those of the lay community (Lyons and Hayes, 1993) and students are less likely to select work with this population (Ezersky et al., 1989). Ann Mosey (1981, p. 1), referring to the art of practice, once said that, in our art, "we touch if only for a moment the realness of each other." The ability to touch the "realness" allows therapists to transcend the challenges of difficult clients and reach them through meaningful interaction. As students enter mental health settings, to reach their potential to touch the realness, they must often first work through layers of fear, ignorance, and stereotypical attitudes. Fear and anxiety are rarely the ideal medium for learning delicate lessons of empathy, sensitive interpersonal intervention, client-centered reasoning, and reflective thinking. Students are less likely to have had prior clinical exposure to people with psychosocial issues. These basic skills are best cultivated through frequent exposure and opportunity to engage with them, and then stepping back from engagement to process the interaction.

How well can a textbook on psychosocial issues prepare students for the difficult challenges of the clinical setting? It is, after all, the *practice* that is important to students. Practice makes perfect, and students in the health professions need to be "hands-on" learners. Remarkably, this book rises to the challenge like no other text available. *Client-Centered Reasoning: Narratives of People with Mental Illness* offers a unique format that allows us to enter into the private thoughts of students on fieldwork and clients in treatment. It is like having an opportunity to watch a story unfold through a two-way mirror, a silent witness to the hidden thoughts, feelings, doubts, and concerns that emerge in the course of everyday practice. This unique volume represents a rich collection of dozens of students' logs, revealing the silent dialogue that accompanies the students' journey of evolution and maturation, from a point of fear or uncertainty in the beginning of their experience to a place of confidence, compassion, and meaningful engagement with people struggling with psychosocial issues. Equally compelling are the many narratives offered by people at various points on the continuum described by Yalom (1985) from "coping to collapse."

Putting a face on the people and their unique circumstances helps diffuse some of the stereotypes and prejudices that are all too common.

But it is not the rich tapestry of the narratives alone that provides the vehicle for negotiating mastery. The author gives students exactly what they need, the opportunity to practice repeatedly on clients at a safe distance. Firsthand exposure to the full continuum of mental health issues is proffered in the context of real people struggling with real problems and real students dealing with mastery of techniques and knowledge to provide client-centered care. The student bears witness to the impact of symptoms of schizophrenia, depression, manic-depressive illness, substance abuse, dementia, AIDS, and other psychiatric conditions. The potential consequences of denial and lack of insight, boundary issues, aggression, violence, hypersexuality, reactions to medication and electroconvulsive therapy (ECT), the role of clients' rights in intervention, and many more significant areas are explored.

The author has a gift for shaping probing questions and assignments to plumb the depths of student learning and raise sensitivity. The therapeutic use of self is rendered a real phenomenon as students explore various possibilities and outcomes in the workbook sections on client-centered reasoning and client-centered activities that are offered throughout the text. Students are given the opportunity for exploration and rehearsal of treatment interventions and outcomes through these and a variety of other exercises and assignments. Reasoning skills are honed as the student expands or rewrites narratives; writes between the lines, interspersing his or her own thoughts and perspectives; and develops approaches to assessment, group protocols, discharge planning, and aftercare activities in a full spectrum of settings with a large variety of clients. Students' insight is gradually deepened through many activities that require them to probe client-centered care through many student and client narratives. These exploratory exercises offer the opportunity for repetition and reinforcement in building a solid framework for a more grounded grasp of mental health practice.

Educators recognize the value of peer support and shared learning. However, most students navigate what they perceive as a treacherous journey alone as a solo student on a psychosocial fieldwork placement. This textbook empowers students to work with fellow classmates in exploring the challenges of mental health practice through various group activities and assignments. Students become role models for each other. The student voices in this book enable future students the opportunity to see the growth process firsthand. They bear witness to these peers' ability to gather the courage to confront the unknown, the sometimes inaccessible and incomprehensible, and begin to help ease the spiritual torment, to mend fractured minds and lives through client-sensitive care. Last, as literature, the many stories by students and persons with mental illness are compelling and moving reading—once started it is difficult to put down—not many texts will make this claim. This book is a necessity for the classroom and equally appropriate for the clinical supervisor and fieldwork student.

Anne Hiller Scott, Ph.D., O.T.R., F.A.O.T.A.

REFERENCES

Ezersky S, Havazelet L, Scott A, Zettler C. Specialty preference in occupational therapy. *American Journal of Occupational Therapy* 1989;43(4): 227–233.

Lyons M, Hayes R. Student perceptions of persons with psychiatric and other disorders. *American Journal of Occupational Therapy* 1993;47(6):541–548.

Mosey AC. Introduction: The art of practice. In B Abreu (ed), *A Manual for Physical Disabilities.* New York: Raven Press, 1981;1–3.

Yalom I. *The Theory and Practice of Group Psychotherapy*, 3rd ed. New York: Basic Books, 1985.

Preface

PURPOSE AND OBJECTIVES OF THIS BOOK

This book was written to help students prepare for their clinical internships while still in the classroom; more specifically, to foster development of necessary clinical reasoning and problem-solving skills to begin their work with people who have barriers that inhibit occupational performance and engagement due to mental health issues or substance abuse. Occupational performance is the ability to perform the activities of daily living and tasks in the areas of play and leisure, self-care, work and productive activities; and engagement is the act of enhancing or enabling occupational performance (American Occupational Therapy Association Commission on Practice, 2000). This book attempts to motivate and prepare students for the complex process of learning effective mental health intervention. This process includes overcoming prejudices and fears associated with this population; gaining a holistic understanding of people in context who live with psychological issues; learning ways to build rapport with people who are resistant or lack insight into their psychosocial barriers; identifying barriers to occupational performance; identifying issues and problems of substance abuse and how they affect occupational performance; applying theory and conscious use of self to clients in context and activity; identifying and working with countertransference issues; setting limits and boundaries; avoiding burnout; dealing with violence, hypersexuality, and aggression; becoming familiar with psychosocial intervention settings and becoming aware of what may be expected during a psychosocial affiliation.

To accomplish these objectives, the book utilizes stories written by clients (client narratives), stories written by occupational therapy (OT) interns about their clients (intern narratives), and daily logs written by OT interns about their internship experiences in mental health (logs). In addition, some of these writings are analyzed by an experienced clinical mental health OT, the author (analyses). Finally, reflective questions written by the author and related to the narratives are used to enhance the thinking processes necessary in developing clinical reasoning and problem-solving skills (client-centered reasoning questions and activities).

Drawing on client-centered intervention, this book attempts to develop clinical reasoning skills through active engagement with the client, viewed as a whole person in context and activity; hence, the title *Client-Centered Reasoning: Narratives of People with Mental Illness.*

HOW THIS BOOK CAME ABOUT

In my work with over 100 interns from 25 different schools, I found that, no matter how well the student curriculum is written, taught, and learned, when students begin their psychosocial internships they are often apprehensive, anxious, and fearful. The images conjured up at the mere mention of psychosocial barriers are often terrifying to new students. Preconceived images of "psychiatric" clients have been described as horrifying, unpredictable, uncontrollable, malodorous, crazy, dirty, disgusting, belligerent, angry, hostile, sex-crazed, fragile, bizarre, and scary. Many negative preconceived prejudices about people with psychosocial issues accompany interns to their internship placements. These prejudices are held not only by interns but also often by their significant others and family members. Some of these negative stereotypes include homeless, criminals, bums, drug addicts, drunks, rapists, prostitutes, molesters, monsters, people to avoid, subway pushers, murderers, and serial killers.

When interns begin their psychosocial internships they are usually in shock for the first couple of weeks. I remember my first day, when I hid in the chart room. Here are quotes from two different interns' logs:

> I remember the first time I went onto the unit. When I walked through the door and spotted a client, I began to feel very nervous. The butterflies in my stomach were tremendous; I thought I might be sick. Clients' faces flew by me as we walked to the nursing station. I could not process what I was seeing. Everything looked so bizarre to me. It was a surreal experience. (Anonymous)

A second intern writes,

> Upon entering the unit, I quickly noticed the number of clients lingering in the hallways. I remember taking a big sigh and began walking with the other interns. . . . I was suddenly distracted by a loud voice, "I am not crazy, I am not crazy, I am not crazy." I jerked my neck around and found a disturbed client talking to himself while he rapidly walked down the hall. As we proceeded down the hall to the intersection of a corridor, a client that did not seem to know that I was right in front of her cut me off. She gave a menacing stare. I observed a man in a hospital gown standing tremulous in front of the nurse's station. I can describe him as looking like a shaking zombie. All of this happened within my first five minutes on the unit. I was now terrified and having feelings of insecurity. I felt unsure of myself. I did not know if I was going to be able to handle the pressure and stress of the unit and the clients. I thought that I was going to drown. (Sheena Sethi)

The interns' anxiety levels can be so high that they inhibit their use of theory and techniques gained in the classroom.

In general, interns often feel more comfortable talking to each other about their fears, their insecurities, and their intense reactions toward clients instead of admitting them to their supervisors. Interns' feedback from each other can also be effective in resolving some of these fears and inadequacies on the unit. Unfortunately, most internship sites have only one intern from a specific discipline at a time, or the workload may be so heavy that too little time is allotted for such discussions.

For his student project, Vladimir Sychev, one of my interns, wrote about his internship experiences. Future interns at the same intervention site read his experiences. The new interns were then better prepared to face similar challenges, felt more confident in their work, felt less isolated, and had a much easier time admitting that they had similar fears, anxieties, and prejudices. Vladimir's paper also enabled new interns to open up early communication with their supervisors by giving the new interns permission to feel, experience, and express what they were going through. Vladimir's paper was published in a two-volume journal (Sychev, 1998a) and as a chapter of a book (Sychev, 1998b), so that other interns may benefit from his experiences.

Because Vladimir's writings were so helpful, I began to assign all of my interns similar writing exercises. After a few years, I had collected many narratives and logs containing valuable internship experiences. I organized them into chapters that each emphasized a certain point or theme necessary to learn in order to provide clinically sound intervention to people with psychosocial issues. This book is the result of these writings and clients' writings organized into a meaningful collection of experiences for anyone wishing to increase his or her knowledge and practice of working with psychosocially challenged clients.

HOW THIS BOOK IS UNIQUE

Most books on clinical reasoning are heavily laden with theoretical aspects of clinical judgment. In addition to these theoretical texts, a clinically-based, self-reflective approach (such as this text) provides rich personal material in which to utilize these theories. Lewin and Reed's (1998) book uses some clinical material with a variety of creative exercises for the learner to sharpen such problem-solving skills as story writing, crossword puzzles, flowcharts, dictionaries, maps, reflective journal entries, word searches, and self-assessments. However, this work is not specific to mental health. To date, few books devote themselves entirely to increasing clinical judgment in the area of mental health. Mental health practices can be more difficult to learn than other areas of practice, due to the nature of psychosocial barriers that do not lend themselves to concrete, well-defined intervention procedures.

Many articles have been written on how journal (log) writing can be helpful to therapists during their psychosocial internships (Baldwin, 1991; Buchanan, Moore, and Niekerk, 1998; Crepeau, 1991; Delve, Mintz, and Stewart, 1990; Greene, 1997; Hurtig et al., 1989; Landeen, Byrne, and Brown, 1992; Lyons and Hayes, 1993; Manen, 1990; Myerhoff, 1992; Peloquin and Davidson, 1993; Progoff, 1975; Sedlak, 1992; Tryssenaar, 1995). However, little has been written on how reading someone else's logs can be helpful. I believe that studying logs (written by other interns about their internship experiences) before beginning their own internship will aid students in acquiring clinical judgment and problem-solving skills, help them integrate theory and practice, and better prepare them for the experience before they actually begin it.

This book uses clinical material to teach clinical reasoning through a learner's perspective, instead of through highly intellectualized theoretical frames of reference. This book fosters the development of clinical reasoning skills through the use of narratives, logs, activities, questions, and critical and clinical analyses by the author. The clinical material in this book is unabashed, honest, all-inclusive, and laden with prejudices and mistakes made by people learning to work with clients that have psychosocial issues. The reader becomes intimately involved with the personal stories of clients and those who have been interacting with them. It tells real stories about real people in pain. In unadorned fashion, this book gives the reader a glimpse of the struggles, disappointments, joys, mistakes, prejudices, misconceptions, and fears surrounding psychosocial issues; and the interactions are fraught with emotional intensity, on the part of both the client and the helper.

All the interns who contributed to this book had internships on locked inpatient psychiatric units handling clients with mixed diagnoses, with the exception of a few interns who worked with people in a five- to seven-day inpatient drug and alcohol detoxification unit. These sites were chosen because they provide intervention for people whose psychosocial issues are extremely severe and who are difficult to work with, especially for novices. While not everyone will be working with people whose issues are so severe, the knowledge and clinical reasoning gained while reading about this population may benefit students assigned to other sites. Although these sites tend to be medically modeled, the narratives provide a rich array of material that can and must include other intervention sites, such as the client's home, community, and follow-up intervention sites. The theme of substance abuse occurs with some regularity and is the topic of a chapter because of its frequent comorbidity with psychosocial issues. Fifty percent of people being treated for psychosocial issues also have had a substance abuse or dependence problem (Helzer and Przybeck, 1988; Kosten and Kleber, 1888; Miller, 1993; Regier et al., 1990). Many more occurrences of substance abuse go undetected or untreated. Unless intervention is given for the substance abuse, the person will most likely continue to experience ongoing psychosocial barriers (Precin, 1999).

Acquiring and teaching clinical judgment in mental health have always been challenges, as have bridging theory and practice. Integration of problem-based learning (PBL) and other techniques into the classroom to better prepare students for clinical internships has been successful. However, students are still entering their internships with doubts about applying their acquired knowledge and fear about working with psychosocial clients, fear that impedes them from using their acquired skills. This book helps enlighten students about the realities of working with psychosocial clients and helps them solve problems, before they begin their internships, concerning personally difficult issues that may arise while working with clients.

REFERENCES

American Occupational Therapy Association (AOTA) Commission on Practice. *Occupational Therapy Practice Framework: Engagement and Participation in Occupation*, Draft IV. Bethesda, MD: AOTA, 2000:9.

Baldwin C. *One to One Self-Understanding Through Journal Writing.* New York: M. Evans, 1991.

Buchanan H, Moore R, Niekerk L Van. The fieldwork case study: Writing for clinical reasoning. *American Journal of Occupational Therapy* 1998;52: 291–295.

Crepeau EB. Achieving intersubjective understanding: Examples from an occupational therapy treatment session. *American Journal of Occupational Therapy* 1991;45:1016–1025.

Delve CI, Mintz SD, Stewart GM. Promoting values development through community service: A design. *New Directions for Student Services* 1990; 50:7–29.

Greene D. The use of service learning in client environments to enhance ethical reasoning in students. *American Journal of Occupational Therapy* 1997;51:844–852.

Helzer JE, Przybeck TR. The co-occurrence of alcoholism with other psychiatric disorders in general population and its impact on treatment. *Journal of Studying Alcohol* 1988;49:219–224.

Hurtig W, Yonge O, Bodnar D, Berg M. The interactive journal: A clinical teaching tool. *Nurse Educator* 1989;14(6):17,31,35.

Kosten TR, Kleber HD. Differential diagnosis of psychiatric comorbidity in substance abusers. *Journal of Substance Abuse Treatment* 1988;5:201–206.

Landeen J, Byrne C, Brown B. Journal keeping as an educational strategy in teaching psychiatric nursing. *Journal of Advanced Nursing* 1992;17:347–355.

Lewin JE, Reed AC. *Creative Problem Solving in Occupational Therapy.* Philadelphia: Lippincott Williams and Wilkins, 1998.

Lyons M, Hayes R. Student perceptions of persons with psychiatric and other disorders. *American Journal of Occupational Therapy* 1993;47:541–548.

Manen M van. *Researching Lived Experience: Human Science for an Action Sensitive Pedagogy.* London, Ontario: Althouse, 1990.

Miller NS. Comorbidity of psychiatric and alcohol/drug disorders: Interactions and independent status. *Journal of Addictive Diseases* 1993;12(3): 5–16. Also published in: Miller NS, Stimmel B (eds). *Comorbidity of Addictive and Psychiatric Disorders.* Binghampton, NY: Haworth Press, 1993: 5–16.

Myerhoff B. *Remembered Lives: The Work of Ritual, Storytelling and Growing Older.* Ann Arbor: University of Michigan Press, 1992.

Peloquin SM, Davidson DA. Brief or new—interpersonal skills for practice: An elective course. *American Journal of Occupational Therapy* 1993;47: 260–264.

Precin P. *Living Skills Recovery Workbook.* Boston: Butterworth–Heinemann, 1999:xiv.

Progoff I. *At a Journal Workshop: The Basic Text and Guide for Using the Intensive Journal.* New York: Dialogue House Library, 1975.

Regier DA, Farmer ME, Rae DS, et al. Comorbidity of mental disorders with alcohol and other drug abuse. *JAMA* 1990;264(19):2511–2518.

Sedlak CA. Use of clinical logs by beginning nursing students and faculty to identify learning needs. *Journal of Advanced Nursing* 1992;31(1):24–28.

Sychev V. Memoirs from a mental health affiliation. *Occupational Therapy in Mental Health: A Journal of Psychosocial Practice and Research.* 1998a: 129–142.

Sychev V. Memoirs from a mental health affiliation. In: AH Scott (ed), *New Frontiers in Psychosocial Occupational Therapy.* Binghamton, NY: Haworth Press, 1998b:129–142.

Tryssenaar J. Interactive journals: An educational strategy to promote reflection. *American Journal of Occupational Therapy* 1995;49:695–702.

Acknowledgments

I would like to acknowledge St. Lukes-Roosevelt Hospital's inpatient psychiatric and detoxification units in New York City, where most of these narratives were written, and the units' staff for their clinical expertise and receptivity to the training of interns: Steve Reibel (unit chief); Robert Fletcher and Antoinette Mitchell (occupational therapy aids), and Frauke Glaubitz (dance therapist) for helping supervise; Elisabeth Refn (occupational therapist) and Sarah Nazimova-Baum (art therapist) for conducting weekly intern seminars; and Marie Sarano, Maria Rios, and Catherine Plum (social workers) for their collaboration with interdisciplinary intern groups.

My sincere appreciation goes to all the clients who shared their stories: Jennifer Lane, Wesley Morrow, Mr. Leavy, Thomas Daniel, Stephen Domina, Lurlene Williams, Julie Taylor, Marc Wolsky, Joyce Chatman, Kathryn Fazio, Vladimir Ramirez, Mark Jules, Corey Simmelkjaer, Clifton Winston, Mandy Fernandez, Jerome Bowens, Carl James, and all the anonymous client writers. I am grateful to the interns who, through individual sessions and creative writing groups, encouraged these clients to write.

I thank the interns who contributed their experiences through writing narratives or logs for this book: Nancy Moritz-Farajun, Keri Reilly, Liliana Mosquera, Laura Bella-Bryant, Eileen Tierney, Elodie Montivero, Aviva Graber, Francia Brito, Rebecca Philip, Marsha Eiserman, Kate Harrington, Kelly Morales, Christine Weiss, Philip Macri, Sheena Sethi, and Gina DeMeo. I thank Jennifer Werner of Hewlett High School's creative writing class, instructed by Dr. Marilyn Maxwell, for her fictional narrative. I also thank Dr. Marilyn Maxwell for her contributions to Chapters 1 and 2.

The following schools in the New York area were responsible for sending high-quality interns to St. Lukes-Roosevelt Hospital: Columbia University, SUNY Health Science Center at Brooklyn, LaGuardia Community College, Kean College, Dominican College, Long Island University, Mercy College, New York Institute of Technology, Philadelphia College of Pharmacy and Science, University of Scranton, Stony Brook School of Health Technology and Management, Suffolk County Community College, Touro College, York College, and New York University. Their fieldwork coordinators Pam Miller, Janet Falk-Kessler, Emily Raphael, Jan Garbarini, David Pallister, Jude De Prospo, Carlotta Kip, Naomi Greenberg, Anne Hiller Scott, Albert Wong, Kathleen Golisz, Phyllis Mirenberg, Lisa Gordon, Susan Haiman,

Acknowledgments

Marty Hill, Rhonda Waskiewicz, Eva Rodreguez, Pei-Fen Chang, Michelle Egan, Catherine Serpico, Lydia Borges, Robin Katz, Ariela Neuman, Tina Barth, Elyse Pimsler, Diane Tewfik, Gloria Graham, and Paula McCreedy were integral in the collaborative process between school and clinic, necessary for interns to emerge as therapists.

I am fortunate to have worked with Leslie Forman and Jennifer Rhuda from Butterworth–Heinemann a second time in the production of this current book. I am thankful for the helpful feedback from Rosanna Tufano, Suzanne White, Diane Tewfik, Anne Hiller Scott, and other readers who reviewed the proposal and to Anne Hiller Scott for providing a Foreword. I am grateful to Peter LaBarbera for emotional support and Cheryl King for being a wonderful boss.

Client-Centered Reasoning

Client-Centered Reasoning Ingredients

Pat Precin and Marilyn Maxwell

CLINICAL REASONING

Mastery of the various techniques of clinical reasoning can prove beneficial to those professionals working with people who have barriers to occupational performance (clients). Many theories and techniques have been advanced to aid in the development of sound clinical reasoning and problem solving (Barris and Kielhofner, 1985; Burke and Depoy, 1991; Crepeau, 1991; Elstein, 1976; Elstein, Schulman, and Sprafka, 1978; Fleming, 1991a, 1991b; Gillette and Mattingly, 1987; Higgs and Jones, 2000; Kassirer, Kuipers, and Gorry, 1982; Krefting, 1985; Law, 1998; Law and McColl, 1989; Mattingly, 1989, 1991a, 1991b; Mattingly and Fleming, 1994; Neuhaus, 1988; Parham 1987; Reed, 1984; Rogers, 1983, 1986; Rogers and Masagatani, 1982; Schell and Cervero, 1993; Schwartz, 1991). Several recent books (Benamy, 1999; Bridge, 1999; Halloran and Lowenstein, 2000; Lewin and Reed, 1998) have been written as tools to help increase clinical judgment in students entering the field of occupational therapy in the areas of physical disabilities, pediatrics, and geriatrics.

CLIENT-CENTERED INTERVENTION

Client-centered intervention is a method of practice in which the person receiving services directs the focus and nature of the intervention (Fearing and Clark, 2000; Law, 1998). The person works with the therapist to develop goals and solve problems he or she faces. The role of the therapist is to help elicit goals and solutions from the person so they are meaningful and relevant to the person's life. While Fearing and Clark (2000) and Law (1998) recently wrote books dedicated to this subject matter, the historical roots of client-centered intervention reside with Carl Rogers (1939), who was against the idea that the therapist was more of an expert than the person receiving services. Instead, he believed that it was important for the therapist to listen closely and spend an ample amount of time with the client to learn about the client's life experiences. The differences among individuals are acknowledged in client-centered practice, but Rogers did not address how to work with such diversities. Strong clinical reasoning skills are necessary to treat each person as the unique individual he or she is in context and activity.

The title of this book includes the words *client-centered reasoning*, because the reader can get to know these clients intimately through the descriptive narratives so that their clinical reasoning truly reflects clients as whole people with specific wants and needs in their environment. The clients should come alive in the readers' minds as they read the narratives because of the straightforward, bar-nothing, honest way in which they are written. The true essence of the client comes out of the narratives, more so than in case studies, a popular style of writing that imparts clinical information about clients and is not used in this book. The narratives read like an unfolding story of a client's life, where gaps of information may be abundant. This is a realistic picture of how clients often present themselves. Clients do not present themselves in the concise, organized manner in which case studies impart information. In fact, much redirection, limit setting, and artful questioning may be necessary to elicit any information at all. At times, material has been purposefully omitted from the narratives and logs, material such as intervention plans, assessments used, and details about the clients' lives in order for students to develop and use their own clinical reasoning skills.

FORMAT OF THIS BOOK

This book includes

1. Client narratives.
2. Intern narratives.
3. Logs.
4. Client-centered reasoning questions and activities.
5. Analyses.

This text format reflects an emphasis on narratives, logs, and clinical and critical analyses as vehicles by which students become conversant with the tools of clinical reasoning. Here, a narrative is a story that describes a client's situation; it can be written by clients or interns. For the purposes of this book, interns are people acquiring on-the-job experience in their area of study; that is, fieldwork, internship, and/or affiliation. Students are people still learning in the classroom. Logs are a set of journal entries that describe interns' thoughts, feelings, actions, and reflections as they work with clients throughout their internship. Clients' names have been changed in all the narratives and logs written by interns to protect anonymity.

This material is organized into chapters based on a particular theme or lesson to be learned. Such lessons include learning that people with psychosocial issues have basic wants and needs similar to other people; mental illness can happen to anyone at any time; due to such strong defenses or denial, some people have to lose just about everything they have before they can acquire insight into their barriers and accept the help they need; recovery from substance abuse is an on-going life process; and people with psychosocial issues usually experience many losses, such as the loss of functioning, identity, family, friends, support systems, jobs, significant others, children, or hope. Additional objectives are listed in the Preface. The material in each chapter emphasizes and supports its lesson, so that multiple examples of the lesson are given from the client's point of view, from the intern's point of view, from the student's (reader's) point of view, and from the author's point of view.

NARRATIVES

Like a set of fingerprints, a personal narrative is unique to that individual. The story each of us tells invites the reader or listener into that unique arena of the self where our fears, hopes and desires, moral constructs, and spiritual concerns reside, often presenting themselves to the reader or listener in the various technical garbs of metaphor, simile, narrative discontinuities, leitmotifs, or recurring themes. The perceptive reader, the sensitive and alert listener, will hear the various rhythms of speech and the nuances of language, will recognize the significance of silences and gaps in the story, will discern the despair or hope embedded in a thematic repetition, and will enter into the story-teller's life. Readers or listeners who falter, who tune out and miss signs and cues in a narrative that would take them into the interior of another self, will remain sightseers, nonparticipants in the empathic journey of storytelling.

The use of personal narrative in education and the health sciences has become widespread. People rely on the genre of storytelling to gain access to the deeper layers of the psyche, mine the veins of the unconscious, and unearth the often hidden fears, motives, and desires of both the storyteller and the listener. In his seminal study of the importance of narrative to the medical and teaching professions, Robert Coles cites his longtime friend and mentor, William Carlos Williams, poet and physician: "'We have to pay the closest attention to what we say. What patients say tells us what to think about what hurts them; and what we say tells us what is happening to us—what we are thinking and what may be wrong with us'" (Coles, 1989). Acknowledging his indebtedness to the poet-physician, Coles came to rely more and more on "doctor stories," those personal, confessional narratives that, unlike the psychiatric profiles of patients scripted in the shorthand of technical jargon, are "meant to evoke the various events, moods, impasses a doctor experiences" (Coles, 1989). Luria (1972, 1987) uses narratives to help his readers get into the minds of his cognitively challenged clients, so they might experience the disabilities as the clients experience them. Bruner (1986) states that, to understand the com-

3

plexities of a client's barriers, one must comprehend the narrative of the client's life story; one must be able to "understand the ways human beings construct their worlds." Sacks (1985) uses "clinical tales" to demonstrate the connection between a disease and a client's personhood. The use of narrative to learn about others and ourselves, to capture the mysteries, moods, passions, and conflicts of the individual storyteller and listener, reflects, as Coles states, a "respect for narrative as everyone's rock-bottom capacity" (Coles, 1989), a respect that pays homage to the journey of the individual self.

The last 15 years have seen an increased interest by health professions in eliciting narratives from clients (Coles, 1989; Kleinman, 1988; Mattingly, 1991a). The use of narratives in occupational therapy has been explored and utilized as a tool to understand people as whole human beings, their values, beliefs, motivation, and how people's disabilities affect their current and future life roles (Fleming, 1991a, 1991b; Taylor, 1989). Mattingly (1991a) writes, "To effectively treat persons with long-term disabilities, one must treat the whole patient, which involves looking beyond the disease to how that disease is experienced by that particular patient."

As Peloquin and Davidson (1993) note, by calling on the ability to empathize, narratives help to place the intern in touch with the "therapeutic use of the self" in dealing with clients; similarly, interns begin to understand both the complexities of psychosocial issues and the significant role they can play as caring people. The narratives nudged the intern writers into the position of identifying with the client, sensing the pain and alienation experienced by someone living with psychosocial issues, and envisioning strategies of intervention.

Narrative reasoning, one of several well-defined types of clinical reasoning in occupational therapy literature (Clark, 1993; Fleming, 1991a, 1991b; Mattingly 1991a, 1991b; Mattingly and Fleming, 1994; Neistadt, 1995; Neuhaus, 1988; Rogers and Holm, 1991; Schell and Cervero, 1993), utilizes narratives to gain insight into a client's life and imagine a future for the client. Reading and analyzing literature about barriers and client experiences (Crepeau, 1991; Kautzmann, 1993; Peloquin, 1989, 1995; Peloquin and Davidson, 1993) have been used to develop narrative clinical reasoning. Reading, analyzing, and reflecting on narrative stories about clients before students begin their internship is invaluable in learning to work with clients that have psychosocial issues.

LOGS

In addition to narratives, interns can benefit from keeping logs of their experiences working with clients. The interns' logs help them gain insight into their own motivations, beliefs, values, and behavior. Interns' life experiences affect their understanding and treatment of their clients (Crepeau, 1991; Hooper, 1996; Schutz, 1967; Tannen and Wallat, 1987). By studying the logs of other interns' experiences while still in the classroom, students may learn of other interns' honest renditions of fears, prejudices, thoughts, and feelings about their internship; how they solved problems around them; and their growth and change and how these occurred.

The logs in this book trace the maturation of thought processes, reactions, emotions, application of knowledge base, clinical judgment, and empathy acquired through interaction and intervention with individual clients. In my experience training interns, I found them to go through stages somewhat in the order listed in #5 of the Client-Centered Reasoning Questions and Activities section of this chapter.

These stages must happen during the two- to three-month training period (for certified occupational therapy assistant [COTA] interns and OT interns, respectively) in order for the intern to become an unbiased entry-level therapist who can effectively treat a variety of severe problems associated with mental health and substance abuse. Needless to say, it is an intense experience, for both the clients and the interns. Since the narratives and logs are told from the interns' point of view, the writings contain elements of and movement through these stages. It is easy to trace the interns' maturation in the understanding of each client as an individual. An author's analysis and client-centered reasoning activities aid in this process.

CLIENT-CENTERED REASONING QUESTIONS AND ACTIVITIES

Client-centered reasoning questions and activities appear throughout the book, referring to a specific narrative or log. Their purpose is to foster the development of many types of clinical reasoning skills. They include a wide variety of activities, such as debates; court scenes; in-service presentations; contractual partnerships; identifying elements of countertransference, clinical reasoning, and intern maturation within the narratives and logs; writing between the lines; documentation; role playing; planning interventions; analyses; developing questions; research; frames of references; writing a journal; self-reflective exercises; creating assessments; futuristic imaging; and group work. They help the student contemplate and devise possible strategies of assessment and intervention, develop an empathetic understanding of both the client's and intern's situations, get in touch with issues that may affect their work with psychosocial clients, and offer the opportunity to solve problems and interventions that maximize each client's occupational performance and quality of life. Professors may wish to alter or adapt these exercises to fit classroom needs. Discussing the answers to the questions in class may maximize the learning experience. The clinical material may be used in a variety of ways, in addition to using the questions and activities provided.

The 15 client-centered reasoning questions and activities common to multiple narratives follow. For brevity, only the name of the activity is given in the text. Refer back to the explanations here when necessary.

1. *Write between the lines.* Write your thoughts, feelings, reactions, perceptions, attitudes, comments, questions, and reasoning in between the double-spaced lines as you read the narrative or log for the first time. It is important to write as you read the material the first time to get your first impressions before you know how the story will turn out. Hence, the "write between the lines" activities are always identified before each narrative to which they pertain. After you have written between the lines, categorize your comments into major themes or issues. Compare your themes with those of your classmates. Which ones are similar and which are different? Do similar themes emerge for you in other "write between the lines" activities throughout the book? If so, what are your recurring themes? This activity is meant to foster an ongoing thought process as you read the information presented. This thought process should include identifying areas in which to pursue further questioning, formulating those specific questions in your head, becoming aware of your own reactions to the material, and determining what material is most necessary to your interventions with the client and what next steps in the intervention process to take and why. This thought process is a skill necessary to have when looking through a chart, listening in a team meeting, interviewing a client, formulating questions for supervision, learning how to facilitate group process, or listening with a third ear. Writing between the lines is an exercise in active judgment (Fleming and Mattingly, 2000), where you actively respond to the written therapeutic dance of the client and the intern in each narrative.

2. *Finish the narrative.* Complete the narrative by writing another narrative in which you imagine the future life of the client. What would you do to help the client get to this point in the life you imagined? Finishing the narrative is an exercise in narrative reasoning (Mattingly, 1991a, 1994), where you must envision interventions that lead the client to a desired outcome based on the client in context and activity.

3. *Identify types of clinical reasoning.* As you read through the narrative or log, identify the types of clinical reasoning the intern has used. There are many types of clinical reasoning; some are mentioned in the following text. Quite frequently, a particular action or thought by an intern contains more than one type of clinical reasoning. Each of the client-centered reasoning questions and activities contains many types of clinical reasoning. The activity of identifying types of clinical reasoning has been graded. The first time it appears, the author has already identified the type of clinical reasoning as an example. The second time it appears, the author has starred (*) some examples of clinical reasoning to be identified by you. The third and following times this activity appears, you must identify the occurrence and the type of clinical reasoning yourself.

Different Types of Clinical Reasoning

In the following pages, the types of clinical reasoning are not mutually exclusive of each other—some overlap or contain elements of others.

Some blatantly contradict each other. It is difficult to separate them. The major characteristics of each are listed. In reality, clinical judgment contains many types of clinical reasoning used together to solve a particular problem. For learning purposes, they have been separated here. Types of clinical reasoning continue to grow and change, as shown in the literature, out of necessity to explain and teach effective and complicated thought processes.

Content (Knowledge) Reasoning

This type of reasoning uses an acquired knowledge base that is large, in-depth, organized, and clinical in order to solve problems. It is based on the idea that effective clinical reasoning requires a voluminous store of relevant knowledge (Higgs and Jones, 2000). This model of clinical reasoning was defined by Boshuizen and Schmidt in 1992 but has been the basic model for studying medicine under the medical model in prior years. Custers, Boshuizen, and Schmidt (1993) state that the element that distinguishes experienced from inexperienced physicians is the ability to access relevant knowledge and apply it to situational demands, not the use of strategies in problem solving and not the completeness of an investigation. Elstein, Schulman, and Sprafka (1978) find that experience in clinical reasoning depends on practitioners' knowledge and emphasize the importance of the practitioners' organization of knowledge instead of the reasoning processes. Hislop (1985) states that this knowledge should be easily understood, recalled, and frequently encountered to be successfully used in the problem-solving process by practitioners. A psychosocial practitioner's knowledge base usually includes but is not limited to the knowledge of biomedicine, basic science, life experience, social interactions, the clinic, psychology, self, and the tacit knowledge of the profession.

An example of content/knowledge reasoning is found in intern Aviva Graber's narrative as follows: "It was noted that her depression was worsening. A discussion on the various antidepressants ensued and the attending psychiatrist changed her medication from a monoamine oxidase inhibitor (MAOI) to a selective serotonin reuptake inhibitor (SSRI)."

Procedural Reasoning

Procedural reasoning attempts to identify problems and interventions on the basis of clients' disabilities; that is, the cause and nature of their functional problems (Fleming, 1991a). According to Mattingly and Fleming (1994), in procedural reasoning models, the clinician develops several hypotheses to explain the nature and cause of functional problems and develops hypotheses for interventions. These hypotheses must be tested using critical reflection to judge the basis on which they rest. Cervero (1988) states that procedural reasoning does not involve just the recall of information but the transformation of information that includes deliberate action and ongoing critical analysis. Cervero emphasizes that content knowledge and procedural knowledge are both necessary for sound clinical reasoning. Procedural reasoning refers to making intervention decisions (such as choosing one intervention procedure over another) and refers to the frequency, intensity, and progression of the intervention.

An example of procedural reasoning is from the text of Elodie Montivero, "I began to work on his concentration skills so that he could focus on one task at a time instead of jumping from one activity to another." Elodie chose to intervene at the level of concentration because the client's inability to concentrate is a manic symptom that affects his ability to complete a task in daily life.

Diagnostic Reasoning

Diagnostic reasoning aims to reveal impairments and etiologies by making decisions based on information required to make a working diagnosis (Edwards et al., 1998). Diagnostic reasoning may begin even before the practitioner meets a client (Rogers and Holm, 1991) by using existing information about the client to identify a general problem. The general problem can include the pathophysiology, the disability and resulting impairments, the structures at fault, and/or the elements that add to the development and maintenance of the dysfunction (Jones, Jensen, and Edwards, 2000).

In the following example of diagnostic reasoning, Marsha Eiserman describes why she thinks that her client is not delusional.

> Many staff members consider Brian to be delusional. Based on his verbal and nonverbal communication during my evaluation, I suspect he is putting on a show in order to get free room and board. He is a little too well focused and organized during the interview, choosing an image for his delusion and supplying answers to fit the image. Brian's physical appearance is also very good. He is well groomed and stands tall and erect when walking. He displays appropriate social interaction with other clients. Additionally, he has good eye contact during the entire interview unless he discusses the delusion.

Interactive Reasoning

Interactive reasoning utilizes dialogue between the client and the therapist with the goal to facilitate the assessment or intervention process (Crepeau, 1991; Fleming, 1991a, 1994). This dialogue is an "interactive system of skilled communication" (Ranka and Chapparo, 2000, p. 193). Interactive reasoning is important to test or justify the validity of prior assumptions or presuppositions about the client made by the practitioner or other clinicians but, more important, to enhance the practitioner's understanding of the client in the context in which the client's difficulties exist (Jones et al., 2000) and to build rapport with the client (Fleming, 1994). Interactive reasoning helps build new knowledge by building on and redefining previous ideas about the client (Eggen and Kauchak, 1988).

Narrative Reasoning

Narrative reasoning is the use of stories about clients to enhance understanding of the clients' unique situations (past, present, and future) in order to manage a clinical situation (Clark, 1993; Fleming, 1991a;

Mattingly and Fleming, 1994). More specifically, the understanding of the client gained through these stories helps the practitioner and the client set up intervention goals that reflect what the client conceives is important in life. For the practitioner to envision intervention strategies that would maximize the client's participation and motivation, the practitioner must be able to imagine a futuristic story of the client that takes into consideration the client's current and past stories. In this way, narrative reasoning goes beyond the telling and interpreting of the client's narrative by guiding future actions of both the practitioner and the client. Narrative reasoning involves searching for motives that will result in certain actions that may lead to certain consequences. When using narrative reasoning, practitioners ask themselves several questions to judge how to act in certain situations, taking into account the desires and motives of themselves, their clients, and other relevant people: Who is this client? What story is the client acting out? How can I enhance the client's commitment to the intervention process? And which intervention goals and activities would be deemed the most appealing and helpful, keeping in mind how the client's life may be after therapy? Sensitive narrative reasoning by the practitioner can help clients link their past (a time before their illness) to their current situation and to a future worth living (Fleming and Mattingly, 2000).

Most of the stories in this text are examples of narrative reasoning, but a specific example can be found in intern Aviva Graber's text, which follows: "Sharon told me that her mother was an unwed teenager when she gave birth to her. She put her in Angel Guardian Home, an orphanage for abandoned infants. At age 1, Sharon . . ." The text continues to describe Sharon's life story.

Ethical Reasoning
Ethical reasoning is the thought process involved in making economic, moral, and political decisions. These decisions usually require the practitioner to achieve a balance between meeting the duty of beneficence and allowing the clients (who are competent to do so) make their own decisions (Smith and Bodurtha, 1995). Beneficence is the obligation to do good things and act in the best interest of the client over and above anything else. This balancing may occur consciously or unconsciously, but when it does occur, it usually affects decision making throughout the course of the intervention; and the practitioners' own moral and ethical values usually affect their decisions. There are many other ethical dilemmas in which the practitioner must balance one value against another. Knowledge, clinical skills, and sound judgment are inadequate if there is not enough money, time, or resources to improve a client's quality of life. When not enough intervention is available to all of the clients who require it, a moral dilemma occurs that must be solved using the best ethical reasoning possible (Neuhaus, 1988).

Interns often experience difficulties with reasoning that lead to decisions regarding the intensity, type, and amount of intervention versus the intervention that takes place at their fieldwork sites. As a result, interns report feeling angry at the system, supervisors, and the intervention site or feeling ineffective. They have not yet fully developed their own ethical reasoning skills, experiences, facts, and wisdom to work with the idea that one decision may be better than a less desirable decision, since there is not always a "correct and achievable" way to proceed (Neuhaus, 1988).

An example of ethical reasoning and an intern who was able to remain flexible during an ethical dilemma is found in intern Nancy Moritz-Farajun's following narrative about Brian:

> Since Brian would not reveal his personal goals to me until the day of his discharge, I based my intervention plan on team rounds and biographical data. It seemed almost unethical for me to compose the above intervention plan without consulting Brain. However, I knew that I had limited time to work with Brian before his insurance expired, so I prioritized goals that would prepare him for discharge.

Teaching as Reasoning

Teaching as reasoning is the willful use of advice, guidance, or instruction to aid in the process of client intervention. Teaching as reasoning can occur on different levels. It can involve giving simple advice to a client; counseling clients in how to modify their lifestyle (Sluijs, 1991a); making judgments about the amount, the level, and the type of teaching necessary and appropriate for each individual client; and assessing the level of understanding of what has been taught (Sluijs, 1991b). Teaching as reasoning also occurs each time practitioners use advice, guidance, or instruction from other practitioners, supervisors, instructors, inservice supervisors, and so forth, to make decisions about the intervention process of their clients.

An example of teaching as reasoning comes from intern Nancy Moritz-Farajun's following narrative: "I gave Brian an educational packet about stress management techniques to read and then discussed the information." Marsha Eiserman provides another example: "Using suggestions made by fellow interns, I am almost able to glide through documentation."

Inductive Reasoning

In inductive reasoning, many specific observations are gathered before making a generalization (Ridderikhoff, 1989). Inductive reasoning is used to generate a hypothesis. An example from the text is intern Elodie Montivero's statement, "From his body language and expression, I could tell that he did not want to be bothered." And, "From his tone of voice and discussion in rounds, I knew not to push him too far. I decided to leave him for the time being and possibly return when he was less irritable."

Deductive Reasoning

Deductive reasoning is almost the opposite of inductive reasoning in that a hypothesis is generated before many observations are made. After the hypothesis is made, in-depth data gathering is conducted to test the hypothesis and further the investigation (Ridderikhoff, 1989). Deductive reasoning includes "if-then" statements where *if* refers to a supporting statement and *then* refers to the related conclusion.

Deductive reasoning has its origins in medical research (Barrows et al., 1978; Elstein et al., 1978; Feltovich et al., 1984; Gale, 1982), but has also been used in physiotherapy (Jones, 1992), nursing (Padrick et al., 1987), and occupational therapy, where it has been linked to procedural reasoning (Fleming, 1991a).

An example of deductive reasoning in a clinical situation is intern Nancy Moritz-Farajun's reasoning on why one of her clients did not want to shave:

> When I encouraged him to shave and offered my supervision, Brian would politely decline or respond that he would shave later in the day. When contemplating why he continuously refused to shave, I reconsidered Brian's comfort level. Maybe he felt uneasy being watched by a female staff member almost identical in age to himself? Brain admitted that my hypothesis was correct. In order to increase Brian's comfort level as well as his independence with self-care, I suggested that he request assistance from a male nursing attendant as needed. Brian followed my advice, and within two weeks, Brain became completely independent with all self-care activities.

The "if" statement in this example is, if Brian felt uneasy in the presence of a female while he was shaving. The "then" statement in this example is, then he would not shave. This hypothesis turned out to be correct.

Categorization Reasoning
Categorization reasoning is when similarities between things are recognized and grouped together in categories with the same label; for example, diagnoses, intervention outcomes, objects, events, signs, or symptoms (Brooks, Norman, and Allen, 1991; Schmidt, Norman, and Boshuizen, 1990). The link made by the practitioner between the current situation or person and past situations or people is important (Medin and Schafter, 1978). The more experience a clinician has, the easier and more accurate will be the comparisons, groupings, and resultant interventions. Prototypes are especially helpful to the beginning clinician in recognizing a clinical pattern, since the clinician can compare the current situation or person with learned abstractions (Bordage and Zacks, 1984) instead of prior clinical cases.

Categorization reasoning has many functions. It may help a clinician go beyond the information presented in a particular case. It can also break down a vast amount of information into usable and pertinent themes. It may allow a practitioner to form predictions regarding symptoms and functioning that are usually present with a diagnosis but may not have been noticed in a client to date (Mumma, 1993). It may also allow predictions to be made regarding the course of the condition and thereby guide intervention strategies (Blashfeld et al., 1989). Finally, it may help practitioners become aware of commonalities in cases that otherwise appear not to be related (Hayes and Adams, 2000).

Some practitioners have believed that categorization reasoning limits the ability to fully understand an individual; however, categorical labels have been used to describe many complex areas, such as psychiatric diagnoses (Genero and Cantor, 1987), personality profiles and biographical descriptions (Lingle, Altom, and Medin, 1983), and semantic concepts (Lakoff, 1986).

Pragmatic Reasoning

Pragmatic reasoning is clinical reasoning that focuses on practical action. Therapists consider what is realistically achievable given their own and the client's world (Chapparo and Ranka, 2000). Pragmatic reasoning issues include but are not limited to reimbursement, practice trends, organizational constraints, intervention settings, therapist's level of expertise, and values and resources; and these issues are taken into consideration when developing an intervention plan (Creighton et al., 1995; Neuhaus, 1988; Schell and Cervero, 1993). Chapparo (1997) and Strong et al. (1995) found that practitioners' thinking is influenced by their practice world.

Conditional or Predicative Reasoning

Conditional or predicative reasoning is a type of reasoning in which the therapist envisions the future of the client, taking into consideration the client's current and past social, psychological, work, or recreational profile and the total context to predict various interventions and outcomes for the future (Fleming, 1991b; Hagedorn, 1996). The therapist then shares these intervention procedures and possible outcomes with the client so that both agree on a way to proceed in therapy. Success or failure depends on the client's level of participation. Conditional reasoning is based on the premise that intervention must be modified continuously for the client to function in the future and hence leads to an overall flexible therapy program.

An example of conditional or predicative reasoning from the text of Elodie Montivero is, "Hector and I came to a realization that he wanted to get his general education diploma (GED) so that he could find a better job."

Integration of Knowledge and Reasoning

Knowledge and reasoning are integrated when the acquisition of knowledge and clinical reasoning occurs at the same time. These two processes affect each other: As knowledge is learned, it is shaped by clinical material; and clinical reasoning guides the type of knowledge pursued (Boshuizen and Schmidt, 1992). As these two are developed, changes in knowledge structure occur. Current health science research has shown clinical reasoning not to be a distinct skill that can be acquired separately from pertinent professional knowledge or other clinical skills (Schmidt et al., 1990). Others (Elstein et al., 1990; Hassebrock et al., 1993; Patel and Groen, 1986; Patel, Groen, and Arocha, 1990; Schmidt et al., 1990) have supported the importance of an organized content knowledge base in effective problem solving. Cognitive skills such as analytic thinking, logic, creativity, reflection, critiquing, and metacognition have also been found to be necessary for effective problem solving and thinking (Alexander and Judy, 1988) and must be integrated with reasoning as well as knowledge.

Intern Marsha Eiserman provides the following example of integrated knowledge and reasoning from her narrative:

> Jean, during a group session, mentioned that she wants to leave the hospital so that she could go back to her business. In order to find out whether it is a real business (it is possible for people with psychosocial issues to run a business) or a symptom of an illness, I decided to approach Jean rather than read her chart. Within five minutes of speaking with her, it was quite obvious she is in either a hypomanic or manic state. This conclusion is based on the fact that the business begins after she is hospitalized, the orders are from staff members, and her goal is to have a wreath hanging on every front door in America.

Here Marsha has integrated her knowledge of manic symptomatology into how the client describes her business.

Interpretive Reasoning

Interpretive reasoning is the process by which a practitioner gains an in-depth understanding of the client's perspectives and the influence of their contextual factors (Benner, 1984; Crepeau, 1991; Fleming, 1991b; Jensen, Shepard, and Hack, 1992). This process is usually but not limited to speaking with the client while listening with a "third ear" and observing closely. Rich descriptive data are necessary to understand the context of behavior. Without this context, human action cannot be interpreted in a meaningful way (Patel and Arocha, 2000). The practitioner's task is to interpret the client's true situation (behaviors, thoughts, actions, drives, functioning, and so forth) as accurately as possible. Gaining an in-depth understanding of clients' perspectives is relevant for many reasons. Research has shown that intervention outcomes are influenced by the meaning that clients give to their problems (Borkan et al., 1991; Feuerstein and Beattie, 1995; Malt and Olafson, 1995). As the field of clinical reasoning progresses, it becomes evident that traditional models do not encompass the vast array of client diversity nor are they applicable to all the health care professions.

An example of interpretive reasoning from the text by intern Elodie Montivero is, "Hector had great interest in weight lifting as well. He felt that he needed to become stronger so that nobody would hurt him." For Elodie to interpret that Hector was lifting weights because he wanted to become stronger to avoid being hurt, she had to engage in several one-to-one conversations with Hector to build rapport so that he would allow her to get to know him more closely.

Collaborative Reasoning

Collaborative reasoning occurs when decision making is shared between a practitioner and a client. The practitioner actively seeks information from the client about the problem and the client's opinions (Higgs and Jones, 2000). An example from the text is given by Elodie Montivero, "Hector and I talked about his future plans and what he wanted to do upon discharge."

4. *Write your own client-centered reasoning questions and activities.* Write a set of questions and activities that relate to the material you will have just read in the preceding narrative or log as the author has done for the other narratives and logs throughout this book. This activity forces you to pay attention to subtle details and helps you develop, organize, and utilize your ongoing personal dialogue in response to the material in a meaningful way. Photocopy your questions and activities for your classmates to complete.

5. *Trace the intern's maturation.* As you read the log, identify through bubble writing the stage of maturation that the intern is exhibiting. The stages of maturation are listed below and have been described under the Log section of this chapter. This activity has been graded, in that the first time this activity is presented, the author identifies the stages of maturation and summarizes them for you as an example. In the logs to follow, you are to find and identify the stages yourself and summarize your findings. The stages of maturation are

1. Prejudice (preconceived ideas about clients).
2. Fear.
3. Shock.
4. Inadequacy.
5. Underestimating pathology.
6. Overidentification.
7. Sympathy.
8. Empathy.
9. Rescue fantasies.
10. Becoming aware of the limitations of interventions, the intervention center, the staff, the supervisor, and sometimes society as a whole.
11. Anger when the rescue fantasies are not possible and limitations are not solvable.
12. Focus.
13. Intervention.
14. Hope.
15. Discouragement around lack of progress, regression, and/or recidivism.
16. Understanding barriers (including symptomatology and pathology) as they relate to diagnoses and functioning.
17. Integrating theory and practice.
18. Consolidation.
19. Feelings of loss around termination.

6. *Write an occupational profile.* Write an occupational profile for the client identified in the narrative or log using the information given. An occupational profile is a description of the client's past and current daily living routines, skills, roles, motivators, interests, aspirations, values, needs, priorities, demographics, and occupational history as defined by the client. It should also include a list of issues and concerns that the client has about participating in meaningful activities. For a more in-depth description of what is included in an occupational profile, see Table 1-1.

Table 1-1 Occupational Profile

Definition and Assumptions

- **Occupational profile**—a profile that describes the client's occupational history, interests, needs, and patterns of daily living. It is elicited from the client and aimed at understanding what is important and meaningful to the client and identifying occupational needs/issues, aspirations, and priorities.

- **Assumptions about the occupational profile:**
  —Occupations can only be defined by the client.
  —Meaning resides in the client and is influenced by society and culture.
  —Clients have the right to determine the occupations, activities, and priorities that will give meaning to their existence.
  —"Some occupations and patterns of occupation are health promoting; others may be health compromising" (Clark, Wood, and Larson, 1998, p. 18).
  —Information about the occupational profile is collected at the beginning of contact with the client. However, additional information is collected and refined throughout contact with the client.

Process

- **Identify the client and the demographics of the client.**

- **Identify the client's concerns relative to participation in occupation:**
  —Why is client seeking service?
  —What are the occupational issues/problems? These could include problems in the areas of competence, identity, occupational performance (problems of efficiency, effectiveness, adequacy, safety, desire, support), satisfaction, meaning/purpose, health status/wellness, life balance, interdependence, and independence.
  —Why are these issues/problems of concern?
  —What has been done to address them?
  —What future directions/results are desired, needed, or required?
  —What are the client's priorities and goals?
  —What is the client willing to do (motivation/active participation)?

- **Elicit current and past occupational history** (identify past and current occupations and their activities that client wants, needs, and expects to do, including facilitators and barriers to participation).
  —Types of occupations and their activities (. . . occupations may be categorized in a variety of ways).
  —Patterns of time use and patterns of occupation.
  —Skills.
  —Roles.
  —Habits and routines.

- **Identify aspects of occupations and their activities that provide meaning:**
  —What are client's interests?
  —What are client's values?
  —What are motivators for client?
  —What are the importance and meaning attached to various roles, occupations, and activities?

- **Identify contexts for participation:**
  —Cultural environment
  —Physical environment
  —Social environment
  —Virtual environment

Source: Occupational Therapy Practice Framework: Engagement and Participation in Occupation, Draft IV, page 7. Bethesda, MD: American Occupational Therapy Association. By: The AOTA Commission on Practice. (2000) by the American Occupational Therapy Association, Inc. Reprinted with permission.

7. *Write a questionnaire.* Write a questionnaire for the client identified in the narrative or log to obtain missing information needed to complete the occupational profile.

8. *List additional assessments.* List assessments or additional assessments you would use for the client in the log or narrative and state why you selected them. What does each one measure? Are they standardized? What are their reliability and validity coefficients? In many cases, the interns have not mentioned which assessments they used with the clients, or this information has been purposely left out in order for you to use your reasoning skills to decide what is needed and why.

9. *Write an occupational performance analysis.* Write an occupational performance analysis for the client identified in the narrative or log using the information given. An occupational performance analysis should include a list of the client's facilitators and barriers to engagement in meaningful activities. For a more in-depth description of what is included in an occupational performance analysis, see Table 1-2.

10. *Write an intervention plan.* Write an intervention plan for the client identified in the narrative or log. The intervention plan should include approaches that will be used to help clients achieve their meaningful goals and outcomes. Identify the frame(s) of reference, theoretical base, evidence, or practice model used for each approach. Provide support for why each is appropriate for this person's needs. Include time frames and how the services will be provided. For a more in-depth description of what is included in an intervention plan, see Tables 1-3 and 1-4.

11. *Readjust the intervention plans for different treatment settings.* Reconstruct a new intervention plan (as in activity #10 above) for the same client in a different setting as defined in the client-centered reasoning activity. Note how the intervention plan changes and why. The following list provides sites and forms of intervention for various types of psychosocial and substance abuse problems. Research each, include the average length of stay, a description of the facility, the facility's mission statement, criteria for admission, funding source, types of interventions offered, types of clients served, number of clients served, average staff to client ratio, and staff qualifications to help you write your new intervention plan. For your new intervention plan, choose one type or site of intervention, research it as described, and then present it to the class as if you are the director describing your facility to the class.

- Assertive community treatment (ACT) teams.
- Day treatment programs.
- Clients' homes.
- Day hospitals or partial hospitals.
- Intensive psychiatric rehabilitation treatments (IPRTs).
- Inpatient psychiatric units.
- Continuing day treatment programs (CDTPs).
- Inpatient detoxification.
- State hospitals.
- 28-day rehabilitation facilities.

Table 1-2 Analysis of Occupational Performance: Consideration of Factors That Facilitate or Hinder Participation in Occupation

Definition and Assumptions

Occupational performance—the ability to carry out tasks and activities of daily life. Includes ADLs and IADLs in the occupational categories of self-care, work/productive activities, and play/leisure activities. Occupational performance is conceived as the transaction between the individual, the environment (context), and the activity that results in behaviors that lead to the accomplishment of the selected activity/task/occupation. Improving or enabling occupational performance leads to occupational engagement (adapted in part from Law et al., 1996, p. 16).

Assumptions:
- The selection of the occupations and their activities that are analyzed in this section are based on wants, needs, expectations, and priorities of the client as identified in the occupational profile.
- Analysis of performance will identify factors that facilitate or act as barriers to participation in occupation.
- An intervention plan can only be established after the factors that support and/or inhibit performance are understood.
- Occupations are performed at the intersection between the client, the activity, and the context.
- The occupational profile provides direction in selection of assessment tools and methods that are evidence-based whenever possible.

Process

Contexts factors that act as facilitators or barriers:

- Physical environment: Temporal, seasonal, structural, architectural, natural factors (weather, air), geographical, products and technology, resources.
- Social environment: Transportation, economics, networks/supports/relationships, politics, housing, systems, institutions, services, policies.
- Cultural environment: Religion, race, family, attitudes/values/beliefs.
- Virtual environment.

Activity demands:

The activity analysis process used in this section focused on understanding the demands that the activity makes on the performer.

Activity demands include—
Equipment/tools/materials; space/environmental requirements; sequence of major step; precautions and contraindications; skills needed (cognitive, sensorimotor, emotional, social); amount of experience required; prerequisite skills

Client (groups, organizations, person, caregivers, communities) factors that act as facilitators or barriers:

- Roles (i.e., father, student, boy scout).
- Routines (i.e., work routine, getting ready for bed routine).
- Habits (i.e., nail biting, putting on seatbelt immediately upon entering a car).
- Skills (i.e., dressing, shopping, walking, completing a task).
- Capacities (i.e., sensory processing, neuromuscular flexibility, temperament).

Summary

Data gathered through a variety of methods specifically identifies facilitators and barriers within contexts, activity, and client.

Source: Occupational Therapy Practice Framework: Engagement and Participation in Occupation, Draft IV, page 9. Bethesda, MD: American Occupational Therapy Association. By: The AOTA Commission on Practice. (2000) by the American Occupational Therapy Association, Inc. Reprinted with permission.

Table 1-3   Intervention Plan

Definition and Assumptions

Intervention plan—an outline of selected approaches to reach the client's identified goals and outcomes.

Assumptions:
- The design of the intervention plan is influenced by
  —The interaction between the client and context.
  —The setting or circumstances in which the intervention is provided (i.e., caregiver expectations, organization's purpose, payer's requirements).
  —The health and well-being of the client.
  —The client's goals.
- Interventions are designed to facilitate performance, engagement, and goal achievement.
- Intervention plans are developed in collaboration with the client and are client centered.
- The selection and design of the intervention plan and goals are directed toward allowing the client to develop the learning strategies and skills that are necessary to independently address ongoing and emerging problems in participation in occupation.

Process

- **Goal setting:**
  —Developed in collaboration with the client and client centered.
  —Are meaningful and acceptable to client.
  —Are related to previously identified occupational issues and needs.

- **Select intervention approach:**
  —Examine available options, theories, practice models, frames of reference, and evidence.
  —Choose strategy(ies). Strategies describe the aspect of performance (client, activity, environment) that the intervention will impact and how.
    - Establish/restore.
    - Modify.
    - Prevent.
    - Create/promote.
    - Maintain.
  —Determine method of delivery.
    - Who will provide.
    - How service will be provided.
    - Where services will be provided.
    - How often and how long.

Source: Occupational Therapy Practice Framework: Engagement and Participation in Occupation, Draft IV, page 10. Bethesda, MD: American Occupational Therapy Association. By: The AOTA Commission on Practice. (2000) by the American Occupational Therapy Association, Inc. Reprinted with permission.

Table 1-4 Intervention Implementation

Definition and Assumptions

Intervention [implementation]—one or more actions taken in order to affect a desired outcome (adapted from *Taber's Cyclopedic Medical Dictionary*, 1997).

Assumptions:
- The intervention process engages the client in tasks, activities, and occupations when a direct or monitor service delivery model is used.
- Implementation of interventions does not occur in isolation from assessment.
- Dynamic assessment occurs throughout the implementation process and includes continuous observation, selected experimentation to gain information about the supportive cues that improve performance, and continual analysis of results.
- Monitoring ongoing change occurs
  —Throughout the evaluation, intervention, and re-evaluation process when working with clients.
  —Throughout the client's life cycle to identify changes in occupational performance due to shifts in occupational profile, context, or personal variables that may signal the need for additional occupational therapy intervention.
- Simultaneously monitor all three factors that influence engagement (i.e., client, activity, context). Practitioners recognize that change in one factor may influence each other in a continual dynamic process.

Process

Occupational therapy interventions:
- **Conscious use of self**—the planning of one's personal responses to help a client (adapted from Mosey, 1981, p. 95).
- **Select and use activities based on analysis and synthesis**—During intervention, implementation activities are specifically selected that are goal directed, support the purpose of the intervention, and have meaning to the client. The unique term occupational therapy uses for these activities is "purposeful activities."

Activity analysis is the examination of an activity to distinguish its component parts, and activity synthesis is the combining of the component parts of the human and non-human environment to design an activity related to occupational performance components. The process is a tool that is used initially in the planning part of intervention to make initial selections of appropriate activity interventions, but it is also used throughout the implementation to adjust interventions.

- **Select and use contexts**—conscious structuring or planning of the context in which performance occurs in order to facilitate or support performance. Includes the choice and structuring of the physical context (e.g., objects, temperature, lighting, location), the social context (number and types of people and interactions), and the cultural context.

- **Teaching and education**—utilization of teaching, training, or collaboration processes (adapted from Punwar and Peloquin, 2000, p. 42).

- **Select and use techniques, if needed, to prepare for engagement in activity and occupation.**

- **Monitor client's responses** to evaluate the selection and use of activities, tools, and techniques (dynamic assessment).

Source: Occupational Therapy Practice Framework: Engagement and Participation in Occupation, Draft IV, page 11. Bethesda, MD: American Occupational Therapy Association. By: The AOTA Commission on Practice. (2000) by the American Occupational Therapy Association, Inc. Reprinted with permission.

- Outpatient clinics (walk-in clinics, clinics for battered women, sleep disorders clinics, anxiety clinics, obsessive-compulsive disorders clinics, eating disorders clinics, private clinics).
- Self-help programs (12-step programs, peer counseling, train the trainer programs).
- Places of religious practice.
- Holistic healing centers (yoga institutes, acupuncture, Asian herbal treatment centers, creative arts therapy centers, and so forth).
- High schools.
- Therapeutic communities (TCs).
- Welfare to work programs.
- Prevocational programs.
- Residences for the mentally ill or chemically addicted (MICA).
- Vocational rehabilitation programs.
- Community integration programs.
- Prevention programs.
- Adolescent after-school programs.
- Business employee assistance programs (EAPs).
- Family therapy centers.
- Acquired immunodeficiency syndrome (AIDS) programs.
- Peer support groups.
- MICA outpatient programs.

12. *Write a progress note.* Write a progress note for the client identified in the narrative or log using the information given. The progress note should contain a subjective section, an objective section, the results of assessments or interventions, a comparison to past behavior, a statement on whether or not the current goals were attained and why or why not, and a plan for further intervention.

13. *Write a discharge note.* Write a discharge note for the client described in the narrative or log. The discharge note should include the goals that the client was able to achieve during the current period of intervention, which intervention strategies helped and why, the goals that the client was not able to achieve during the current period of intervention, which intervention strategies did not work well and why, future goals, the types of follow-up interventions recommended and how they could be helpful in attaining the desired outcomes, and the type of housing recommended and why. A list of housing options for people with psychosocial or substance abuse issues follows to help you write an accurate discharge note. Research each housing option until you feel comfortable making accurate referrals. To do this, work in groups, where each member researches one type of housing and presents it to the class. In addition, if possible, visit a few facilities to get a sense of the level of occupational performance necessary to live there.

- Supported housing programs.
- Residence for adults (RFAs).
- Adult homes and private proprietary homes for adults.

- Therapeutic communities (TCs).
- Single-room occupancy (SRO) buildings.
- Supportive SRO buildings.
- Shelters.
- Supervised community residences.
- Intensive supportive apartments ("scatter site" apartments).
- Low-demand supervised community residences.
- MICA community residences (MICA CRs).
- Single-room/community residences (SR/CRs).
- Residential care center for adults (RCCA).
- Adult foster care.
- Unserviced apartments.
- Residential health care facilities.

14. *Make referrals to other services.* Identify additional services necessary to help clients achieve their outcomes. These could be medical services, community services or activities, and so forth. Be specific by listing agencies in your area.

15. *Write a group protocol.* Write a group protocol for a particular client or group of clients. A group protocol should contain the title of the group; the time, duration, location, and frequency of the group; the purpose of the group; the population served by the group; admission, exclusionary, and discharge criteria; goals of the group; materials required to run the group; role of the group leader; methods for carrying out the group; and methods for evaluating the group's effectiveness.

ANALYSES

After the students have responded to the client-centered reasoning questions and activities provided at the beginning or end of each narrative, the students may go on to read the author's analysis of that narrative. They then may compare their own responses with that of the author, resulting in a comprehensive understanding of how to intervene with the client. The first few chapters of the book have more extensive analyses and less extensive client-centered reasoning questions and activities. As the chapters progress, the analyses become small to nonexistent so that students can analyze more on their own through the client-centered reasoning questions and activities that become more extensive.

REFERENCES

Alexander PA, Judy JE. The interaction of domain-specific and strategic knowledge in academic performance. *Review of Educational Research* 1988;58:375–404.

Barris R, Kielhofner G. Generating and using knowledge in occupational therapy: Implications for professional education. *Occupational Therapy Journal of Research* 1985;5:113–124.

Barrows HS, Feightner JW, Neufield VR, Norman GR. *An Analysis of the Clinical Methods of Medical Students and Physicians. Report to the Province of Ontario Department of Health.* Hamilton, Ontario: McMaster University, 1978.

Benamy BC. *Developing Clinical Reasoning Skills: Strategies for the Occupational Therapist.* San Antonio: Therapy Skill Builders, 1999.

Benner P. *From Novice to Expert: Excellence and Power in Clinical Nursing Practice.* London: Addison-Wesley, 1984.

Blashfeld RK, Sprock J, Haymaker MA, Hodgin J. The family resemblance hypothesis applied to psychiatric classification. *Journal of Nervous and Mental Disease* 1989;177:492–497.

Bordage G, Zacks R. The structure of medical knowledge in the memories of medical students and general practitioners: Categories and prototypes. *Medical Education* 1984;18:406–416.

Borkan JM, Quirk M, Sullivan M. Finding meaning after the fall: Injury narratives from elderly hip fracture clients. *Social Science and Medicine* 1991;33:947–957.

Boshuizen HPA, Schmidt HG. On the role of biomedical knowledge in clinical reasoning by experts, intermediates and novices. *Cognitive Science* 1992;16:53–184.

Boshuizen HPA, Schmidt HG. The development of clinical reasoning expertise. In: J Higgs, M Jones (eds), *Clinical Reasoning in the Health Professions*, 2nd ed. Oxford: Butterworth–Heinemann, 2000:15–22.

Bridge K. *Clinical and Professional Reasoning in Occupational Therapy.* Thorofare, NJ: Slack, 1999.

Brooks LR, Norman GR, Allen SW. Role of specific similarity in a medical diagnostic task. *Journal of Experimental Psychology General* 1991;120: 278–287.

Bruner J. *Actual Minds, Possible Worlds.* Cambridge, MA: Harvard University Press, 1986.

Burke JP, Depoy E. An emerging view of mastery, excellence, and leadership in occupational therapy practice. *American Journal of Occupational Therapy* 1991;45:1027–1032.

Cervero RM. *Effective Continuing Education for Professionals.* San Francisco: Jossey-Bass, 1988.

Chapparo C. Influences on clinical reasoning in occupation therapy. Ph.D. thesis. Sydney: Macquarie University, 1997.

Chapparo C, Ranka J. Clinical reasoning in occupational therapy. In: J Higgs, M Jones (eds), *Clinical Reasoning in the Health Professions*, 2nd ed. Oxford: Butterworth–Heinemann, 2000:128–137.

Clark F. Occupation embedded in a real life: Interweaving occupational science and occupational therapy, 1993 Eleanor Clarke Slagle Lecture. *American Journal of Occupational Therapy* 1993;47:1067–1078.

Clark FA, Wood W, Larson E. Occupational science: Occupational therapy's legacy for the 21st century. In: M Neistadt, EB Crepeau (eds), *Willard and Spackman's Occupational Therapy*, 9th ed. Philadelphia: J. B. Lippincott, 1998:13–21.

Coles R. *The Call of Stories.* Boston: Houghton Mifflin, 1989.

Creighton C, Dijkers M, Bennett N, Brown K. Reasoning and the art of therapy for spinal cord injury. *American Journal of Occupational Therapy* 1995; 49:311–317.

Crepeau EB. Achieving intersubjective understanding: Examples from an occupational therapy treatment session. *American Journal of Occupational Therapy* 1991;45:1016–1025.

Custers EJFM, Boshuizen HPA, Schmidt HG. The influence of typicality of case descriptions on subjective disease probability estimations. Paper presented at the Annual Meeting of the American Educational Research Association, Atlanta, 1993.

Edwards IC, Jones MA, Carr J, Jensen GM. Clinical reasoning in three different fields of physiotherapy—A qualitative study. In: *Proceedings Fifth International Congress.* Melbourne: Australian Physiotherpay Association 1998:289–300.

Eggen P, Kauchak D. *Strategies for Teachers: Teaching Content and Thinking Skills,* 2nd ed. Englewood Cliffs, NJ: Prentice-Hall, 1988.

Elstein A. Clinical judgment: Psychological research and medical practice. *Science* 1976;194:696–700.

Elstein A, Schulman LS, Sprafka SA. *Medical Problem Solving: An Analysis of Clinical Reasoning.* Cambridge, MA: Harvard University Press, 1978.

Elstein A, Schulman LS, Sprafka SA. Medical problem solving: A ten-year retrospective. *Evaluation and the Health Professions* 1990;13:5–36.

Fearing VG, Clark J. *Individuals in Context: A Practical Guide to Client-Centered Practice.* Thorofare, NJ: Slack, 2000.

Feltovich PJ, Johnson PE, Moller JH, Swanson DB. LCS: The role and development of medical knowledge in diagnostic expertise. In: WJ Clancey, EH Shortliffe (eds), *Readings in Medical Artificial Intelligence: The First Decade.* Reading, MA: Addison-Wesley, 1984:275–319.

Feuerstein M, Beattie P. Biobehavioral factors affecting pain and disability in low back pain: Mechanisms and assessment. *Physical Therapy* 1995;75: 267–280.

Fleming MH. Clinical reasoning in medicine compared with clinical reasoning in occupational therapy. *American Journal of Occupational Therapy* 1991a;45:988–996.

Fleming MH. The therapist with the three-track mind. *American Journal of Occupational Therapy* 1991b;45:1007–1014. Also published in: Mattingly C, Gleming MH (eds), *Clinical Reasoning: Forms of Inquiry in a Therapeutic Practice.* Philadelphia: F. A. Davis, 1994:119–139.

Fleming MH, Mattingly C. Action and narrative: Two dynamics of clinical reasoning. In: J Higgs, M Jones (eds), *Clinical Reasoning in the Health Professions,* 2nd ed. Oxford: Butterworth–Heinemann, 2000:54–61.

Gale J. Some cognitive components of the diagnostic thinking process. *British Journal of Educational Psychology* 1982;52:64–76.

Gillette NP, Mattingly C. The foundation—Clinical reasoning in occupational therapy. *American Journal of Occupational Therapy* 1987;41:399–400.

Genero N, Cantor, N. Exemplar prototypes and clinical diagnosis: Toward a cognitive economy. *Journal of Social and Clinical Psychology* 1987;5:59–78.

Hagedorn R. Clinical decision making in familiar cases: A model of the process and implications for practice. *British Journal of Occupational Therapy* 1996;59:217–222.

Halloran P, Lowenstein N. *Case Studies Through the Healthcare Continuum: A Workbook for the Occupational Therapy Student.* Thorofare, NJ: Slack, 2000.

Hassebrock F, Johnson PE, Bullemer P, Fox PW, Moller JH. When less is more: Representation and selective memory in expert problem solving. *American Journal of Psychology* 1993;106:155–189.

Hayes B, Adams R. Parallels between clinical reasoning and categorization. In: J Higgs, M Jones (eds), *Clinical Reasoning in the Health Professions,* 2nd ed. Oxford: Butterworth–Heinemann, 2000:45–53.

Higgs J, Jones M (eds). *Clinical Reasoning in the Health Professions,* 2nd ed. Oxford: Butterworth–Heinemann, 2000.

Higgs J, Jones M. Clinical reasoning in the health professions. In: J Higgs, M Jones (ed.). *Clinical Reasoning in the Health Professions,* 2nd ed. Oxford: Butterworth–Heinemann, 2000:3–14.

Hislop HJ. Clinical decision making: Educational, data, and risk factors. In: SL Wolf (ed), *Clinical Decision Making in Physical Therapy.* Philadelphia: F. A. Davis, 1985:25–60.

Hooper B. The relationship between pretheoretical assumptions and clinical reasoning. *American Journal of Occupational Therapy* 1996;51:328–338.

Jensen GM, Shepard KF, Hack LM. Attribute dimensions that distinguish master and novice physical therapy clinicians in orthopedic settings. *Physical Therapy* 1992;72:711–722.

Jones MA. Clinical reasoning in manual therapy. *Physical Therapy* 1992;72: 875–884.

Jones M, Jensen G, Edwards I. Clinical reasoning in physiotherapy. In: J Higgs, M Jones (eds), *Clinical Reasoning in the Health Professions*, 2nd ed. Oxford: Butterworth–Heinemann, 2000:117–127.

Kassirer J, Kuipers B, Gorry A. Toward a theory of clinical expertise. *American Journal of Medicine* 1982;73:251–259.

Kautzmann LN. Linking patient and family stories to caregivers' use of clinical reasoning. *American Journal of Occupational Therapy* 1993;47: 169–173.

Kleiman A. *The Illness Narratives: Suffering, Healing and the Human Condition.* New York: Basic Books, 1988.

Krefting LH. The use of conceptual models in clinical practice. *Canadian Journal of Occupational Therapy* 1985;52(4):173–178.

Lakoff G. *Women, Fire and Dangerous Things: What Categories Tell Us About the Nature of Thought.* Chicago: University of Chicago Press, 1986.

Law M (ed). *Client-Centered Occupational Therapy.* Thorofare, NJ: Slack, 1998.

Law M, Cooper B, Strong S, Stewart D, Rigby P, Letts L. Person-environment-occupation model: A transactive approach to occupational performance. *Canadian Journal of Occupational Therapy* 1996;63:9–23.

Law M, McColl MA. Knowledge and use of theory among occupational therapists: Canadian survey. *Canadian Journal of Occupational Therapy* 1989;56(4):198–204.

Lewin JE, Reed AC. *Creative Problem Solving in Occupational Therapy,* Philadelphia: Lippincott Williams and Wilkins, 1998.

Lingle JH, Altom MW, Medin DL. Of cabbages and kings: Assessing the extensibility of natural object concept models to social things. In: R Wyer, T Srull, J Hartwick (eds), *Handbook of Social Cognition.* Hillsdale, NJ: Lawrence Erlbaum, 1983:71–116.

Luria AR. *The Man with a Shattered World: The History of a Brain Wound.* Cambridge, MA: Harvard University Press, 1972.

Luria AR. *The Mind of a Mnemonist: A Little Book About a Vast Memory.* Cambridge, MA: Harvard University Press, 1987.

Malt UF, Olafson OM. Psychological appraisal and emotional response to physical injury: A clinical, phenomenological study of 109 adults. *Psychiatric Medicine* 1995;10:117–134.

Mattingly C. Thinking with stories: story and experience in a clinical practice. Unpublished doctoral dissertation. Cambridge: Massachusetts Institute of Technology, 1989.

Mattingly C. The narrative nature of clinical reasoning. *American Journal of Occupational Therapy* 1991a;45:998–1005.

Mattingly C. What is clinical reasoning? *American Journal of Occupational Therapy* 1991b;45:979–986.

Mattingly C, Fleming MH. *Clinical Reasoning: Forms of Inquiry in a Therapeutic Practice*, Philadelphia: F. A. Davis, 1994.

Medin DL, Schaffer MM. A context theory of classification learning. *Psychological Review* 1978;85:207–238.

Mosey AC. Legitimate tools of occupational therapy. In: A Mosey (ed), *Occupational Therapy: Configuration of a Profession*. New York: Raven Press, 1981:89–118.

Mumma GH. Categorization and rule induction in clinical diagnosis and assessment. In: GV Nakamura, DL Medin, R Taraban (eds), *The Psychology of Learning and Motivation,* vol. 29. New York: Academic Press,1993: 283–326.

Neistadt ME. Teaching strategies for the development of clinical reasoning. *American Journal of Occupational Therapy* 1995;50:676–684.

Neuhaus B. Ethical considerations in clinical reasoning: The impact of technology and cost containment. *American Journal of Occupational Therapy* 1988;42:288–294.

Padrick K, Tanner C, Putzier D, Westfall U. Hypothesis evaluation: A component of diagnostic reasoning. In: A McClane (ed), *Classification of Nursing Diagnosis: Proceedings of the Seventh Conference.* Toronto: Mosby, 1987:299–305.

Patel VL, Arocha JF. Methods in the study of clinical reasoning. In: J Higgs, M Jones (eds), *Clinical Reasoning in the Health Professions*, 2nd ed. Oxford: Butterworth–Heinemann, 2000:78–91.

Patel VL, Groen GJ. Knowledge-based solution strategies in medical reasoning. C*ognitive Science* 1986;10:91–116.

Patel VL, Groen GJ, Arocha JF. Medical expertise as a function of task difficulty. *Memory and Cognition* 1990;18:394–406.

Parham D. Nationally speaking—Toward professionalism: The reflective therapist. *American Journal of Occupational Therapy* 1987;41:555–561.

Peloquin SM. Sustaining the art of practice in occupational therapy. *American Journal of Occupational Therapy* 1989;43:219–226.

Peloquin SM. The fullness of empathy: Reflections and illustrations. *American Journal of Occupational Therapy* 1995;49:24–31.

Peloquin SM, Davidson DA. Brief or new—Interpersonal skills for practice: An elective course. *American Journal of Occupational Therapy* 1993;47: 260–264.

Punwar AJ, Peloquin SM. *Occupational Therapy Principles and Practice*, 3rd ed. Philadelphia: Lippincott Williams and Wilkins, 2000.

Ranka J, Chapparo C. Teaching clinical reasoning to occupational therapists. In: J Higgs, M Jones (eds), *Clinical Reasoning in the Health Professions*, 2nd ed. Oxford: Butterworth–Heinemann, 2000:191–197.

Reed KL. *Models of Practice in Occupational Therapy.* Baltimore: Williams and Wilkins, 1984.

Ridderikhoff J. *Methods in Medicine: A Descriptive Study of Physicians' Behaviour.* Dordrecht, the Netherlands: Kluwer, 1989.

Rogers CR. *The Clinical Treatment of the Problem Child.* Boston: Houghton-Mifflin, 1939.

Rogers JC. Clinical reasoning: The ethics, science, and art. 1983 Eleanor Clarke Slagle Lecture. *American Journal of Occupational Therapy* 1983;37:601–616.

Rogers JC. Clinical judgment: The bridge between theory and practice. In: *Target 2000: Occupational Therapy Education.* Rockville, MD: American Occupational Therapy Association, 1986.

Rogers JC, Holm MB. Occupational therapy diagnostic reasoning: A component of clinical reasoning. *American Journal of Occupational Therapy* 1991;45:1045–1053.

Rogers JC, Masagatani G. Clinical reasoning of occupational therapists during the initial assessment of physically disabled patients. *Occupational Therapy Journal of Research* 1982;2:195–219.

Sacks O. *The Man Who Mistook His Wife for a Hat.* New York: Summit, 1985.

Schell BA, Cervero RM. Clinical reasoning in occupational therapy: An integrative review. *American Journal of Occupational Therapy* 1993;47:605–610.

Schmidt HG, Norman GR, Boshuizen HPA. A cognitive perspective on medical expertise: Theory and implications. *Academic Medicine* 1990; 65:611–621.

Schutz A. *The Phenomenology of the Social World* (G. Walsh, F. Lehnert, trans). Evanston, IL: Northwestern University Press, 1967.

Schwartz KB. Clinical reasoning and new ideas on intelligence: Implications for teaching and learning. *American Journal of Occupational Therapy* 1991;45:1033–1037.

Sluijs EM. Client education in physiotherapy: Towards a planned approach. *Physiotherapy* 1991a;77:503–508.

Sluijs EM. A checklist to assess client education in physical therapy practice: Development and reliability. *Physiotherapy* 1991b;71:561–569.

Smith TJ, Bodurtha JN. Ethical considerations in oncology: Balancing the interests of clients, oncologists and society. *Journal of Clinical Oncology* 1995;13:2464–2470.

Strong J, Gilbert J, Cassidy S, Bennett S. Expert clinicians' and students' views on clinical reasoning in occupational therapy. *British Journal of Occupational Therapy* 1995;58:119–123.

Taber's Cyclopedic Medical Dictionary. Philadelphia: F. A. Davis, 1997.

Tannen D, Wallat C. Interactive frames and knowledge schemes in interaction: Examples from a medical examination interview. *Social Psychology Quarterly* 1987;50:205–216.

Taylor SE. *Positive Illusions: Creative Self-Deception and the Healthy Mind.* New York: Basic Books, 1989.

2

Suicide: It Could Happen to You

Marilyn Maxwell and Pat Precin

Whenever Richard Cory went downtown
We people on the pavement looked at him;
He was a gentleman from sole to crown,
Clean favored, and imperially slim.
And he was always quietly arrayed,
And he was always human when he talked;
But still he fluttered pulses when he said,
"Good morning," and he glittered when he walked.
And he was rich—yes, richer than a king—
And admirably schooled in every grace;
In fine we thought that he was everything
To make us wish that we were in his place.
So on we worked, and waited for the light,
And went without the meat, and cursed the bread;
And Richard Cory, one calm summer night,
Went home and put a bullet through his head.

("Richard Cory," by Edward Arlington Robinson)

Edward Arlington Robinson captures the plight of the individual who appears to be psychologically stable but in fact suffers such inner torment and anguish that he ends his own life. Blessed with every material comfort imaginable and with admiration and respect from those with whom he comes into contact, Richard Cory nonetheless falls prey to depression so severe that he can envision no way out other than suicide.

Psychosocial issues show no prejudice. They can afflict the wealthy, the poor, the popular, the reclusive, the young, the old, and the successful. They traverse cultures, races, ethnicities, and religions. Although they can afflict anyone, psychosocial issues may sometimes go undetected due to the frequent disparity between the way a person appears to others and the way the person actually feels inside.

Like "Richard Cory," the following fictional narrative and true-life stories alert us to the dangers of remaining uneducated about the barriers and indicators of psychosocial issues. In addition, these narratives and stories provide us firsthand accounts of the fears and conflicts that face both the afflicted and the helper and strategies for resolution.

NEVER JUDGE A BOOK BY ITS COVER . . .

ANONYMOUS

My cover does not always reflect all of my pages. My cover is not fake; it is just not always consistent to what is inside. Ever since I can remember, people have given me too much credit. "Oh do not worry, you always land on your feet," or "you have survived the worst, you can get through this," or—my favorite—"you are a fighter—nothing can keep you down." Guess what? It is happening again here: "She seems stable. She seems to be able to keep it together. So what if she has had one therapy session in the last 13 days, she is not showing any signs of self-destruction. Let's see how far we can go. She is not a priority." They do not understand that everything they are seeing is surviving techniques. I am surrounded by people who are supposed to help me and more than half of them are unequipped to help me. They do not understand that I am sitting on a pinhead in limbo because I do not know when my transfer is going to come through.

I tried to end my life because there was not a place in this world for me. There is not even a place for me in this hospital and no one cares!

Client-Centered Reasoning Questions

1. What one phrase do you find most disturbing in this story and why?
2. Give an example of a discrepancy in your own life between the way you appear to others and the way you actually feel inside. When do you think your discrepancy ceases being a healthy defense and becomes detrimental to your mental well-being?
3. Assume that someone wrote this story during your therapeutic group and asked you to read it after the group was over. What would you do after reading it and why?
4. How would you begin to develop a rapport with this client? Why did you choose this technique?
5. What would be your first intervention priority with this client? Why did you select this to be the most important?
6. Read the following analysis. How does the analysis add to your understanding of the plight of the storyteller?

Analysis

In this story, the client is aware of the difference between her outer persona and functional abilities and her inner state of mind. In addition, she brings forth four other themes that she is experiencing during her inpatient psychiatric stay for depression and borderline personality disorder: (1) professionals do not know how to help her, (2) no one cares about her, (3) there is no place in the world for her, (4) and she feels immobilized in her treatment because she is awaiting a transfer to another facility.

Let us first examine the difference between this client's outer persona and occupational performance and her inner state of mind. She tells us of her outward appearance: "My cover does not always reflect all of my pages. Some of them do, but a lot of them do not. My cover is not fake, it is just not always consistent to what is inside." She is also able to give examples of how people see her differently than she really is: "Ever since I can remember, people have given me too much credit, 'Oh do not worry, you always land on your feet,' 'you have survived the worst,' 'you can get through this,' or 'you are just a fighter—nothing can keep you down.'"

Even though this client has an awareness of this discrepancy, it still results in her feeling misunderstood. She feels that professionals do not know how to help her (first theme): "I am surrounded by people who are supposed to help me and more than half of them are unequipped to help me." "They do not understand that everything they are seeing is survival techniques."

Some clients devalue therapists who are trying to help them because these clients feel so bad inside themselves. They may have built up anger that they displace onto the therapist. Or it may be not that professionals are unable to help clients but that some clients do not know how to receive the help offered. Clients can reject help, even though they appear to be asking for help. They may have difficulty responding to interventions.

This client gives examples of statements that lead her to believe that no one cares about her (second theme): "'She seems stable—she seems able to keep it together. So what if she has only had one therapy session in the last 13 days. She is not showing any signs of self-destruction. Let's see how far we can go. She is not a priority.'" This client may be feeling so bad about herself and unable to care for herself that she feels that no one cares about her. If she has not experienced a nurturing environment in the past, she may not be able to receive support and care from her current environment. If her internal state is so painful, she may experience the same pain in her environment no matter how good her situation looks on the outside. In addition, her depression may be causing her to shut out people and interventions around her.

Some clients can be so affected by their psychosocial barriers that they do not understand certain intervention procedures or decisions. Instead, they misunderstand them as being cruel or contrary to their welfare. It is good to work with the clients to develop interventions and outcomes together. But it is rare that clients understand all the rationales behind interventions.

From the team's perspective and in today's times of health care reformation, people are admitted to an inpatient psychiatric unit only if they are in danger of harming themselves or others. Most other people are treated in an outpatient setting, such as a day treatment program, clinic, or a therapy or prevocational program. Once on the inpatient unit, people are discharged as soon as they are no longer in danger of hurting themselves or others and have a place to return to with follow-up treatment. Their stay may be a matter of days or months, depending on the individual, but no one is discharged feeling 100% better. People are discharged as soon as the immediate danger is over, but they still may suffer from psychosocial barriers. Ongoing intervention occurs on an outpatient basis. If people can be maintained as outpatients, they are usually kept out of the hospital. For this reason our storyteller has been told that "'she is not showing any signs of self-destructive behavior. Let's see how far we [the treating team] can go. She is not a priority.'" However, this person attempted suicide without the usual signs.

Sometimes people are chronically suicidal and not admitted to the hospital in hopes that they can be better managed out of the hospital. Outpatient intervention allows them to keep functioning as much as possible in their life roles and gives them the possibility of having more support from family and friends, all of which can be necessary for preventing further decrease in occupational performance. Often it is difficult to decide whether or not to admit someone to the hospital. But if certain signs and symptoms arise, there should be no hesitation for referral for professional intervention, either to outpatient care or to the emergency room. The professionals there will decide the necessary intervention.

This client feels that there is no place in the world for her (third theme): "I tried to end my life because there was not a place in this world for me. There is not even a place for me in this hospital and no one cares!" Even though she is able to express her hopelessness and helplessness, she is unable to feel relief at this time.

This client describes herself as "sitting on a pinhead" waiting for her "transfer to come through." She refers to a transfer from this inpatient unit to a state hospital. Further intervention in a state hospital will give her more time to get over her suicidality while still safe as an inpatient. She is looking forward to being in a state hospital because she is afraid that she will not be able to cope with the stress of living independently and will try to kill herself again. Her image of "sitting on a pinhead" alludes to the idea that she cannot move at all or she will fall. This situation is very uncomfortable for her. Much of her discomfort stems from the fact that she feels passive in this situation (fourth theme) and that others are failing her.

Sometimes people feel so uncomfortable dealing with the issues that brought them into the hospital or caused them to try to commit suicide, that they focus on other things, like their discharge or their transfer (as with this client). They can become unwilling or unable to discuss the issues that brought them into the hospital in the first place. If they cannot discuss these important issues, then they will be unable to receive the intervention they need the most. Perseveration on other issues can be a defense against dealing with the more difficult issues. It is important for therapists to realize that clients need to utilize their strengths while working on their barriers. Intervention must be balanced and checked frequently as one observes the client's reaction to the use of the intervention. It is also important to recognize when a behavior is a defense mechanism. This defensive behavior is individual (particular to each client), but its recognition will aid the helper to proceed with further intervention and give the clients insight into their own defenses, if possible, so they can break through some of them and deal with their painful issues.

People can look good on the outside but feel bad on the inside. They can have all the right support systems in place; appear to be doing well in school, family, and work; have many friends; and still feel bad inside—bad enough to try to kill themselves.

People can be in therapy and still feel bad. Sometimes when people first open up to a therapist, they feel worse because they are now getting in touch with painful feelings of which they may not have been previously aware. People can be in an inpatient hospital for weeks and still feel that no one cares and that no place exists for them to feel comfortable in. People can read all the right books and be treated by the most highly trained professionals and still feel miserable. They may speak aloud of their bad feelings, asking for help and get a response that they are not a high priority.

For these people, change can be slow, intervention may take years, and there is no magic pill to make them permanently feel better. It takes ongoing hard work for them to deal with their painful issues and feel better about themselves.

It is important for therapists not to underestimate people's pain. It may not be obviously affecting their occupational performance, but if they are suicidal, it may end their lives.

WHY?

JENNIFER WERNER (Fictional Student Narrative)

Great, Gabrielle Miller sighed as she walked into the locker room and thought about the sweat that was covering her body as a result of the gym tennis game. The dingy locker room smelled of deodorant blanketed over a thick layer of sweat and perfume. The noisy room was cluttered with girls in Gabrielle's gym class, most of them rushing to get redressed before the bell rang, signaling the last period of the day.

She swung open the locker that she shared with her best friend, Morgan, who had been out sick from school for the past week. The thought of enduring one more day of gym without Morgan was depressing; Gabrielle needed someone to be tennis doubles with, and Morgan was the only one who would tolerate her terrible serve.

The locker room had started to clear out by the time that Gabrielle had laced up her sneakers, when she walked over to the mirror to recomb her tangled ponytail. She stood behind Jolene Morris, a tall volleyball player who was dominating most of the mirror, patiently waiting her turn. When the bell rang and Jolene rushed to grab her loose-leaf and duffel, Gabrielle stepped up to the mirror, silently reproaching herself for not getting dressed sooner and reminding herself that she could not be late for next period's Chemistry test.

Standing in front of the mirror, Gabrielle heard a soft whimpering come from the far corner of the locker room on the other side of the wall. She glanced over there and saw nothing. "Is there a cat in here?" she thought to herself, for the whimpering was soft enough to belong to a delicate feline. She checked her hair again and was ready to tell Mrs. Nattos that there was some animal in the locker room when she heard footsteps. She stepped away from the mirror and peered around the wall only to suppress a gasp when she saw Marielle Less sitting on the bench. She was straddling the bench, her hands pressed down in front of her, with her head hanging down. Her long blond hair cascaded in waves around her shoulders, and Gabby could smell the faint tinge of strawberries in the air, a definite indication that Marielle Less was in the room. *She always smells like fresh strawberries,* Gabby thought disdainfully.

It seemed odd to her that Marielle was crying; she had never seen Marielle's face contorted into such an unhappy expression. Because she was the captain of the cheerleading team, the president of the senior class, and the lead dancer on the dance team, Marielle's face was often plastered around the school. She had two beautiful rows of pearly whites, and Gabrielle was not used to seeing them in any position other than a smile.

Gabrielle tried to recall if she liked Marielle or not and decided that she did not. "Mixed Reviews," Morgan always said. "Either you love Marielle, or you hate her." "It all depends on whether she likes you. Just because she is really nice to her boyfriend and her best friends and she is an angel with her teachers does not mean that she is really a nice person." Gabrielle recalled Morgan's words of advice to her when she first moved here. "Marielle is like this perfect façade thing; like a plum which is shiny and black on the outside. It is such a fake because when you bite in and it is all sour, it seems necessary to hate it for being such a tease."

She pulled her head from around the wall and stood in front of the mirror, looking at her own figure and comparing it to that of Marielle. She compared her own pale, freckled legs to Marielle's long, tanned ones; her curly red ponytail to Marielle's shiny, silky blond halo of hair. She felt a pang of jealousy and decided that she did not care why Marielle was crying. *Just walk back to your books, and go to your Chemistry test. You are going to need as much time as you can get.*

She ignored herself and glanced around the wall once more. Somewhere in the distance Gabrielle heard the second bell ring, signaling the beginning of class and of her Chemistry test, but the shrill ring paled in comparison to Marielle's faint sobs, which

Gabby was straining to hear. Suddenly, as if the picture had just come into focus, Gabby saw Marielle raise her left wrist from the bench. The rest of her body dimmed and Gabby's eyes focused on three long red scars up the side of her arm.

Gabby threw her body back against the wall, fearing that Marielle would have heard her. She quickly scanned her mind to find what could cause such deep marks on the side of her arm. *Pencil marks, cat scratches,* she wracked her brain, but knew that only a razor blade could make such marks.

Did a relative die? Did she break up with Steve? Does her Mom have cancer? Gabrielle thought of what could possibly force Marielle to slice her left arm with a razor blade. *Maybe it was an accident. But, no, an accident would not result in such perfect parallel lines.*

I should talk to her. I should ask her what is wrong; maybe I could help. No, I cannot ask her, I have never spoken to her. But she is human; maybe she just really needs someone to talk to. No, no, no, she is mean, she is a mean person, she is a phony and a fake, and I do not want to help her. She deserves whatever she is upset about. No, she does not deserve anything that forces her to shove a razor blade into her arm. I have a Chemistry test, and I am worried about Marielle Less. This is ridiculous. I have to get to my test.

She walked around the wall and stood in a few feet away from Marielle; the scent of fresh strawberries had become almost drugging. *How does she manage to smell so sweet?* Gabrielle wondered. *Just say her name. Just say it. Marielle. Marielle.*

"Marielle?" No response.

"Marielle?" Marielle's head snapped up, her eyes on fire. Her small features were pulled tightly into an angry expression, and she pulled her sleeves down before throwing her arms behind her back.

"What do you want? How long have you been in here? I did not know anyone was in here."

"I know, I was looking in the mirror and I heard you—I heard you—here. I just, I mean I was not like listening I just wanted to make sure—"

"Like, are you going to say something, or what?" Marielle asked in a bitter, superior tone.

"Nothing. You know what, just forget it. Sorry I bothered you." Gabrielle started to walk away, scolding herself for making such a stupid mistake by assuming that Marielle Less was actually in need of compassion.

"No wait."

"What?"

"No, I mean I did not mean to be so nasty. I am sorry. I am fine."

Gabrielle turned around and looked at Marielle. *She looks so small. . . .*

"I just heard you crying and I thought that you—were not all right."

"Gabby"—Gabrielle was shocked that Marielle knew her name, much less to call her by such a familiar nickname. She started wondering if Marielle had always known her name and never bothered to say hello. *I never should have come back here. I should have just walked away. I never make the right choices in situations like this. Morgan would kill me.*

"—because I could not go to a clinic, and I just got so frustrated with myself and with Steve and with everything, that I did this." Gabrielle looked up and realized that Marielle was still talking, and as she caught the last bit of the conversation, she saw Marielle lift up her sleeves and expose her naked flesh. The red lines seemed to jump out at Gabrielle, making her nauseous and confusing her. *Clinic? Why would she go to a clinic? And what does Steve have to do with anything?*

"—but the worst part of everything is that his Mom wants us to keep the baby!" Gabrielle's jaw dropped open and she sat down on the bench next to Marielle, who was sobbing hysterically now. *Baby? Marielle has a baby?* The thought of the girl next to her carrying a secret baby overwhelmed Gabrielle. All of a sudden she did not want to touch her; she did not want to touch this "infected" girl. The idea of Marielle Less carrying a baby made her nervous to even be next to her. *Marielle Less is having a baby?*

"—and she was like I am having a baby. And I said to the doctor—"

The doctor must be wrong!

"—but my mom knew, she just *knew* when I went to tell her. I said Mom, I do not know how to tell you this, but she just *knew*! She said—"

Marielle? You are having a baby?

"—oh and I could not help it; I have seen my psychiatrist and we have discussed the razor problems; my fucking psychiatrist always promises it is confidential, she always lies! She always tells me—"

This is a secret! I cannot tell anyone that Marielle Less is having a baby and that she makes razor marks up her arm because her boyfriend's mother wants her to keep the baby. . . .

"And, Gabrielle, I do not know what to do! I just cannot do this and I cannot tell anyone and none of my friends would understand! There is no one who knows and I just know you would not tell anyone, I know that you are a good person and I know that I can trust you with this, you are a good person and you came over to talk to me and I know that was hard because I know who I am and I know what I am and I know what you must think but you came over and you are listening and I will never forget that. . . ." At this point, Marielle's rushed choked voice completely broke and her sobs took over. Gabrielle just sat next to her, at a loss for what to do. She looked at herself and looked at Marielle and looked at her own beautiful, smooth arms and then at Gab(Ma)rielle's arms which now, up close, revealed a group of scars that skin had grown over, and she was suddenly so grateful to have her own body.

I have to do something. I cannot just sit here. I will just . . . will just touch her. I will just reach out to her, because at least if I reach out to her, just touch her arm or her shoulder or her hand or her leg or her hair then she will know that I want to help her. Then maybe this poor shuddering girl will not feel alone, this girl who I have never spoken to before this day and who is harboring the worst of secrets is not alone. Marielle is not alone, because I am sitting next to her and I can just touch her. I will touch her and that will help her. I can touch her.

And she did.

Client-Centered Reasoning Activities

1. Working in dyads, role-play the Marielle/Gabrielle interaction by creating a new dialogue that reflects your own personality and personal experiences.
2. Shortly after the interaction role-played in the previous activity, you now find yourself in your therapy session. Discuss with your therapist your thoughts and feelings regarding the interaction.
3. Create a hypothetical situation in which Marielle has just confided in you as a therapist. Working in dyads, role-play a dialogue between Marielle and the therapist. How did you define your boundaries as a therapist in this situation? What kinds of confidentiality issues arise here?
4. Finish the narrative.

Analysis

Jennifer's narrative is a poignant portrayal of a young woman whose unplanned pregnancy leaves her vulnerable to depression, despair, and thoughts of suicide. Captain of the cheerleaders, president of the senior class, and an attractive girl, Marielle Less is the last person Gabrielle Miller would expect to find upset in the girls' locker room. Indeed, Gabrielle is shocked as she secretly observes Marielle crying and notices the scar lines running up Marielle's arm, clear indicators to Gabrielle that Marielle has attempted suicide. After a brief internal struggle, Gabby decides to bypass her jealousy of this popular girl and offer her assistance.

The narrative reveals much about a layperson's perceptions of suicide; of our need and desire to empathize with another person's pain; about our ambivalence, fears, and at times, overidentification with those in trouble. Like many narratives of people in distress, Jennifer's story invites the reader to enter into the discourse of pain, to listen carefully to everything that is said and not said, to pay attention to the manner in which language is used and conclusions reached.

One striking aspect of Jennifer's story deals with her choice of a narrative point of view. Filtered through Gabrielle's consciousness, the story begins to unfold from an omniscient narrative point of view that presents events to the reader as Gabrielle experiences them. Interestingly enough, the narrative point of view slips into a first-person stream of consciousness when Gabby allows herself to get closer to Marielle and listen to her story. The author, however, never allows this shifting narrative lens to project events through Marielle's consciousness or to reveal Marielle's feelings through her first-person voice. Consequently, the reader gets to know Gabrielle more intimately than Marielle, so that the narrative, while ostensibly focused upon a young girl's suicide attempt, is primarily about an observer's attempt to deal with her own feelings when confronting someone in deep psychological trouble. Because of the narrative strategy in this story, Marielle remains somewhat impenetrable to the reader. What we learn about Marielle is confined to what she says and does not say and depends on the extent to which Gabrielle is a reliable narrator. Seeing Marielle through Gabrielle's eyes, the reader can only hypothesize as to the real motives and source of pain that would prompt a suicide attempt—is it just her pregnancy, her boyfriend's mother's insistence upon her keeping the child? Yes, we learn something about Marielle, but we learn far more about Gabrielle because of the narrative shift into a first-person stream of consciousness and, perhaps, because we identify with the "I," we learn much about ourselves and our perceptions and feelings about suicide and dealing with people in crisis.

Jennifer's choice of a shifting narrative stance is fascinating and reveals, perhaps, some of the ambivalence that her character, Gabrielle, feels toward Marielle, perhaps some of the ambivalence that many of us feel when getting too close to someone in pain, especially someone who is very much like us. While we initially see the events through Gabrielle's eyes, we are prevented from completely identifying with Gabrielle because of the narrative distance affected by the omniscient point of view. We learn about Gabrielle's jealousy of and disdain for Marielle, but we do not feel these emotions intimately because we have not yet been invited into the interior of Gabrielle's consciousness through a first-person perspective. The writer has chosen to differentiate the internal musings of Gabrielle from the rest of the narrative by using italics, but interestingly enough, the initial internal musings—"*She always smells like fresh strawberries*"—focuses on Marielle and not on the feelings of the observer, Gabrielle. When Gabrielle is trying to decide whether she should offer Marielle assistance or go to her Chemistry test, the narrative slips into an italicized internal debate, in which Gabrielle splits into two personas, one voice addressing her "other" self in the second person: "*Just walk back to your books and go to your Chemistry test.*" Now, we are pulled in a bit closer to the feelings of the observer, specifically her ambivalence and antithetical feelings, which are captured so well in the split consciousness. What is striking about this narrative strategy, whether conscious or unconscious in origin, is the avoidance of a full-blown first-person narrative voice—there is no "I" yet; it is as if the writer is approaching Marielle, the subject in distress, with extreme caution as a matter of self-protection, as if Marielle might be contagious—indeed, Gabrielle later recoils from touching Marielle for fear of becoming "infected" by the latter's pregnancy.

Not until halfway through the story does the narrative lens risk revealing the "I" of the observer, and even though the internal debate continues and tries to resolve the ambivalence, we now are invited to identify with the observer more fully, as we hear her muse about her emotional state in the first person: *"I should talk to her."* It is significant that the shift to a first-person voice and all the attendant issues of risk taking, intimacy, empathy, and identification occur at the point in the story in which Gabrielle resolves her ambivalence and decides to reach out to Marielle.

In addition to the interesting and revealing narrative structure of the story, the choice of character names raises issues of psychological import. The writer has chosen two names for her characters that are strikingly similar, Gabrielle and Marielle, suggesting perhaps a commonality that flirts with overidentification. We have already seen how the narrative distance between observer and observed is gradually bridged as Gabrielle overcomes her fears and gets closer to someone in trouble. The shift from omniscient to second-person to first-person narration is consonant with Gabrielle's jettisoning of her own resistance as she risks feeling compassion and empathy for Marielle. The danger, of course, is that such emotional closeness and intimacy can lead to an overidentification and dissolution of ego boundaries that threaten the integrity of the self.

The fear of such a blurring of ego boundaries perhaps explains Gabrielle's inability to process Marielle's complete story all at once. In an apparently self-protective maneuver, Gabrielle allows the details of Marielle's story to penetrate her awareness only by degrees. When Marielle begins to relate her tale of pain, Gabrielle retreats into her own thoughts and does not hear everything Marielle says: *"I never should have come back here. I should have just walked away."* Almost as a defense mechanism, Gabrielle blocks the painful tale from entering her consciousness all at once. When she does reattune herself to Marielle and start to listen, Gabrielle is somewhat lost as to the full meaning of Marielle's story and must reassemble the narrative from the fragments of sentences and words that did penetrate her awareness. As if to protect herself from overidentifying with someone else's pain, losing herself in someone else's despair, Gabrielle tunes in and out to the information being given by Marielle, thereby allowing herself to assimilate the potentially tragic import of the situation by degrees.

The author manages to avoid typographical "slips" and does not confuse Marielle with Gabrielle until the very end of the story when she writes: "She [Gabrielle] looked at herself and looked at Marielle and looked at her own beautiful, smooth arms and then at Gab(Ma)rielle's arms. . . ." The error at this point in the story is very telling: Gabrielle has just been let in on Marielle's secret—her pregnancy and attempted suicide—and she has just expressed her own fear of becoming "infected" by Marielle's situation. Has Gabrielle gotten too close? As an observer, Gabrielle cannot control what Marielle tells her and perhaps by getting close to and listening to the pain of the popular, intelligent coed, someone like herself, Gabrielle suddenly realizes that she too is not immune to the "accidents" of life, to the unexpected exigencies that challenge all of us at times; Gabrielle suddenly feels vulnerable to the "infections" of the unpredictable and unplanned contingencies of life, that is, she viscerally intuits that "this could happen to her."

In walking that fine emotional line between empathy and over-identification, Gabrielle has perhaps recouped herself and acknowledged the ego boundaries necessary to maintain a healthy distance between Marielle and herself, for she concludes that paragraph by telling us "she was suddenly so grateful to have her own body." Clearly demarcated ego boundaries allow Gabrielle to reach across to Marielle and touch her compassionately, to let Marielle know that she is not alone, that someone else cares.

In touching her, Gabrielle has overcome her fear and resistance and opened up a new world for both of them. Gabrielle has overcome her jealousy and ambivalence to reach out in compassion. She will hear Marielle's tale and piece it together in an acceptable form, one her ego can tolerate, one that will allow Gabrielle to protect herself while not rejecting Marielle.

SEALING OVER

ANONYMOUS INTERN

Eighteen-year-old Samantha was admitted into the hospital for an attempted suicide. She was at school and attempted to jump out a window. She is now on the psychiatric ward and is the youngest client here. She is a very pretty, slim African American girl who is well groomed, in fashionable clothes, and has good hygiene. I have seen her around the unit today with other young female clients and she appears scared and nervous.

We discussed Samantha in our team meeting. It was agreed that she needs a good follow-up program, but otherwise she should be discharged soon. Today is Friday, and on Fridays I run a discharge-planning group. I select the clients who are nearing discharge and those I feel can benefit from this group. Samantha seemed like she was a good candidate for the group today, so I made a point of inviting her to join us. She accepted and arrived with two of the other female clients.

The group was productive. The clients offered their concerns about discharge and their hopes, too. Samantha was relatively quiet while all of these topics were being discussed; she sat and politely listened to everyone else's ideas but did not offer any of her own. I decided to try to engage her in the conversation. I asked her if she had any concerns about her discharge and being back home again. She looked at me with big eyes and said, "I am afraid of what people are going to think. My friends at school are going to think I am crazy or something. I am afraid that people at school are going to treat me differently. I do not want them to have a security guard following me around school, afraid that I am going to do something else." This was a response I have never heard before on this unit. Most of the other clients have been dealing with their illnesses much longer. It appears to me that many have given up on the idea that anyone would ever view them normal again. This is not a commonly expressed concern around here. Samantha got a little misty eyed when she was telling us this, and I immediately felt for her. She does present much differently than most of the other clients. Her thoughts are much more organized, her activities of daily living skills are completely intact, and she has pretty good time management skills at home. These thoughts of hers are so incredibly potent at her age. As a senior in high school, she is prey to all of the other trappings of adolescence. She explained that the reason she almost jumped out of a window was because she did poorly on a college entrance exam. The most important thing to her right now is getting into a college. Now, after attempting to jump, she is faced with even more stressful situations. It can be emotionally scarring to go into school if you are having a bad hair day or a boy says something bad about you. But, imagine having to return to school after a trip to the psychiatric unit of the local hospital. She is having very valid fears, and it was hard for us to answer her. In fact, we could not. Our group (discharge planning) is the clients' group. They are supposed to offer ideas and work out their problems together. We are just facilitating this exchange. So, we asked the group to respond to Samantha's situation. The group basically decided that the best answer is that, "If they are your friends, they will not care or think any less of you." It was one of those "looks good on paper" ideas, and to be honest, I could not have come up with anything better at the time.

We as a group launched into a discussion of stigmas, and it was interesting how these clients often called themselves "crazy," even though they were talking about how much it hurts to hear the term "crazy."

Samantha is experiencing very real, very scary feelings for a person of any age, but she is 18 years old and image is everything. A possible cry for attention may be getting her just the opposite of what she was looking for. Or, the first onset of an illness is causing her to enter a life that no one is ready for. If the latter is true, chances are she will not be viewed the same, and her life is going to be very different. It will be a hard road.

Client-Centered Reasoning Questions

1. What are your personal feelings toward Samantha?
2. What are your personal reactions to the intern?

Client-Centered Reasoning Activities

1. Form a group of people and role-play the interactions among Samantha, the intern, and the other clients. Switch roles, paying particular attention to the different techniques one could use as the intern.
2. Finish the narrative.

Analysis

Here is another example of someone who appears to be doing well on the outside but has many problems on the inside. Samantha has been described as an 18-year-old, pretty, slim, well-groomed, fashionable, young female high school student. Samantha was "admitted into the hospital [psychiatric] for an attempted suicide. She was at school and attempted to jump out a window."

This story is also a good example of the stigma that arises around psychosocial issues. Samantha obviously feels much peer pressure at school and is concerned about what people will think about her when she returns. These concerns are "normal" for someone in Samantha's situation. People have many different reactions to a suicide attempt, depression, or a stay in the psychiatric ward. Things will probably be different for her when she goes back to school. She did a serious thing. Most people at school may not know how to deal with it.

The intern deals with Samantha's fear of stigma in several ways. She engages her in conversation about her discharge. She empathizes with her fears. She relates to Samantha's situation by recalling what it was like during her own high school days.

She imagines herself in Samantha's situation. She validates Samantha's fears to herself. Then the intern gets stuck. She does not know how to respond verbally to Samantha.

All the preceding techniques—eliciting information after having set up a safe environment to speak, forming a rapport, empathizing, identifying, transposing, and validating—are very hard to implement in a group setting. The intern uses them all, yet does not know what to say to Samantha.

The intern's solution is to elicit a group response. The group comes up with an answer. The intern then utilizes the group to discuss stigmas of psychosocial issues. This is a very powerful technique because it gives Samantha a group to fit into, since she now feels that she will not fit in at school. This "therapeutic" group helps her normalize her situation so that she no longer feels like she is the only person dealing with stigma. This technique, called *universality*, can be a good reason for conducting interventions in a group setting. The technique is also powerful because it shifts the emphasis from a particular client to the rest of the group. Group members help solve the problems at hand. In doing so, they relate and empathize, then bring in a similar problem that they may be having. Clients often respond more when another client gives them feedback than when the therapist offers the feedback. One of the therapist's goals in a group is to get the clients themselves to say what the therapist would like to say in the group. The group discussions around Samantha's feelings about returning to school are probably helpful to Samantha and helpful to the intern, who now has a better rapport with Samantha because of the discussions. However, the issue of "sealing over" needs to be addressed.

Sealing over is a term used in psychosocial rehabilitation to describe a situation in which a client feels so uncomfortable discussing painful feelings that he or she would rather not discuss them at all, despite support and help from others. Instead, the client discusses issues that are not as difficult to talk about.

In this case, Samantha chooses to discuss how she may be feeling once out of the hospital, instead of how she is currently feeling or processing what led her to try to kill herself. She may have already discussed the reasons for her attempted suicide with other staff members, since the team feels comfortable making the decision to discharge her soon. However, her issues probably require much further discussion. (Samantha's stay in the hospital was less than a week.) This inability to confront painful feelings appeared in the previous story, in which the client felt immobilized because she was waiting for a transfer. Both cases exhibit the process of sealing over.

The intern may benefit from knowing more information concerning the suicide attempt. Why did Samantha try to kill herself at school if she was so worried about what her peers would think of her? Was it a call for attention? Was she impulsive? Why did she not complete the jump? Did someone stop her or did she stop herself? What did she respond to that changed her mind? Has she had any past attempts? How serious was this attempt? Samantha does state that she "almost jumped out of a window because she did poorly on a college entrance exam" and because "the most important thing to her right now is getting into a college." What is the source of the pressure to go to college? Parents? Samantha? What expectations are put on her? Why did she do poorly? Did she do poorly? Could she apply to a college that has lower admission requirements? Why is college the most important thing to her right now? What else was going on in Samantha's life that may have led up to her attempt?

Suicide rarely happens out of the blue. Usually many factors lead up to it over a long period of time. Many people perform poorly on college entrance exams, but most people do not try to kill themselves because of it. What makes Samantha different? Was she depressed to start with? The intern described her as "very pretty, slim, and well groomed, in fashionable clothes, and has good hygiene." Was she depressed underneath? Does she have to be perfect? What happens if she is not?

Whatever Samantha's problems were before admission, have they been resolved? If so, how? Was Samantha empowered during the process, or did someone solve her problem for her? How has her situation changed so she can return home and to school without the same pressures and stress that led to her admission? What else still needs to change? How much insight does Samantha have about what she still needs to work on, about how to get help, and about the seriousness of what she has done? Has the family received psycho-education about suicide? How involved is the family? What are her support systems in addition to follow-up intervention? Has she ever had intervention before?

It seems as though there may have been reluctance on the part of Samantha, the intern, and the team to discuss some of these issues. We already discussed some of the reasons why Samantha may have "sealed over"; that is, resisted dealing with difficult feelings. In addition, sometimes young people who try to commit suicide do not know why they tried it. They may never have been in therapy and have little insight about their situation. Sometimes, they feel embarrassed about what they have done and do not want to discuss it. Sometimes, they feel exposed and wish to cover it all up by stating that everything is fine now. Sometimes, there is pressure from family members to "keep the whole thing a secret."

There are many reasons why an intern may experience difficulty discussing thoughts, feelings, and behaviors that lead to a suicide attempt. Perhaps the intern overidentifies with the client or is afraid to cry in front of the client. There may be a fear that talking about the attempt would so upset the client that he or she would fall apart, and the intern would be blamed for "damaging" the client. There may be a fear that the client would become so upset that he or she would attempt suicide in the hospital. The intern may feel responsible. The intern may be afraid of becoming depressed and unable to think of appropriate interventions for the client. The intern may have had suicidal thoughts or have unresolved issues with family or friends who tried or succeeded in killing themselves. The intern, like many lay people, might have difficulty understanding why a client who is young, beautiful, and apparently protected from the harshness of society would want to end her life.

The intern brings her preconceived experiences, thoughts, reactions, and beliefs about suicide into the therapeutic relationship. This is a normal phenomenon but must be consciously examined by the intern in order to distinguish her own feelings from those of the client. The intern can then step away from the client, step away from her own feelings, and examine the situation clearly to determine, with the help of the supervisor, the best possible intervention. Over time, interns learn how to listen to and deal with the upsetting stories they will inevitably hear from their clients.

The team's lack of communication about the details of the suicide attempt may be due to a time limit and to the expertise of each member. If, in dealing with a suicidal client individually, a team member feels that the client is no longer suicidal, that team member will bring this to the attention of coworkers. If no other team members disagree, a discharge date is set that will allow for both intervention and housing dispositions to be in place. The details of a particular case are not always discussed among team members. Interns must assert themselves by posing questions to interdisciplinary members during and after team meetings. If these questions do not elicit satisfactory answers, the interns must speak directly with the clients.

The most secure place for clients to discuss their most difficult problems is in the hospital, where many staff members work around the clock, providing intervention and making sure the client remains safe. It is important for clients to deal with their issues before they are discharged from the hospital, so that they may attain some insight and resolution. Problem solving can then occur with the help of the intern; and together, the client and intern can set and achieve goals.

In Samantha's case, it would be helpful to know why she did not score well on the college entrance exam. If she lacks the ability at this time, she should know this, so she can avoid another low score if repeating the test. Her parents may be told that she lacks the ability at this time, so that they may take some of the pressure off her (if they are creating high expectations). The social worker and intern could help the parents understand and accept their child's limitations. The intern could administer aptitude tests, measure test anxiety, and determine if Samantha could make any improvements or adjustments that could help her score higher next time. Perhaps Samantha possesses the ability but was not used to taking standardized tests, in which case both practice and the knowledge that she could do better might help to improve her score. Much of this work can take place out of the hospital, but the intern should make some kind of recommendation based on the assessments of what the next step should be regarding college.

Samantha's concern about what other people will think about her is valid, but it also may be a projection. She may be worried about what she thinks about herself and what has happened to her. She states, "'I do not want them [school faculty] to have a security guard following me around school afraid that I am going to do something else.'" She may actually wish that she had more "security" at school. She may be afraid that she might "do something else." It is important for interns to learn to listen with a third ear, especially when clients are not completely forthcoming about their situations. To listen with a third ear means not only to listen to the exact word the client is saying but also observe all body language and discern his or her unconscious issues as well. In this case it may be helpful to ask Samantha how she would like things to be at school when she returns.

UNANSWERED QUESTIONS

NANCY MORITZ-FARAJUN

To climb steep hills requires slow pace at first.

—WILLIAM SHAKESPEARE, *Henry VIII*, Act I, Scene I

It is 9:00 A.M., the standard hour for team rounds, when clinicians discuss and present cases on the inpatient psychiatric unit. In the third week of my 12-week internship, I was just beginning to fully understand evaluation and intervention of an individual with psychosocial issues. The psychiatry resident opened a chart and reported the admitting information about the new client, Brian. Brian was brought to the hospital after his suicide attempt from the sixth floor of his father's apartment building, fortunate to have only injured his foot. Suicide attempts were not uncommon to this unit. In order to be admitted, clients must be in danger of hurting themselves or others.

Brian was a 26-year-old man, over 6 feet tall, a former basketball player, a graduate from a respectable university; prior to admission he resided in his own apartment in a city distant from his immediate family, worked full time, and had no apparent psychosocial issues or family psychosocial history. Brian was a good student, popular, and a well-known basketball player at his university. Prior to admission, Brian worked as a promoter for a sports company after graduating from college. In that time, his company suffered a difficult financial period, in which Brian blamed himself for poor sales. The transition from being an accomplished man on campus to working for an unsuccessful business was a key stressor for Brian. In addition, his parents were divorced and his father was very demanding and controlling toward Brian and others involved in his son's intervention. Before his suicide attempt, Brian admitted to having paranoid thoughts that his father was planning to castrate him and that his coworkers were speaking critically about him in private. Brian was diagnosed with major depression with psychotic features and prescribed antipsychotic and antidepressant medications. Upon admission, Brian was selectively mute and would remain so for about two weeks.

Several questions were running through my mind. How would I get Brian to talk if experienced professionals were unsuccessful? What could occupational therapy do for him? Furthermore, a change of environment and controlling parents were factors for many individuals in their twenties. I, myself, had transitioned from university to internship and soon to the role of a worker and wife. Stress was an everyday word in my lexicon of life. I realized Brian demonstrated psychotic symptoms in addition to his depression. Still, many people with Brian's identical problems never attempt to end their own lives. It frightened me to think about what could have pushed this well-liked, bright, handsome young man off the edge of a sixth-floor building.

Since Brian would not reveal his personal goals to me until the day of his discharge, I based my intervention plan on team rounds and biographical data. It seemed almost unethical for me to compose the above intervention plan without consulting Brian. However, I knew that I had limited time to work with Brian before his insurance expired, so I prioritized goals that would prepare him for discharge. My goals focused on Brian's independence with hygiene, activities of daily living, concentration on tasks, time management, leisure, socialization skills, stress management, and effective problem solving in order for him to eventually return to work or graduate school and independent living. These were all sensible goals on paper, but how would I be able to have Brian put them into practice? The answer was *gradually*—over approximately a six-week period of time.

The first step was attempting to develop a rapport with an individual who was voluntarily not speaking. Brian was my contemporary—he could have been my classmate, star player on my college basketball team, or a coworker. Knowing that he enjoyed basketball and reading, I would deliver the *New York Times* Sports Section and later ask Brian questions about the articles. I felt that, before Brian would speak to me about his problems, he needed to feel that he could trust me. In addition, the purpose of these visits was not to acquire knowledge of athletics but three-fold in nature: (1) to develop rapport by working with something interesting to him, (2) to increase his ability to attend to task, and (3) to improve socialization.

Once Brian trusted me and realized that I genuinely wanted to help him, he slowly began attending therapeutic activity groups, focusing on personal hygiene with minimal cues, and reading in his free time. When I encouraged him to shave and offered my supervision, Brian would politely decline or respond that he would shave later in the day. When contemplating why he continuously refused to shave, I reconsidered Brian's comfort level. Maybe he felt uneasy being watched by a female staff member almost identical in age to himself? Brian admitted that my hypothesis was correct. In order to increase Brian's comfort level as well as his independence with self-care, I suggested that he request assistance from a male nursing attendant as needed. Brian followed my advice, and within two weeks, Brian became completely independent in all self-care activities.

To increase not only Brian's attendance but also his participation in group activities, I led a basketball activity during a Leisure Skills group. I acknowledged Brian's experience, asked him to explain my typed game rules and assist with refereeing. Brian's verbalization and eye contact increased, and he demonstrated a more appropriate affect. Brian even laughed when a 64-year-old woman patient defeated him in a shooting match. Eventually, Brian's time management improved and he required no reminders to attend therapeutic groups, complete activities of daily living (ADLs), or incorporate leisure into his daily schedule.

At this point, I felt Brian was ready to discuss the factors leading up to his suicide attempt and better ways of coping with these stresses. Brian remained somewhat guarded but revealed that his job was a key stressor that caused him to neglect his ADLs and become isolated. Living away from his relatives (namely, his sister) and close friends did not seem to help this situation. Brian's controlling father seemed to be a source of aggravation rather than relief for Brian. I acknowledged that Brian's feelings were valid responses to the above stresses but his solutions to these problems were ineffective. Psychosocial barriers are nothing to be ashamed of—according to the National Institute of Mental Health's 1998 report; 17 million Americans develop depression each year. I gave Brian an educational packet about stress management techniques to read and then discussed the information. When I asked Brian about his future goals, he stated that he would eventually like to return to work or graduate school to pursue a field in which he could work with children. Brian may have chosen this goal in part due to his feelings of being an inadequate role model for his younger brother. He also wanted to begin playing basketball again and eventually live on his own. I encouraged Brian to join a community basketball league with his friends and volunteer as a basketball coach for younger children to explore his expressed interest in working with them. In addition to incorporating leisure into his daily schedule, these suggestions would also improve Brian's ability to socialize appropriately—a skill necessary for him to return to work or school.

The day of Brian's discharge was an emotional one for me as well as for the other interns. In the field of mental health, you do not always directly witness improvement in the people with whom you have worked. It is not uncommon that some clients are readmitted in the same week of their discharge, secondary to non-compliance with medications, psychiatric follow-up, or lack of insight into their illness. I am not a gambler, but on that day, I would have bet a million dollars that Brian would eventually attain the goal of independent living.

Clinicians in the field of mental health do not always see the results of their work with their clients and do not always receive feedback from them. Brian was able to express his gratitude, pinpoint the ways in which staff assisted him, and state realistic future goals. He was now open to the idea of seeking further help and eventually returning to work.

So, where is Brian now? He is soon to be discharged from his outpatient day treatment program to a private clinician. He is returning to his old job, own apartment, and has expressed an interest in applying to law school. Presently, Brian is on a low dose of antidepressants but refuses to continue taking his antipsychotic medication secondary to Parkinson-like symptoms (stiffness) and because he denies his past psychotic state, characteristic of schizophrenia. Overall, Brian is a success story from an occupational therapy standpoint, for he is able to return to independent living. If his delusions reappear, I hope that Brian will seek the counseling and medication he requires.

One question in Brian's case was left unanswered for me: What ultimately pushed him—who could have been my classmate, friend, basketball team star player, or coworker—to attempt suicide? And what makes the rest of us maintain our sanity in this stressful world? I guess this piece of the puzzle will remain unsolved for me as well as for so many others who work with the mentally ill.

Client-Centered Reasoning Questions

1. Compare and contrast the interns' level of involvement with their clients in this story and the previous story. How does each intern go about building rapport? How does each intern's rapport with the client affect the depth of the discussion about suicide?

2. Let us assume that Marielle (the character from Jennifer Werner's narrative) has been hospitalized in a psychiatric inpatient unit. What kind of effective interventions do you think one of these interns could provide for Marielle?

Client-Centered Reasoning Activities

1. Finish the narrative.
2. Write an occupational profile.
3. Write a questionnaire.
4. List additional assessments you would use with this client.
5. Write an occupational performance analysis.
6. Write an intervention plan.
7. Readjust the intervention plan if you were to treat Brian in (a) an employee assistance program at his job after his return and (b) once-a-week family therapy with his father after discharge.
8. Write two progress notes for Brian at different intervals during his work with Nancy.
9. Write a discharge note.
10. Make referrals to other services.
11. Write a group protocol for an ongoing group that would address the majority of Brian's goals.
12. What types of clinical reasoning have you applied when writing Brian's assessment, occupational profile, occupational performance analysis, intervention plan, discharge plan, referrals, and group protocol?
13. What frame of reference or theory have you applied in creating Brian's assessment, occupational profile, occupational performance analysis, intervention plan, discharge plan, referrals, and group protocol? Provide support for why this theory is appropriate for Brian's needs. What other frames of reference might be appropriate and why?

Analysis

This story about Brian is another example of someone appearing functional on the outside but feeling hopeless and helpless on the inside. Brian is a 26-year-old basketball player and college graduate, who is living independently and working full time. He was a good student and socially popular. Prior to admission, neither he nor his family had any history of psychosocial issues. However, he was admitted to the psychiatric inpatient unit after attempting to jump from the sixth floor of his father's apartment building.

This story talks about how to deal with suicidal people who do not wish to open up and discuss their thoughts, feelings, and situation. It shows how Nancy built rapport with Brian and then was able to discuss his stresses that led to the suicide attempt. Nancy feels empathetic and relates to Brian's situation and, in addition, feels comfortable talking about Brian's suicide attempt. Unlike the intern who worked with Samantha, Nancy is able to offer interventions without Brian sealing over. Brian's intervention progresses further than Samantha's because Brian's suicide attempt is addressed in more depth than Samantha's. Many interns are uncomfortable asking about details of clients' symptoms, even though the symptoms may be interfering with the clients' occupational performance. It is difficult to help people improve their functioning if their emotions are in the way. Some people with psychosocial issues have skills but cannot apply them, due to an exacerbation of their symptoms. Reasons why interns may be reluctant to discuss symptoms have been mentioned in the previous story.

Nancy uses a variety of graded techniques to build an effective rapport over time with this "selectively mute" person. Nancy begins by bringing the daily newspaper to Brian's room (where he spent most of his time during his first two weeks in the hospital) with encouragement to read the sports section. This intervention is nonthreatening, normalizing, and matches Brian's interest. After learning that Brian was reading the articles, Nancy spent time discussing sports with Brian, who now feels comfortable enough to speak about sports in the news. Because it becomes apparent that Brian enjoys reading, Nancy brings him books to read in his free time. Bringing the books is also a nonthreatening intervention, since Brian has control over when and what he will read and the material is of general interest and not yet about suicide. As Nancy senses that Brian is beginning to trust that she genuinely wants to help him, she encourages Brian to attend therapeutic activities. Once he does well in the hygiene group, Nancy encourages him to take care of his hygiene independent of the group setting. Nancy then notices his lack of follow-through and postulates that it may be because she had offered to help him with his shaving. The fact that she is a young woman, close to his age, may have embarrassed him. Nancy responds to her own intuition by being sensitive to his needs and, therefore, arranged for a man to help him with his shaving. Overall, Nancy, unlike Brian's father, tries to interact with Brian in a noncontrolling, nonthreatening way. She tries to respect Brian's wishes, needs, and fears by working with him and letting him regain some control over his life.

Having gained a rapport with Brian, Nancy is able to use the following intervention techniques to help him. She validates his feelings but points out that there are other, healthier ways to deal with them: "I acknowledged that Brian's feelings were valid responses to the above stresses but his solutions to these problems were ineffective." Nancy empowers Brian by providing him educational packets on stress management. She provides the family with psycho-educational material on depression to help him and his family understand and accept what has happened to him. She fosters in Brian problem solving and independence. She uses his interest in basketball to create a therapeutic activity that she grades to match his occupational performance.

Some people have a difficult time doing something in the hospital that they used to be good at on the outside, especially if the hospital activity is an easier simulation. Clients' egos can be fragile. They may think the new activity is childish or they may be afraid to fail. In this case, the graded activity works with Brian. How did Nancy know to try this? What were her cues? She helped him modify and pursue his interests on the outside (community basketball league and volunteer basketball coach for children), allowing him to have a balanced day of work, socialization, and his own leisure time. After these interventions, Nancy and Brian are both ready to deal with his suicidality.

At the end of her story, Nancy says that there is one question that she still cannot answer: "What ultimately pushed Brian—who could have been my classmate, friend, basketball team star player, or coworker—to attempt suicide? And, what makes the rest of us maintain our sanity in this stressful world?" Suicide does not usually happen capriciously. Brian's relationship with his father probably had long-standing problems that may have played a role in contributing to his suicide attempt. There may have been other contributing factors.

Let us examine the cues found in the intern's story, cues that indicate underlying problems. Let us also examine how to read between the important lines in the story to develop deeper insight into Brian's pain. Prior to admission, Brian became more socially isolated and began to neglect his ADLs. He made a life transition from being a successful university student to an employee at a business that was not doing well. His parents are divorced. Both he and the staff experience his father as demanding and controlling. Prior to admission, Brian thought his father was going to castrate him. Even though Brian was in a psychotic depression, the content of his psychosis, the castration fantasy, can provide insight into his underlying problems. He also believed that his coworkers were criticizing him behind his back. Brian blamed himself for his company's financial problems. He may or may not have been responsible, but the fact that he blames himself may illustrate Brian's exaggerated sense of failure. Not only is he hard on himself, he also feels that others are hard on him. But why the suicide attempt now? He made it through college. He made it through living with a difficult father and his parents' divorce.

The fact that Brian jumped out of his *father's* sixth-floor apartment building in a suicide attempt is important. It may be indicative of a strong tie or bond (good or bad) with his father. People's choice of the place and type of death is always meaningful. Suicide acts are often carefully planned. The person attempting suicide usually wishes to affect someone who would frequent the place of the attempt. In Brian's case, it is his father. Notice that Brian does not jump from his workplace, even though we know he feels responsible for the business' poor sales. No, something deeper was affecting him, something more long-standing.

An important part of Brian's intervention would be to explore the relationship with his father, so that Brian may experience less pressure in his life and be able to set alternative goals for himself graded to his current level of functioning, so that he feels good about what he can do instead of feeling bad about what he cannot do. Brian also needs help testing the reality of his work skills. Did Brian make mistakes at work that led to the company's difficulty or did Brian just feel responsible? What were his feelings based on? Could he make improvements if he were to return? Will he be able to return? What are his skills at work, problem solving, and reality testing now? How could he be less hard on himself now?

Depression often leads to a narrowing of perception. People who are depressed may not see reality clearly. They may feel guilty or responsible for things that do not directly or exclusively involve them.

Therefore, reality testing may be of help. They often do not see many options for themselves. They can become more and more depressed until they can see no way out. This may have happened to Brian.

In intervening with a depressed person, the cycle of depression must be broken. It can be broken through a variety of methods, but the method(s) selected must be particular to the depressed person. For Brian, it could be a combination of the following, in addition to the intervention provided by Nancy: (1) testing the reality of his work performance skills; (2) helping set realistic, measurable, graded goals that provide structure (as did college) and enable him to regain control of his life, to feel productive and successful; and (3) encouraging discussions about his feelings toward his father and how his father may influence his behavior and decisions.

CLIENT-CENTERED REASONING QUESTIONS
FOR CHAPTER 2

1. What are some of the cues of suicidality?
2. What concerns might you have about working with or treating someone who has attempted suicide?
3. A recurring theme in Jennifer Werner's and both of the interns' narratives is that no one is immune to psychosocial distress. In particular, all three writers express shock that seemingly normal people can become desperate enough to attempt suicide. What are some issues that arise for you when you consider the postulate that psychosocial issues can afflict anyone?

CLIENT-CENTERED REASONING ACTIVITIES
FOR CHAPTER 2

1. Choose a character from Jennifer's short story or one of the clinical narratives and write a first-person journal entry as that character in which you reveal your more intimate thoughts and feelings about your situation.
2. Describe any precautions you would take while working with Catherine, Marielle, Samantha, and Brian.

3

We Are People Too, Same Wants and Needs as You

Waltzing through the looking glass I see a perfect picture of a hand filled with love and understanding. Every person in this land has a mirror, a twin that reflects every side within. The twin has a distinctive way about his whim. They are one, which allows the other to know of that within. (Jennifer Lane)

Client-Centered Reasoning Questions

1. In this epigraph Jennifer effortlessly waltzes through a looking glass out of reality into a perfect world that satisfies "every person's" wants and needs. According to Jennifer what are these wants and needs? How are they similar to yours? What would you say are the wants and needs of all people?

Often people are prejudiced against working with people that have psychosocial issues, especially those who never encountered anyone with them. The more you get to know your clients as individuals yet understand that their wants and needs are similar to those others have, the more effective your interventions will be. The following narratives describe how three interns moved through their preconceived ideas to achieve a more mature understanding of their clients.

OVERVIEW OF THE FIRST FIVE WEEKS

LAURA BELLA-BRYANT

I am currently an intern at a major metropolitan hospital in New York City. When I was assigned to the inpatient psychiatric unit of the hospital, I was extremely anxious and somewhat scared. I thought that I was going to dislike my experience because I had preconceived ideas about people with psychosocial issues. I thought that all the clients were going to be deranged or insane and that there would be little or no hope for their future. Five weeks later, I can now say that my thoughts and fears were extremely prejudiced, and my experience has been incredible.

The first day when I walked onto the unit after my orientation, I was scared of the clients and staff. I was sure that I was going to be miserable because the unit was so intimidating. I was so negative in the beginning that I am almost embarrassed to admit how I felt. I was sure that I was not going to enjoy working with this population. I observed several clients wandering the halls and some were talking to themselves, but for the most part, the unit seemed to be calm, quiet, and well under control. I was surprised to notice how bright and clean the unit was, because I had imagined it to be dark, gloomy, and depressing.

For the entire first week, I observed the clients and reviewed most of their charts. This eye-opening experience revealed that they are real people who have lives outside of the hospital, just as I do. When I realized this, I felt guilty about my previous thoughts regarding people with psychosocial issues.

When I went home on Friday at the end of the first week, I began to think about the clients whom I had just met or learned about by reviewing their charts. I felt depressed. I had a tough time dealing with these sad feelings. I was sad for the lives some of the clients have lived. I knew that I might become extremely depressed if I continued to let the clients' lives affect my own. On the other hand, I did not want to appear to be a cold-hearted person. This was my first real struggle that I had to overcome to ensure my well-being. Sometimes, it is still difficult to control my emotions when a client's life has been so terrible, but somehow I learned to express my sympathy and empathy to the clients in a professional manner. When the clients spoke about their lives, I would listen and they would have my full attention. I wanted them to know that I cared.

By the end of my second week, I was exhausted because there was an abundant amount of paperwork to be completed. I felt that I was not getting to know the clients as well as I should have. However, this changed by the middle of the third week. I managed to structure my time in a more organized manner in order to intervene more effectively and complete my evaluations and progress notes.

During the third week, many clients were being discharged; therefore, new clients were admitted to the unit. I knew that this was my time to observe the new people from admission until discharge. I began interviewing and learning about their lives and difficult struggles.

I specifically remember interviewing a young girl, whom I will call Maria. Maria is a Hispanic teenager who was admitted to the hospital for homicidal ideation and threats against a friend who was having an affair with Maria's boyfriend. Maria has a 3-year-old daughter who lives with her boyfriend's mother. When I asked Maria about her daughter, she told me that she loved her, but I did not notice any change in her facial expression. This surprised me because I knew that she had been in the hospital for about two weeks, and due to her belligerent behavior, she was not allowed to see any visitors, including her daughter. From the moment I met Maria, I realized that I wanted to make an impact on her life. I wanted her to talk about her problems, goals, and future, but she did not want to have anything to do with me or anyone else. I began going to her room and knocking on her door before every group to encourage her to come, but she would not acknowledge my requests. I decided that, if she would not join our groups, I would encourage her to talk about her problems privately, but she resisted this as well. One day, when I was walking down the hall to a morning meeting, Maria stopped me in the hallway, said "hello," and asked me what my profession was. I told her that I was an intern who could help her with problems that she may be having and that she could come to me if she ever wanted to talk. Maria began to walk away in the middle of my sentence, but halfway down the hall she turned around and asked me if any groups were being held today. This was an incredible moment because she had not been talking to any other professionals on the unit. When I notified the staff about Maria, they were shocked. They told me to continue my pursuit of her, and I did. Maria began to talk to me more and more every day. She also began coming to and participating in groups.

Maria's affect was flat in the beginning of her hospitalization. Toward the end of her hospital stay, she had a wider range. She began to smile when she mentioned her daughter. When I saw her smile, it made me smile. On the day of her discharge, Maria attended a goals group that I was leading. I asked Maria about her goals immediately following discharge. She told me that she was going to try to control her temper, take a shower every day, and graduate from high school; however, the most important goal for her was to take care of her daughter. Everyone, including the clients, was surprised by her improvement and elated mood. Maria was the last one to leave when the group was over. I encouraged her to continue improving her tolerance for frustration and impulse control, and I wished her luck in the future. Maria thanked me for all my help and told me that I was a caring person. This was a great accomplishment that I will never forget.

I realized that psychosocial issues could affect anyone. In this day and age, teenagers' lives are affected by many different stresses that make it extremely difficult to live in such a hateful world. Maria is just one example of many touching encounters that I have experienced in the past five weeks.

Client-Centered Reasoning Questions

1. What are Maria's wants and needs? What are Laura's?
2. During her first week Laura stated that, "I knew that if I continued to let the clients' lives affect my life, I might become extremely depressed." During her second week, she felt she was not getting to know her clients as well as she should because of the abundance of paperwork to complete. Besides a flight

into paperwork, what are some additional strategies you can do to guard against feeling depressed or letting your clients' lives affect your own life?

3. Laura states, "Somehow I learned to express my sympathy and empathy to the clients in a professional manner." What specific techniques can you use to keep from becoming "too emotional" in front of your clients? List appropriate ways to express emotions to clients. State why each way is acceptable and helpful. List inappropriate ways to express emotions to clients. State why each way is inappropriate and how each could be damaging to your client's well-being.

Client-Centered Reasoning Activities

1. Finish the narrative.
2. Write this narrative from Maria's point of view.
3. Write an occupational profile for Maria.
4. Write an occupational performance analysis. How might each barrier interfere with her ability to care for her daughter?
5. What additional information would you need to help her return to her role as primary caretaker of her daughter? How would you assess Maria's ability to return to this role? How would you determine when she was ready? What accommodations could be made if Maria became psychiatrically stable but was still unable to fully care for her daughter, perhaps due to continuing her high school education?
6. Write an intervention plan for Maria.
7. Write a discharge note.
8. Make referrals to other services.
9. Identify the types of clinical reasoning you applied in writing Maria's assessment, occupational performance analysis, intervention plan, discharge plan, and referrals.
10. What frames of reference or theory have you applied in creating Maria's assessment, occupational performance analysis, intervention plan, discharge plan, and referrals? Provide support for why this theory is appropriate for Maria's needs. What other frame of reference might be appropriate and why?

WE ARE ALL HUMAN

KERI REILLY

It was Tuesday morning. I walked into one of the rooms to see a new client, Dave. He was in bed with all of the lights off and the covers pulled over his head. I could see that he was awake because he was moving and responded when I knocked on the door before I entered. I asked to speak to him. I needed to orient him to his new surroundings and the unit, and I wanted to speak to him regarding his intervention plan that I wished to write with him. I started to introduce myself, but Dave did not take the covers from over his head. I finally asked him to take the covers down and sit up. He did just as I asked. To my surprise, Dave had only one eye and one empty eye socket. I thought to myself, *No wonder he was hiding. I would feel very self-conscious about that myself.*

During our talk, Dave avoided eye contact as much as possible. I stayed with him for only a short period of time. During that time, we spoke about what he wanted to work on while in the hospital and what goals were important to him. Dave stated that he needed help motivating himself. Dave was in the hospital this time because he was sleeping through his morning medications at his shelter. As a result of not taking his medications, he was hearing more voices, getting angry more often, and found himself wandering the streets at night when he was unable to sleep. He knew that this was a dangerous situation for him.

After leaving the room, I went to look over Dave's chart. I found out that he was living in a shelter, was diagnosed with schizoaffective disorder, and had an extensive history of polysubstance abuse with many detoxification attempts. Dave had also been arrested for drug dealing and possession of drugs. He had a long history of being in and out of the hospital. Dave was hearing voices telling him to harm others. I thought of Dave as just another client who needed help.

Dave had some stereotypes that I would associate with a psychosocial client. He was living in a shelter, was a "druggie," and his appearance was less than normal looking. He appeared unclean and unkempt. His missing eye contributed to this stereotype even more. I automatically assumed it had been caused by a fight or health problem resulting from his extensive drug and alcohol use in the past. He also would pace up and down the halls and rock back and forth when sitting. The stereotypes and stigmas attached to people with psychosocial issues can often cause one to disregard the human being behind those stereotypes and the reasons that those stereotypes exist.

It was not until I sat down with Dave and spoke to him for an extended period that I realized who this person really is. Dave is a human being with all the same wants, needs, and goals as the rest of us. I went into the interview with a mindset that this person would not want to talk and would blame his being in the hospital on somebody else. Much to my surprise, he proved otherwise. He spoke about personal issues, goals for himself, and what caused him to come to the hospital. This person was more than just a client.

Dave began our conversation by explaining his fake eye. He had trouble putting in his glass eye the first day at the hospital and was therefore more comfortable in his bed, where nobody could see the empty socket. He continued with an explanation of why he had only one eye. Contrary to what I had thought, he lost his eye when he was 8 years old due to glaucoma and a blood clot that he had in his brain at the age of 7. I could not believe it. I felt horrible that I automatically assumed that he lost his eye by some reason he himself brought on.

Dave then spoke about his appearance. He wanted to get his teeth fixed eventually, because he was missing a few of them. He was also very anxious to shower and groom himself. He told me that he usually keeps himself well groomed, but he did not have any of his toiletries to do this. At that time, Dave was using the toiletries and necessities given to him in the hospital. Dave expressed concern about using the deodorant given to him. He wanted to use his own toiletries. He explained that he usually uses a certain brand of deodorant because it works best with his particular body chemistry. He raised his arm and put his nose close to his armpit. He felt that the brand of deodorant given to him was not working. I asked him if that made him feel uncomfortable being around others. He told me it did.

This man, like the rest of us, was more concerned about what others were going to think of him because he was missing an eye and his deodorant might not be working as best it could. This man wanted to be accepted by his new group of peers and not be stigmatized as an unclean, unkempt man right from the start.

I know that, when I am not in my usual surroundings and do not have my usual necessities, it is more difficult to feel comfortable. I wanted Dave to feel as comfortable as possible in the hospital. I felt that, if he were not comfortable being around others, spending most of his time in his room, his progress would suffer. I asked Dave what his usual deodorant was and I told him that I would look in our cabinets to see if we had any. I went to the drug store that day and bought him his usual brand of deodorant. I went back to him the next day with the deodorant in my hand ready to give to him. He saw the deodorant and recognized the red cap and stripes right away. I did not tell him that I went out to buy it for him, because I did not feel that that was important. What was important was his comfort and creating a rapport with him. Dave took the deodorant and put it on while I was standing there. He shook my hand and kept repeating, "This is so great, thank you." I could not believe the smile on his face. It was the first of many. Dave immediately turned and left the room to attend a therapeutic group. On his way to the group, he turned to me and asked if I would please let him know if the deodorant was not working. I had gained his trust.

Dave seemed to have very real concerns in life and very low self-esteem. He wanted to be accepted by others, he was concerned about his appearance, and he wanted to be a respected member of society. I kept thinking, *who does not*? Was that too much to ask on his part? No. Even though he has had some difficulties in the past and continues to need intervention, he is still human. He deserves all that life is willing to offer and all that he is willing to give. And, from what I could see, this person was willing to give a lot, not just to his intervention process but also to others. He would always help out when possible. He would try to give an explanation of his behavior and barriers when necessary and would help other clients with solving problems or offer his thoughts on a topic when necessary.

Little by little, Dave participated more often in groups, was more visible on the unit, and was more sociable with the other clients and staff. I decided it was time to sit down with Dave to find out more about him. He opened up and began to talk. He spoke about his childhood and his upbringing. Dave told me how his parents would keep him locked up in the house all day long. This, he explained, was how he became claustrophobic. And this claustrophobia causes him to pace the halls and rock back and forth while sitting. He explained that his parents always called him stupid and continuously compared him to his brother. Dave's self-esteem issues appeared to be deep-rooted. Dave told me that, at 38 years old, he still tries to prove to his parents that he is not stupid.

It seems that, at one time or another, we all try to prove something to others. In an ideal world, the only people we would need to impress are ourselves. Unfortunately, this is far from an ideal world. Dave's concerns are very real.

Some of Dave's goals included improving his self-care and hygiene skills, anger management skills, and ultimately his problem-solving abilities. With Dave, I also felt it was important to work on improving his self-esteem because, without this, he may not have the motivation or confidence to attempt to improve these skills.

Dave would be discharged soon because he was doing much better on the unit. Unfortunately, we would have limited time to work on the important things that he needed. We worked on his performing his self-care skills independently and improving his anger management skills and even his problem-solving skills. The self-esteem was more difficult. This was not something tangible. This is something that could be worked on all day, everyday. I tried to integrate it into his entire intervention plan. While working with Dave, I would always have him concentrate on his strengths. He had very good insight into his barriers, was very articulate at expressing himself and his needs, and was very goal oriented. We would try to include this into his therapeutic groups. For instance, during one of the groups, another client was having difficulty with a project. Instead of explaining the project to the client myself, I asked Dave to do it. He was doing the same project, just at a faster rate. Dave approached the task with apprehension but continued anyway. When the other person finished the project after Dave's instruction, the sense of accomplishment showed on both of their faces.

When preparing for discharge, Dave and I talked about why he was brought to the hospital and what he could do to avoid relapse. Since he was sleeping through his morning medications, he thought it would be important to invest in an alarm clock. He was very good at recognizing his signs and symptoms so we made sure he had a list of them handy so he could become aware of his getting sick earlier and avoid coming to the hospital again.

This one client has taught me so much. It is important to create a rapport with people because they are unique, with much more to offer than just what meets the eye. Recognizing what is important to people and realizing what they want out of life can help guide intervention and help develop a good therapeutic relationship. The client's wants and needs may be different from yours or they may be similar, but they are real and should be dealt with during the intervention. I feel that it is very important to listen when individuals speak, but more importantly, hear what they say.

Client-Centered Reasoning Questions

1. What are Dave's wants and needs?
2. Do you believe that Dave's difficulty with getting out of bed and taking his medication in the morning prior to admission was due to not having an alarm clock? Why or why not? Do you think it was due to his self-esteem? Why or why not? If not, do you think the real reason for his "needing help motivating himself" in the morning is solved so that he will not return to his previous setting, only for it to happen again? How do you know? What additional questioning or intervention is necessary?
3. Dave responded positively to the attention and structure this inpatient hospitalization gave him. How could you prevent a regression when he leaves the hospital and returns to the shelter, where he may not get as much structure and attention?

Client-Centered Reasoning Activities

1. Finish the narrative.
2. Write an occupational profile.
3. Write a questionnaire.
4. List additional assessments you would use with this client.
5. Write an occupational performance analysis. Separate David's facilitators and barriers into the following categories:

   - Psychosocial issues.
   - Self-esteem issues.
   - Functional abilities.
   - Cognitive abilities.

6. Write an intervention plan.
7. What kind of intervention would you provide Dave in his shelter?
8. Pick a setting other than a shelter and readjust your intervention plan.
9. Write a discharge note.
10. Make referrals to other services.
11. Write three group protocols that would strengthen Dave's self-care and hygiene skills, anger management, and problem-solving skills.
12. Identify the types of clinical reasoning you applied in writing Dave's assessment, occupational performance analysis, intervention plan, discharge plan, and referrals.

13. What frame of reference or theory have you applied in creating Dave's assessment, occupational performance analysis, intervention plan, discharge plan, and referrals? Provide support for why this theory is appropriate for Dave's needs. What other frame of reference might be appropriate and why?

I DO NOT WANT TO BE DIFFERENT

LILIANA MOSQUERA

As I walked down the hallway toward the room of the client I was supposed to orient and evaluate, I realized I was approaching the special care area on our unit. Brenda had just undergone a relapse and returned to the unit. The therapist gave a brief explanation of her arrival on the unit and a history of her difficulties. Not much else was said about her except that she is inconsistent and unreliable when providing information about herself, paranoid and psychotic. Her placement in special care was due to her suicidal ideation. Her presentation was not very different from other clients admitted to our unit. I wonder what really happened to them? Why would people want to hurt themselves? As a child, my Mom always reminded me that, to love others, you need to love yourself; throughout my education, professors remind us that, to help others, you need to be able to help yourself. *Does not a child learn from others and by teaching others? Does not an adult also know these things? Did their parents or teachers not tell them?*

These issues raced through my mind as I came closer to her room and realized that she was curled up in bed in the fetal position with her back facing the door. I knocked. She did not answer. *Great, should I call out her name, say "hello," or simply walk out and really believe she was asleep and did not hear me knocking?* I had only been on the unit for two weeks and did not know how to approach her. *Just go with your instincts and think about why she would be exhibiting these signs. All right, think back to school. What would you want someone to do if you were in his or her situation?* I knocked on the door again and this time said her name. She answered this time by saying, "Huh huh," but did not turn around to look at me. I entered her room, which had only a bed and one window. I slowly walked to the side of her bed to stand in front of her. She barely looked up and only made minimal eye contact. I introduced myself and asked her if we could speak for a while.

The next couple of minutes, during our conversation, she was as described, inconsistent and paranoid, and she also had a flat affect. However, when I validated some of her feelings about her past and her childhood, the expressions on her face changed and direct eye contact was made. There seemed to be a tear in her eye. I wanted to reach over and just touch her hand. As a person, I would have needed that, too. But then I recalled the whole notion about no physical contact, and I pulled away. I let her say what she was saying. When she was finished I told her that I understood. There were a lot of issues that she had to deal with growing up. She was diagnosed at a point in her life when success meant everything to her, and she could not have wanted anything else but to continue being happy. After all she had gone through, she emerged as a strong woman, one with many accomplishments. As we were speaking, I noticed that her thoughts were once again becoming fragmented. She was able to answer my questions with only a few words, unable to fully express herself. However, I felt I had enough information to write up her evaluation. As I was leaving the room where the interview took place and started walking her back to her room, I thought, *author, creator of words in rhyme, imagination—what happened?*

I continued to stop by her room on a daily basis and check on how she was doing. She was improving slowly. She now had no signs of being psychotic and could hold a conversation for at least five minutes. She expressed to me the need of wanting to shower in her own room and not be under constant observation; this made her feel like her Mom used to. Several times during this conversation, she said to me, "I want my privacy. To some extent, I understand I am in the hospital, but would you not want the same?" I thought, *I certainly would,* but decided to keep the thought to myself.

The next day at team meeting, we decided that she no longer needed to be under special care, and she was moved to a room that she would share with someone else. No longer was she talking to herself, lying in bed listless, afraid about where she was or afraid of herself. Later that day, I saw her, and she said, "Thank you. You understand." I explained to her that her being moved out of special care was a team decision, not one I made on my own. Still, she thanked me again. Her words, "You understand," lingered in my head for hours to come. I did understand. She was in her mid-thirties, an African American woman living independently, making a living for herself, and holding onto a career she loved. Besides this, I could see how someone would want her own things, want privacy, want someone to care, and want to be successful in life and in her career. *I want the same things.*

I was amazed that Brenda could behave so differently within a matter of hours after her move out of special care. She was in a better mood, her affect was brighter, and now, instead of a tear, she had a twinkle in her eye. I was not too sure what brought about the change. I thought our talks and short-term goal setting had helped. *But had they really?*

Now that she had accomplished one of her goals, we decided to work on her reason for being in the hospital. Not every therapist approaches someone's suicide attempt as directly as I did with Brenda. I did so because I felt there was a connection between the two of us. I was confident that she felt it, too, and that one way or another I could help her. First, Brenda was to attend groups, including her group therapy session and her individual session with her psychiatrist. Attending groups was just the beginning. After her first one, which happened to be a group I lead every week, she thought it would be great to not only attend groups but to also participate and listen. I had invited her to my group. It was one that could offer her concrete information about the unit but, at the same time, give her the opportunity to engage with others. I thought this area was important because her prior interactions with others had not been positive.

Brenda and I discussed her feelings. She felt different, as if no one was like her, as if she was in a different category. Many of the reasons for her feeling the way she did were due to her past. *I cannot help with that, I am not a psychologist*, I thought, *so what can I offer her? Offer something she can use again in order not to be in or react to a situation in the same manner that she previously did* [attempt suicide]: *Coping skills such as stress and anger management, relaxation techniques, and education on recognizing her symptoms and understanding her illness?* A lot of ideas crossed my mind in a matter of a few minutes. I knew in which direction I wanted to go, but where would I start? Brenda helped me with that answer. We would start working on her anger and stress management techniques through group and individual interventions. We would then focus on recognizing her signs and symptoms of relapse to prevent another hospitalization. It was a lot to accomplish, but if we worked together it could be a good start.

Brenda and I would work on this plan for about three days. We would work in therapeutic groups, individually, and also every time she stopped me in the middle of the hallway (which was always congested with traffic and loud at times) to let me know how she was doing. Without realizing it, the next day at team meeting, she was one of the clients mentioned for discharge planning. The weekend was coming up so she could not leave then, but early into the next week was a possibility. *That quick? I only got to work on a few goals. I wanted to do so much more. She is better though.*

I decided to see her right after the meeting was over. After a few words were exchanged, she told me that she felt better and that, on her own during the evening hours, she had continued to work on the work sheets I had given her. I took a look at what she had written. *These are the same expectations and desires as anyone of us would have. She had presented her goals just as we had discussed but in her way, through writing.* For the next couple of minutes, we talked about what she had written for herself; and she was glad that she was able to open up and feel that she was a person and not someone (thing) different. One of her biggest fears was having a mental illness and, as a result, not being seen as an individual with the same needs, desires, and wants as anyone else. She confessed this idea to me by saying, "I never really wanted to admit it to myself. It is hard to know you will have to live with this the rest of your life and that it can have such an effect on the way you do things and function in life. It makes you think you are different than everyone else. I do not want to be different. I just do not." I was not at all surprised by the way she expressed herself to me; it was intelligent and well thought through. *Who would have thought she was any different than any other person; she did.* In many ways she was different but not in the way she perceived it. Her difference was a positive one; she was a published author, a poet, and a person with a lot of self-reflection. She simply could not get past the idea of taking medication the rest of her life.

Before I left for the weekend, she quickly approached me and asked if I would be returning the following week. I assured her that I would be there. I asked if she would write some poetry for me to read. Her face lit up and teeth were seen as her lips curled up to form a smile. "Of course," she said, "it will be waiting for you Monday morning." I knew her discharge would be approaching soon, so I thought, *it is time to really see what happens. I am not sure if her emotions and feelings about her illness will be evident in her writing but, if writing is her way of expressing herself, she might be able to see a connection between her writing and her barriers to occupational performance and maybe begin to understand them better.*

Four pieces of paper with writing on them were handed to me as I entered the unit floor. She was already up and dressed. I took them from her, told her we would speak about them later, and that I hoped to see her in group that afternoon. I was on my way to a team meeting. I could not resist the temptation of reading what she had written for me over the weekend. Many ideas rushed to mind. Over the weekend, I had thought of possible scenarios and how I would handle each of them if I needed to. I read one writing—silence consumed me.

That afternoon, as I was leaving an activity room to start rounding up clients for the next group, she held out her hand signaling me to stop. I did. She said to me, "I was always afraid of being different than everyone else after my first break and hospitalization. Now, slowly, I have learned here that I am not different, that I am not the only person in the world who is sick and taking medication. I can do things. I want the same things as anyone else. It is all right that I have a mental illness." As she was speaking to me, I thought, *this is the closest she has come to accepting her psychosocial issues and herself as a person.*

I got all emotional inside. Some of my colleagues overheard our brief conversation. It was the topic for the day. I can still hear myself thinking, *I do not want to be different. No, you are not; having an illness does not separate you and me. You are one of us; I hope you really understand that.*

Client-Centered Reasoning Questions

1. What are Brenda's wants and needs?
2. Liliana states that Brenda, "simply could not get past the idea of taking medication the rest of her life." How did Liliana help Brenda overcome this barrier to wellness?
3. What precautions would you take with Brenda and why?

Client-Centered Reasoning Activities

1. Finish the narrative.
2. Write an occupational profile.
3. Write a questionnaire.
4. List additional assessments you would use with this client.
5. Write an occupational performance analysis.
6. Write an intervention plan.
7. Readjust the intervention plan as if you were working with Brenda in an outpatient day treatment program.
8. Write two progress notes at different periods of time during her intervention.
9. Write a discharge note.
10. Make referrals to other services.
11. Write a group protocol for a group that would address most of Brenda's barriers to occupational performance.
12. Identify the types of clinical reasoning you applied in writing Brenda's assessment, occupational performance analysis, intervention plan, discharge plan, and referrals.
13. What frame of reference or theory have you applied in creating Brenda's assessment, occupational performance analysis, intervention plan, discharge plan, and referrals? Provide support for why this theory is appropriate for Brenda's needs. What other frame of reference might be appropriate and why?
14. Liliana brings up the issue of no physical contact in this narrative. Break up into two-person debate teams. Debate the issue of physical contact, with one team for and one team against the use of physical contact. Each set of two teams is to pick a different type of physical contact—between staff member and psychiatric client, between psychiatric clients, and between staff members. Each set of two teams is to choose a different psychosocial treatment setting where the physical contact may or may not be taking place (see Chapter 1 for a list of intervention settings). Hold a timed debate in front of the class with two teams debating each other at a time. Designate judges; the rest of the class should observe. Write a paper on the conclusions you have drawn from the debates. How would the results be different if the clients were geriatric people? Physically challenged people?

4

Order in the Court: Patients' Rights

People have certain rights that must be honored no matter what form of intervention they are receiving or what type of facility they are receiving it in. Each state in the United States has a list of patients' rights. For hospitals in New York state, the Patients' Bill of Rights is as follows (reprinted courtesy of New York State):

As a patient in a hospital in New York State, you have the right, consistent with law, to:

1. Understand and use these rights. If for any reason you do not understand or you need help, the hospital MUST provide assistance, including an interpreter.
2. Receive treatment without discrimination as to race, color, religion, sex, national origin, disability, sexual orientation or source of payment.
3. Receive considerate and respectful care in a clean and safe environment free of unnecessary restraints.
4. Receive emergency care if you need it.
5. Be informed of the name and position of the doctor who will be in charge of your care in the hospital.
6. Know the names, positions and functions of any hospital staff involved in your care and refuse their treatment, examination or observation.
7. A no-smoking room.
8. Receive complete information about your diagnosis, treatment and prognosis.
9. Receive all the information that you need to give informed consent for any proposed procedure or treatment. This information shall include the possible risks and benefits of the procedure or treatment.
10. Receive all the information you need to give informed consent for an order not to resuscitate. You also have the right to designate an individual to give this consent for you if you are too ill to do so. If you would like additional information, please ask for a copy of the pamphlet "Do

Not Resuscitate Orders: A Guide for Patients and Families."

11. Refuse treatment and be told what effect this may have on your health.

12. Refuse to take part in research. In deciding whether or not to participate, you have the right to a full explanation.

13. Privacy while in the hospital and confidentiality of all information and records regarding your care.

14. Participate in all decisions about your treatment and discharge from the hospital. The hospital must provide you with a written discharge plan and written description of how you can appeal your discharge.

15. Review your medical record without charge. Obtain a copy of your medical record for which the hospital can charge a reasonable fee. You cannot be denied a copy solely because you cannot afford to pay.

16. Receive an itemized bill and explanation of all charges.

17. Complain without fear of reprisals about the care and services you are receiving and to have the hospital's response, you can complain to the New York State Health Department. The hospital must provide you with the Health Department telephone number.

18. Authorize those family members and other adults who will be given priority to visit consistent with your ability to receive visitors.

19. Make known your wishes in regard to anatomical gifts. You may document your wishes in your health care proxy or on a donor card, available from the hospital.

Sometimes there is a fine line between what is therapeutic for people and what appears to be an infringement of their rights. For instance, at what point do you restrict visitation if the visitor is causing the person's condition to worsen? Is it ethical for insurance companies to influence the length and type of intervention? When should medication be administered against someone's will? Can or should a person be hospitalized against his or her will? Under what conditions is it all right to put someone in four-point restraints?

Through experience, practitioners along with state reviewers, consumers, organizations that support family members, client rights advocates, insurance companies, pharmaceutical companies, and government officials have established best practice models for mental health issues. These continue to evolve as clinical, medical, and psychopharmacological research progress.

This chapter presents several currently used mental health practices that have caused controversial thoughts and feelings in interns. Such thoughts and feelings often affect interns' ability to objectively administer the best possible intervention until the interns can resolve some of these issues in their own minds. Such practices include electrical convulsive therapy (ECT), insurance companies influencing intervention, the restriction of certain personal rights during hospitalization, the use of psychotropic medication, hospital retention, and long-term state hospitalization. Different points of view are presented through narratives written by clients and interns. Client-centered reasoning questions and activities are aimed at fostering identification and resolution of students' issues surrounding these practices and may be used as templates for the resolution of concerns regarding other practices as well.

ELECTRICAL CONVULSIVE THERAPY

LILIANA MOSQUERA

Over the course of my studies this past year, I heard of an intervention method used on only a few clients. These clients are severely depressed individuals who fail to improve using pharmacology, among other criteria. As I understand, this intervention was used often in the past but is no longer used as frequently. The attending psychologist on my team tries not to impose or even suggest this form of intervention for clients.

However, one client has shown no sign of improvement even after several changes in his medications. As a team, we decided to wait a couple of weeks to see if this last medication trial would be helpful to him, since he had failed other pharmacological regimens. Now, after some time, nothing has worked. This man is so introverted and devoid of hope for life itself that nothing seems to interest him.

After careful consideration, the suggestion of giving ECT has been brought up, and I do not know how to react to it. In some ways, I am against it, yet I think it can help. For this particular client, because he is at such a low point in his life, I can see how this intervention can help and actually outweigh the side effects. A waiting period to taper off his medication is needed before this intervention can be attempted. I feel that this waiting period can be anxiety provoking to someone knowing what the next step in his intervention would be. The team did not tell him right away. With the anxiety he already has, I can see how he could get even more anxious awaiting ECT.

Client-Centered Reasoning Questions

1. Do you think any parts of the Patients' Bill of Rights in your state have been violated in Liliana's narrative? If so, which ones and why?
2. Are you for, against, or neutral about the administration of ECT? What is your conviction based on?
3. What are some of the positive and negative things you have heard about ECT from films, clinical textbooks, life experiences, or storytelling?

4. Do you think ECT is cruel, barbaric, or unscientific? Do you think it was something done in the past because people did not know any better and should no longer be used?

5. Liliana mentions that ECT is used on only a few clients and that, on her intervention team, the psychologists try not to use this form of intervention at all. Do you think ECT is currently used often, infrequently, or not used at all?

6. Answer the following technical questions about ECT. If you do not already know, research the topic.

   - Liliana also mentions that ECT is used for people who are severely depressed, who fail to improve through psychopharmacology, and who meet other criteria as well. What are the other criteria? When is ECT treatment counterindicated?
   - Is ECT given as an inpatient or an outpatient procedure?
   - Is ECT an effective intervention? If so, what is the neurological mechanism for its effectiveness?
   - What are the side effects of ECT? Are they reversible? What percent of clients who have received ECT have permanent side effects?
   - How long does the usual intervention take to administer? How many times is the intervention given? Can someone have more than one set of ECT? If so, what happens to the effectiveness?
   - How can you tell when enough ECT has been given?
   - Research a case study in which the client received ECT and improved. Briefly record the salient features.
   - Statistically, what percent of clients who have received ECT got better, stayed the same, or got worse?
   - Where did you obtain this information?

7. Now that you have researched more about ECT, has your opinion of this intervention changed? How? What specifically altered your perception? Would you recommend ECT to a family member who met the criteria for administration?

8. Can you treat a person while he or she is receiving ECT? If so, what kind of therapeutic interventions would you give and why?

9. The team decided not to tell this person right away that they would recommend treating him with ECT because they thought it might make him more anxious. Do you agree or disagree and why? When would you tell him? Justify your reasoning.

10. Substitute ECT with another intervention of your choice that you have conflicting thoughts about and answer all of the preceding questions with regards to the intervention you chose.

Client-Centered Reasoning Activities

1. Just as you may have had preconceived ideas about ECT, some of which were probably negative, so too do clients. Write a

paragraph in quotes of what you would say to this client to prepare him for his upcoming ECT. Keep in mind the information that you answered previously that may have altered your own opinion of the intervention. Read your paragraph to the class and allow your classmates to debate your statements. Support your reasoning. Participate in a class discussion to collectively generate one paragraph that would be helpful to this client.

2. The preceding formula (identifying your own preconceived ideas about an intervention, learning more about the particular intervention through as many different avenues as possible, integrating your newly learned information into your previous cognitive set, identifying your new ideas about the intervention, and finally taking someone new to the intervention concept through the learning process as you just did by imagining yourself in their situation, that is, needing the intervention) is helpful and necessary in developing client-centered reasoning. This formula works with many issues in addition to intervention. Learn to question the material in this text in this manner. Develop an ongoing examination of all that you read. If and when you find conflicting information, either within the text or within your own belief system, question it, do some research, and then reexamine your ideas while discussing them with others. What type of clinical reasoning is this?

The following two narratives deal with the influence insurance companies have on intervention. In the first, intern Liliana Mosquera discusses her frustration of working under the time limits set by insurance companies.

INSURANCE

LILIANA MOSQUERA

I feel torn between feeling like a professional member of the staff and department and an intern trying to grasp and understand my role in the field of mental health. There is a lot to learn on the unit I work in. One can have many different experiences and learn from each one. A diversity of mental health issues is addressed on our unit. Family issues, domestic violence, and child and sexual abuse are discussed frequently because it is in the best interest of the client. The best interest of the client is one of the most important factors for some staff members. However, the insurance companies do not always facilitate the process of helping individuals understand or come to terms with their illness and the reason for their hospitalization. At times, it seems that the managed care companies who reimburse us restrict us as therapists who want to help clients. It is frustrating to find yourself wanting to help someone and knowing how to go about it but not being able to because of the restrictions placed on you by someone who does not know the client personally. Sometimes, I feel that I have reached a dead end because I work so hard at helping people recognize their symptoms and come to terms with their illnesses, but at the same time I am unable to provide them with more in-depth intervention. Most clients do not become well enough to even communicate with me after several days, but by this time I need to have already begun a discharge plan because the insurance company requires it and wants the client out as soon as possible. What if the client is really not ready for discharge?

I often ask at team meetings for more time to work with particular clients. If other staff members back me up, then the clients can usually stay for one extra day, after which they need to be discharged. But how much can I really do in such a short amount of time? People do not miraculously get better overnight, although we all wish they would.

During one of our team meetings, a client's discharge plan was discussed. The client would have benefited from staying on the unit a couple of more days, but the insurance company refused to pay any more of the hospital stay. What is the staff to do when working with deadlines such as the ones frequently given by insurance companies regarding people's health and well-being?

Client-Centered Reasoning Questions

1. Do you think any parts of the Patients' Bill of Rights in your state were violated in this narrative? If so, which ones and why?
2. Liliana states that "insurance companies do not always facilitate the process of helping individuals understand or come to terms with their illness and the reason for their hospitalization." Do insurance companies usually reimburse a unit for increasing someone's insight into their illness? What kinds of interventions will they reimburse a unit for? How long does it usually take a person with psychosocial issues to "come to terms with their illness," if ever? Why is it difficult to improve people's occupational performance if they do not understand why they are in the hospital?
3. Liliana mentions that insurance companies impose a time restriction on interventions. List other ways that insurance companies restrict the work of therapists? What can be done about each of these restrictions?
4. Liliana raises the issue that most of her clients are not well enough to communicate with her until a few days into their intervention. What kind of intervention could you give these people within their first few days? What is your rationale for each intervention?

Client-Centered Reasoning Activities

1. Create a brief case study of a person with depression. Write five intervention plans for this depressed person given (a) one day to intervene, (b) three days to intervene, (c) one week to intervene, (d) two weeks to intervene, and (e) one month to in-

tervene. Why did you prioritize your interventions in this way? Note how the client's interventions change with time.

2. For any barriers that you did not have time to address in activity 1, what follow-up services could you refer this client to?

The next narrative goes into detail about trying to find appropriate housing for Meibel before her insurance runs out.

SUITABLE DWELLINGS

LILIANA MOSQUERA

One of my clients, Meibel, was being discharged. I did not feel that she was well enough to be discharged to a drop-in center. This was the only place the caseworker could get for her to live. Ideally, the team would refer her to a residence that could provide her support, but it would take weeks if not months for the paperwork to go through. What was anyone to do in the meantime? No one wanted her to go to a drop-in center, but it felt like all we could do was discharge her there and hope that she would survive.

I was alarmed and shaken at the thought that, although she had greatly improved since her arrival on the unit, her discharge would be earlier than it should be. Even one more day in the hospital would make a difference. I found her to be in such a fragile state that, by not giving her a supportive environment on discharge, she might fall apart and cease to function. She would probably go into a relapse and be in a worse situation than when she arrived almost two months ago.

After much debating, persistence, and the final support of the social worker and her doctor, the team decided that she indeed needed to have somewhere concrete to go before discharge could be an option, but we were allowed only one extra day to accomplish this. This decision did not alleviate the pressure and stress the client was dealing with, knowing she had to find a place quickly, as well as the pressure we felt, knowing that we also had a quick deadline to meet. We lacked the time to figure things out the way we would have preferred. The team decided to give only one extra day because she was psychiatrically stable. An insurance company will no longer pay for a hospitalization once the person is stable. This was of concern to the team.

I worked with her and the others to try to find her a place to live. In the back of my mind, I was scared for her. What if she could not find anything? It was already somewhat out of our control whether she stayed in the hospital or not. I was scared that all the hard work she had done to better herself, the work done with her by me and all of the staff as well, would crumble because she could not have a place that provided enough structure. It was past 5 o'clock and the social worker, doctor, and I were working hard on making her discharge plan feasible and acceptable to her situation. I held my breath and prayed for the best as I left the building that day, knowing that, when I returned the following day, she would have left and, after that, there would be nothing left for me to do but wish her well.

Client-Centered Reasoning Questions

1. Do you think any parts of the Patients' Bill of Rights of your state were violated here? If so, which ones and why?
2. What is a drop-in center?
3. What parameters may Liliana have used to determine that Meibel was not well enough to be discharged to a drop-in center?
4. What are some possible reasons that a drop-in center was the only place the caseworker could get for Meibel to live?
5. What is a residence?
6. What are some feasible reasons why it takes weeks or months for paperwork to go through a residence to secure a bed for a client?
7. If the team had decided to keep Meibel for an extra month to secure her placement in a residence, what kind of therapy would you give her during that month and why, given that she is already stable?
8. Liliana felt that all that could be done for Meibel if she had to go to a drop-in center was to discharge her and hope she would survive. What services other than housing are usually set up before someone leaves a level of intervention?
9. Liliana stated that Meibel's discharge was earlier than it should be and that Meibel was leaving in a fragile state, even though she was stable. What is the difference between being psychiatrically stable and being in a fragile state? Why would a psychiatric hospital discharge people while still in a fragile state? Who sets these parameters? Liliana felt alarmed and shaken; what are your feelings and thoughts about early discharges?
10. Statistics show that most people who have a relapse have it within the first week after discharge and end up back in the hospital. Do most insurance policies and managed care companies reimburse for a relapse within the same year as a psychiatric hospitalization?
11. What is your role in discharge planning? Does your role differ from facility to facility? Should it? Which parts of your role should be constant and why?
12. Why is it important to be knowledgeable about types of housing?

Client-Centered Reasoning Activities

1. Two types of housing centers are mentioned in Liliana's narrative, a drop-in center and a residence. What is the difference between these two? Approximately 12 other types of housing facilities are available to people with mental health issues. What are they? Compare and contrast them on the following points:

types of services provided, rules and regulations, responsibilities of the clients, functional level required of the clients who reside there, types of on-site staffing, dispensing of medication, layout of facilities, average time to wait for an empty bed, and funding sources. Where did you find this information?
2. Identify problems with the systems in Liliana's narrative about Meibel. Set up a program or programs that eliminate or address all of these problems. Keep in mind the good of the client.

Most people would agree that a great amount of personal freedom is lost while in the hospital and some other intervention facilities. People inevitably lose the freedom to do what they want and to carry out their usual lifestyle in exchange for clinical intervention. Decision making is often deferred to others or depends on others' knowledge and experience. In addition, the reasons why people are in the hospital to begin with add to the anxiety and frustration of the whole intervention experience. But where does it stop? When are the restrictions on personal freedom too severe? How do you judge?

WHAT HAPPENED TO MY FREEDOM?

LAURA BELLA-BRYANT

During my three-month internship experience, many clients expressed their thoughts about freedom. I can specifically remember a client whom I will call Anne. Anne is a 39-year-old white woman who had multiple psychiatric hospitalizations. Her brother actually died in a psychiatric hospital. Anne suffers from schizophrenia just as her brother did.

Anne is extremely expressive about her thoughts and feelings at times. Ever since Anne was transferred from another unit in the hospital after ransacking the nurses' station, she has remained under special care. Whenever I talked to Anne, she was concerned about her freedom. She expressed her hatred toward the nurses because they will not leave her alone. She said that she feels that she is in prison because she cannot even wear her own clothing. She does not like wearing the "stupid hospital gown," and she cannot even take a shower without someone letting her into the bathroom. "This place is stupid, these nurses get on my nerves, they treat me like a little baby. How do you think that makes me feel? I hate it here and I want to go home," she pronounced.

One day, an arts and crafts group was being held that Anne wanted to attend. Her primary nurse gave her permission to come, but she was allowed to draw only with crayons and paper. At her nurse's discretion, Anne was not allowed to work with any other materials. Anne was not enthused about this decision. "I cannot do anything, not even crafts. *This is so stupid!* No one cares. It feels terrible when someone tells you what you can do. No one cares." Anne then began talking about a time when she was injected with medication against her will. "When I got here, the woman took off all of my clothes and made me put on this gown. She then injected me with medication just so I would shut up. Well it worked, but it is not right. It is not right how I am treated here."

I felt bad for Anne because she felt like she was being treated like a child. All she wanted to do was arts and crafts but no one would let her. If I were her, I would be upset too because my freedom was taken away. On the other hand, Anne's behavior can be out of control at times. One minute she could be extremely pleasant, but the next minute she could be out of control. In the instances when she is out of control, the staff's reaction is justifiable.

Client-Centered Reasoning Questions

1. Do you think any parts of the Patients' Bill of Rights in your state were violated in Laura's narrative? If so, which ones and why?

2. Are you for, against, or neutral about how Anne was treated in the hospital?

   - Stripped and injected with medication against her will.
   - Having to wear a hospital gown.
   - Requiring an escort to the shower.
   - Not being able to work with craft projects.

3. What are some plausible reasons that Anne would be restricted in each way?

4. For each restriction list what could transpire if Anne had not been restricted.

5. Are all psychiatric clients restricted in this way on the unit and in psychiatric hospitals?

6. What are some of the positive and negative things you have heard about how people are currently treated in psychiatric hospitals from films, clinical textbooks, life experiences, or storytelling?

7. Bella believes that the restrictions are justified when Anne becomes out of control, implying that they are not justified when Anne is in control. Is getting out of control predictable? If a person has a history of being out of control, does this mean that she will become out of control again? How do you know? Are there signs or patterns? What are they? Is it worth a person's sense of personal freedom to err on the safe side? What is the worst-case scenario? Is it worth the risk?

8. What do you *think* about the primary nurse allowing Anne to come to Laura's group? What do you *think* about the primary nurse restricting Anne from using crafts in your group? How do you *feel* about the primary nurse allowing Anne to come to your group? How do you *feel* about the primary nurse restricting Anne from using crafts in your group?

9. How would you, as a therapist, respond if Anne came to you yelling that she hates this place and the nursing staff, no one cares and she wants to leave?

10. Anne suffers from schizophrenia just as her brother did. Is schizophrenia congenital? What are the latest findings about the possibility of a gene for schizophrenia?

Clinical-Reasoning Activities

1. Write a paper on the history of how clients were treated in psychiatric inpatient facilities. How has the milieu changed over time? What factors were responsible for these changes?
2. Describe what you feel, what you would think, and what you would do in each scenario that follows. Justify the rationale for your actions.

   a. You are running a crafts group. Anne is in your group. Her primary nurse told you ahead of time that she could use only paper and crayons.
   b. You are running a crafts group. Anne is in your group. Her primary nurse did not tell you ahead of time that Anne should not be using anything but paper and crayons for her therapy. Anne is safely and fully participating in a craft project of her choice. Her primary nurse comes into your group after it has begun, sees Anne working with scissors and says to you, "Take the scissors away from her. She can use only paper and crayons."
   c. You are running a crafts group. Anne is not in your group because you heard about Anne's out-of-control behavior so you think her behavior might be inappropriate. In the middle of your group, the primary nurse walks into your group with Anne, sits her down in an empty chair, and says to Anne, "Sit here, but you had better not use anything but crayons and paper," then leaves the intervention room.

The following narrative is by an anonymous intern who is able to see some of the negative aspects of taking psychotropic medication.

MEDICATIONS: CON

ANONYMOUS INTERN

Is it Denise's lack of motivation or her medication level that keeps her from participating and keeps her in bed? In team rounds, the doctors warned us that they were increasing the level of one of her medications and that she might be more lethargic. She was doing better on the unit, so why did they increase her medications? I know there is more to it, but do the clients? Not much information is given them about their medications.

One thing that surprised me when I began the internship is how medicated these clients are. When the residents present a new client to the team, and the attending doctor asks about intervention, all that is discussed are medications. How can clients be expected to perform and prove to the staff that they are capable of making it in the community when they can hardly pick their heads up off their pillows? We are encouraged to get them out of bed for groups and monitor their performance. It is like any one of us taking an over-the-counter sleeping pill in the morning and being asked to voluntarily take part in different task groups and very intense conversations about our futures. I know for a fact that I could not do it. Denise can do well on the unit. She knows that her medications affect her occupational performance. She tries to express how medications affect her occupational performance to the doctors, but they do not hear it. It is so ironic that they are warning us that her medications will make her more lethargic but then question why she is in bed all day.

Client-Centered Reasoning Questions

1. Have you ever taken medication that had side effects? Have you ever discontinued a medication because of the side effects?

2. The intern who wrote this narrative is obviously not in favor of so much medication. What is your stance? Are you for, against, or neutral toward the administration of psychotropic medicines? What is your conviction based on?

3. What are some of the positive and negative things you have heard about psychotropic medicines from movies, clinical textbooks, life experiences, and word of mouth?

4. Do you think psychotropic medication is harmful, cruel, or unscientific? Do you think that these medications were used in the past to control and sedate people with psychiatric diagnoses and should no longer be used in this day and age of preventative and occupational therapies?

5. Answer the following technical questions about psychotropic medications. If you do not already know the answers, research the topic.

   - What are the five major categories of psychotropic medicine? Which medicines fall into each category? What are the main effects and side effects of each? What is the difference between a side effect and a main effect?
   - Are the side effects temporary or permanent? Do they last until the person stops taking medication or do they lessen once the person's system adapts to the medication?
   - How long is a typical medication trial for each of the main categories of psychotropic medicines? Why do they vary in length?
   - Are medications effective in treating psychiatric symptoms?
   - What does the term *refractory* mean with regards to medication and psychiatric symptoms?
   - What percent of psychiatric clients are refractory to each of the main categories of psychotropic drugs?

6. What intervention could you as a therapist use to help people better manage the side effects of their medication? Give intervention suggestions for each side effect.
7. Do you think any parts of the Patients' Bill of Rights in your state were violated here? If so, which ones and why?

Client-Centered Reasoning Activity

Write a group protocol for a medication education group addressing the problems mentioned in the preceding narrative.

The following two narratives are from people who take medication and describe their experiences.

MEDICATIONS: PRO

ANONYMOUS

My antipsychotic medication makes me sleep. My mood stabilizer makes me gain weight. My antianxiety medication makes me eat. The antidepressant helps me a lot. All of the medications help me a lot and help to get rid of some of the voices, but not all of them. My antipsychotic helps me sleep at night and the sleeping pills help me sleep at night. I am glad that I am taking medication to really help me.

QUICK

WESLEY MORROW

I want my medication to help me maintain a normal level of activity and attention. I think we are close to a good time and dosage for the medicine. Without the medication I heard so many voices and experienced tactile hallucinations that I thought I was going crazy. On medication, I still have problems with the tactile hallucinations and every so often I feel overwhelmed by the voices, but most of the time I feel the medication is a God-sent blessing. I think that one pill of an antianxiety medication, one pill of an antipsychotic, and one dosage of extrapyramidal medication in the morning would be a good mixture after breakfast. This process should be repeated after dinner. The antipsychotic pills quiet the voices in my head and help me focus. However, sometimes, I experience muscle stiffness as a side effect. The extrapyramidal medication solves the side affects. The antianxiety pills calm my agitation.

If clients refuse to follow the team's interventions and the team feels that they would be in danger to themselves, then the final decision is made in the judicial system after the clients and their doctors present their side of the story. The following narrative is from a client, Mr. Leavy.

COURT

MR. LEAVY

I had never been to court. The experience was new to me. I thought that my lawyer did a good job cross-examining the doctor. I gave an account of how I got there [psychiatric hospital]. I thought I was convincing. I thought the judge would rule in my favor. The other lawyer asked me a few questions. I asked to see the court order, but they would not show me the court order. I thought it would be a traumatic experience, but it was not. I thought the doctor was not bad to me, he took it easy.

I was asked to tell the court why I went to the hospital in the first place and why I did not want to take my medicine. I went to the hospital to get away from things and rest. I thought medicine would not be helpful because not all agree that medicine is the right way to go. I saw an article on how medications can be toxic. I am afraid to take my medicine because I think it is damaging to the mind and body. I feel victimized, angry, and scared about what it is doing to my mind and body. I cannot believe that medicating people against their will is still happening in the year 2000. I feel that I am getting this medicine illegally with a court order. I want to get out of the hospital, and when I am discharged, I will not take my medicine. I do not need any help. I do not need forced hospitalization or medication.

Client-Centered Reasoning Questions

1. Mr. Leavy states that he came to the hospital to "get away from things and rest." Is this realistic? He may have wanted to get away and rest, but what criteria do psychiatric hospitals use for admission?
2. Mr. Leavy is definitely against taking his medication. Do you think he is well informed about his medication? Why or why not?
3. This narrative is a good example of how forcing Mr. Leavy to take his medication may not be effective without providing him with more education about his medication and more work with his resistance. However, there is a way that the court mandate to keep Mr. Leavy in the hospital and taking his medications may help him be compliant with intervention and medication in the future. Can you identify this way?

When a client cannot be present in court, a decision is made after hearing the doctor's case presentation, as in the following narrative.

ABSENT AT THE HEARING

ANONYMOUS INTERN

Today I saw something happen that had more of an effect on me than I thought it would. Larry is a 19-year-old African American man with whom I have not had much contact. He isolates himself in his room or stands staring at the TV for hours, expressionless and motionless. He often fakes being mute to avoid answering questions or acknowledging staff members. He has refused his medications on numerous occasions.

This particular day he was supposed to go to court regarding his status. The doctors feel he is still in danger of hurting himself, so he needs to be in the hospital. These hearings are designed for a judge to make a decision about the best practice for a client when the client and the clients' doctor disagree. Clients present their side of the story. The staff was getting ready to take him to the court hearing, but he refused to go. When a client refuses to appear, the doctor still goes to present the case. The court usually rules in favor of the doctor, which is what happened in this case; Larry lost, so he stays in the hospital.

Client-Centered Reasoning Questions

1. How would you begin to work with Larry, given that he fakes being mute, stands in front of the television for hours, isolates himself in his room, and is 19 years old?
2. The intern begins this narrative by saying that she had seen something that had more of an effect on her than she thought it would, but she does not express what effect this story had on her. What are your feelings about Larry having to stay in the hospital?
3. Thoughts are different from feelings, and when working with people who have mental health issues, it is important to be aware of both your feelings and thoughts. For example, you could intellectually understand the reasons for needing to keep Larry in the hospital because he is still seen as dangerous to himself and others (your thought), yet you could feel sorry for Larry and feel that the decision to keep Larry is unfair since Larry could not get to express himself in front of the judge (your feeling). So, what are your thoughts about Larry having to stay in the hospital?
4. Often a person's thoughts and emotional responses do not match. Are your thoughts different than your feelings about Larry's situation?
5. Do you think any parts of the Patients' Bill of Rights in your state were violated in this narrative above? If so, which ones and why?

Analysis

When working in the area of mental health your feelings and your awareness of them are very important. There are no incorrect feelings. They are whatever they are. You have a right to feel whatever you feel, even if it is not the norm or politically correct. In fact, your feelings about a situation can help inform you and the team about what may really be going on with a client. The more you learn to trust your feelings, the more you will express them when appropriate and the more helpful they will become to your practice and your supervision. If you are able to observe your feelings, you are stepping out of yourself long enough to reflect on the situation. This is a helpful practice that prevents you from acting on your feelings. As mentioned before, you are allowed any feelings you want, but actions count.

If you are not aware of your feelings, you may unconsciously act differently toward a client in a way that may not be helpful. (The next narrative contains an example of how its author, an intern, allows her feelings to affect her interventions with her client.) If you are not aware of your thoughts, you may get too wrapped up in your emotions and not be able to see the logic behind the decision. If you are working with an intervention team, everyone may have different thoughts, feelings, and ideas about a person's intervention, so another element comes into play: the decision of the team. Once the team members express their individual thoughts on the intervention, backed up with concrete examples that justify their decisions, the team must agree on one decision and carry it out. Even if the team's decision is different from yours, as long as you expressed yourself earlier as part of the team decision-making process, that is really all you can do unless you think the team decision would endanger the client in some way. Then, it would be prudent to keep pushing your point. Otherwise, you need to carry out the decision with full conviction when with the client, even if you do not believe in it, in order not to split the team and confuse the client.

A person can be admitted to a psychiatric hospital voluntarily or involuntarily. If people come in of their own free will, their status is voluntary. People who are brought in by a family member, the police, or someone else but refuse admission can be admitted against their will if two psychiatrists' evaluations agree to admit them. Their status is then involuntary. People are admitted into a psychiatric facility only if they are in danger of hurting themselves or others, and as soon as they are no longer in danger of hurting themselves or others and they have a discharge plan, they are discharged.

Client-Centered Reasoning Activity

Research Kendra's law. What is this law? How did it come about? How is it different than the laws before it? How may it affect people with mental health issues? Their families? Intervention centers? Society? Do you think it is fair? Why or why not? What are some good things that could come from having this law? What are some negative things? Where did you find your information?

Interns often need to assert themselves to gain a fuller internship experience. The following intern asked to go to court to learn more about the proceedings. She writes about her day in court in the following narrative.

MY DAY IN COURT

Anonymous Intern

"You are going to court today, Lou. Get up, and get dressed. They will pick you up in one hour," said the nurse.

Lou apparently got up and showered for the first time in two weeks. When I saw him in court a few hours later, he was clean and his hair was combed. He looked down and did not return my greeting as I walked by to get a seat in the courtroom. I felt bad, as if I was one of the people he viewed as out to get him. I used to be one of the few people he spoke to on the unit. I wondered if being in court today was going to affect my future therapeutic relationship with Lou.

The clients wait out in the hall until their case is called. I got to witness all of the cases presented today. Court proceedings in mental health are designed to help the clients receive the care they need. Very often people with mental health issues are unable to make these decisions for themselves. When intervention teams in the hospital suspect that a client is unable to make these decisions and refuses intervention, the hospital schedules a court hearing.

The hospital supplies transportation for the clients to go to court. The hospital also supplies them with their own mental health lawyer. The lawyers are there to cross-examine the doctors and ask favorable questions of the clients and give the clients a chance to express themselves in the best possible light. The purpose of the clients' going to court is to speak on their own behalf and make the court aware of their thoughts on their situations. This also allows the clients to feel that they have a little control over their lives. Clients often feel out of control. They cannot control their illness, they cannot control being brought to the hospital, and most of the time they cannot control when they get out of the hospital. If they were not given the opportunity to go to court, the feeling of helplessness that they experience in their lives would increase. However, allowing clients to make a statement in court and be questioned by their own lawyer demonstrates better than any doctor testimony just what condition the client is really in.

The outcomes of the first few cases were fairly easy for me to predict. Both of the clients had quite violent episodes that culminated in their being hospitalized. Both demonstrated no insight into their illness and, therefore, had no intention of taking their medications when they were released. They had no problem telling the court just that. The hospital was asking for 60-day retention extension and medication. That means that the hospital wants the court order to say that the client must remain in the hospital for an additional 60 days and that the client will be court ordered to take medications. If the client refuses the medications, the hospital now has the right to use intramuscularly injected medications whose effects last for weeks.

The hope of the hospital is that, if the clients stay long enough, they not only will become stable but also will learn the importance of taking their medications and following their intervention plans. During the hospitalization clients will have OT [occupational therapy] intervention to help improve occupational performance. Intervention could include educating clients about their medications and working with them to set up medication schedules. The clients also have many other types of therapeutic sessions, with OT, Psychology, Creative Arts Therapy, and Social Work.

The third case was more complicated. The client was a 32-year-old white woman who had been diagnosed with bipolar disorder. Her elderly, sickly looking father was present in the courtroom and, to my surprise, asked that she be kept in the hospital. Her father felt that she was a danger to herself and to her mother, with whom she has had altercations in the past. I was surprised that the father was asking for retention. In the previous two cases, the parents came in and asked for their child's release. It did not seem to matter to them that their child was extremely psychotic and disorganized. This case continued with the doctors and the father reporting her previous hospitalizations (all of which were out of the state or the country, with no records available). The client's lawyer attempted to object due to the fact that there were no records to prove any of this, but the judge snapped at him and allowed testimony to continue. The client's lawyer also tried to cross-examine the father and the doctors, but the judge kept cutting him off. The lawyer and the client both looked helpless, and the spectators, including me, were dumbfounded. They also reported her having had two violent altercations with her elderly mother. The client would then deny everything or report it in a different way. It was unclear to me whether the client was intentionally lying, honestly remembered it differently due to her illness, or her father was lying for unknown reasons. It was difficult to predict the outcome of this case because there were no records or reports to substantiate anything said by anyone. In the end, the word of doctors and family members carried more weight than those of the client. This could have been due to an underlying bias against the mentally ill. Some people may view doctors and family as more credible just because they are not the ones in the hospital. This judge appeared to have a very strong bias. Without hesitation, the judge ruled against the client. She will stay in the hospital and will be court ordered to take medications. The father sat in his seat and cried.

It was difficult not to notice that the judge was in a horrible mood and absolutely "pro" doctor. He spent much of each case ripping apart the defense lawyers and ruling in favor of the lawyers representing the hospital and intervention team. I could not help but think that he was responding to the front page of every New York newspaper. On this day, the lead story in New

York was about the mentally ill homeless man who pushed a hard-working father of three in front of a speeding subway train. The victim is now clinging to life and had to have both of his legs amputated. It is difficult not to be angry and disgusted by a story like that; the judge is human. But he is a judge and must judge fairly. It appeared to me that this judge was allowing his own personal biases or the current feelings of the public to interfere with his job as a fair and impartial figure. I sat there in stunned silence every time the judge was unnecessarily nasty to a defense lawyer and cruelly handed down each ruling without a word of explanation to the client.

Then, my first of two cases came up. Lou is physically anorexic but does not have anorexia. Anorexia occurs when a person becomes obsessed with the idea of losing weight. Anorexics restrict their intake and increase their activity level so severely that their very lives are threatened by the weight loss. People suffering from anorexia may have a distorted perception of personal appearance, which convinces them that they are obese, although in reality they are emaciated. Lou meets only some of the criteria. Lou restricts his intake but has not increased his activity level. In fact, Lou sits in a chair in his room all day and lies in bed all night. Lou also does not see himself as obese. He knows how thin he is and feels he should be heavier, but he is unable to eat. He does not have the same thought processes as anorexics. The reasons for starving himself lie in his psychosocial issues and are not the same as those suffering from textbook anorexia. Unfortunately, Lou would never share his reasoning with us. When asked about the reasons, he would give very vague answers. Often he would state that it was a personal, religious reason and he would not tell us because we would think he was crazy.

Our attending psychiatrist took the stand and presented our case for retaining Lou in the hospital to prepare for a state hospital transfer. The defense attorney *attempted* to highlight the fact the Lou has gained 17 pounds while in the hospital, but the judge did not allow him to go too far on that line of questioning.

The judge then began to question Lou, "Why are you not eating, sir?"

Lou replied, "I was very overweight, and went on a radical diet. I know now that it was wrong. I do think I need to gain another 15 pounds to be a normal weight. I plan on doing that."

The judge questioned him further, "How do you plan on doing that if you are out of the hospital?"

Lou responded, "I will eat vegetables, fish, and poultry."

"Why are you not eating anything but the protein drinks in the hospital?"

"Well, I ordered a vegetarian meal in the hospital but they sent me something with chicken, and it repulsed me."

I knew that the case was now over. Lou contradicted himself in such a blatant manner that the judge had no difficulty making his ruling. Yet, the way the judge was conducting himself that day, I believe he would have made that decision regardless of what Lou said. "Retention granted," ordered the judge. It was over for Lou. Lou will remain in the hospital until the state hospital transfer is complete.

Bringing the clients to court and allowing them to have their say is supposed to make them feel that they may have a little control over their lives. However, this judge did not do justice to that process. He was out of line in the way he conducted himself. I am not saying that the verdicts were wrong but that the way he treated them was not right. They are people with illnesses; they are not objects to be disregarded. Every verdict could have been handed down with a touch of compassion and tact; instead, the judge made the clients feel powerless and helpless, and that is the part that is just not right.

"We received the acceptance from Rockland State Hospital. Lou can go. They are going to take him. He is going Wednesday morning. The ambulance will pick him up at 8:40 A.M." The social worker gave the team the news that it has been waiting for.

"Does Lou know yet?" asked the nurse.

"No. We will tell him when we make our rounds," the attendant replied.

In the morning, the team meets to discuss client care and progress. After the closed door meeting, we make rounds on all of the clients, which means that we walk around the unit and meet with each client as a team.

Lou sits in a chair next to his bed in the dark, foul-smelling room, staring at the wall all day long. He has a terrible swelling in his feet and ankles due to his lack of physical activity. We entered Lou's darkened room, and he was in his usual position. He looked at all of us but said nothing. My concerns about my court visit affecting our therapeutic relationship may have been correct. Since the court date, Lou has not come to any of our groups and has not spoken to me aside from some superficial conversation.

The attending psychiatrist greeted Lou and asked Lou how he was feeling. Lou gave his usual reply, "I feel fine." Lou has poor eye contact and tends to look at the floor after he says something. The attending then told him that we had received word from Rockland and that everything was set for the next morning. Lou seemed to explode from inside. "I do not want to go to Rockland! I told you I am fine. I told you I will gain weight and that I will start to eat! I do not see why I cannot just stay here a little while longer." The attending explained that staying here was just not possible. Lou continued, "I have seen people here a lot longer than me. Why cannot I stay here?" The attending asked him why he has such strong objections to going to another hospital. Lou responded, "Because they are dangerous places. I just do not belong there. I will not feel safe. Bad things happen there." The attending and the resident expressed that they understand his apprehension, but that it is really the only possibility right now.

I felt so bad for him just then. I put myself in his shoes, and at that moment I would be absolutely terrified. I could not imagine having no control over what happens to me. Lou honestly feels that there is nothing wrong with him that he cannot fix himself, but no one is listening to him.

As we left the room, I turned and looked at Lou, but he had his head down. He looked so pathetic and small in the chair, and the darkness of the room was so depressing. I felt terrible. There was nothing that I could say to him to make him feel better, and I am sure he did not want to hear from me anyway. He views me as one of the people who were responsible for him being transferred to a state hospital.

I wanted to talk to him, but I avoided it almost all day. Normally, I go to his room to invite him to every group that we run, but I did not do it this day. I finally went to invite him to the last group of the day, knowing that I was unable to talk after group because the day is over for me. I was really nervous that he was going to ask me the hard questions that I had no answers for. So, half consciously, half unconsciously, I avoided any situations that could lead to that conversation. I knocked on his door and entered. He was still in the same position we left him in seven hours earlier. He looked up, and I asked him if he would like to come to our yoga group. "No thank you," he replied. He put his head back down. "All right, we are down in the solarium if you change your mind." I lost my nerve. I could not bring myself to ask him if he would like to talk. My heart was pounding as I walked out of his room, and I felt as I had felt the first time that I ever talked to a client. I was so angry with myself for not doing my job.

I think I was really affected by his leaving, partially because he had been there since I started. I was sad to see him go, no matter what. I knew he was going to a place that scared him and that made it all the more difficult to see him go. But I think I would have been upset when he left, even if he was going home and was happy. Lou has been here since I started. I saw him start out in the beginning, just lying in bed all day in a hospital gown. He fought any medication or nutrition drink brought to him, requiring him to be tube fed very often. Then, he began to come to our groups a few times a week. Then, one day, he was in his street clothes. He even smiled a few times. Once his court date came and he was ordered to go to the state hospital he began to isolate himself again, this time sitting in his chair all day. He was very difficult to work with because he really resisted any help offered. I think I really felt sadness over his situation, and I will always wish that we could have done more for him while he was here.

The next day in rounds the attending was reading off the names and he said Lou's name. "Gone. They picked him up this morning." My heart sank.

Client-Centered Reasoning Questions

1. This intern states that Lou would never tell the staff why he did not want to eat food because he thought that the staff would think "that he was crazy." Lou did, however, hint that his not eating had to do with religious and personal reasons. They probably had to do with his delusions. In quotes, write five different things you could say to Lou to find out what his true thoughts behind not eating were. Why is it important to try to find out?

2. Find and describe an example in this narrative where this intern's feelings may have affected her behavior. What could she have done differently, and how could this have helped?

3. Do you think any parts of the Patients' Bill of Rights in your state were violated here? If so, which ones and why?

Client-Centered Reasoning Activity

This intern mentions in her narrative that clients receive therapeutic sessions with occupational therapists, psychologists, social workers, and creative arts therapists. Interview a psychologist, a social worker, or a creative arts therapist to better understand the discipline's role in working in the area of mental health. What kind of intervention does the discipline provide? How is each of their interventions different from occupational therapy? How is it similar? What are creative arts therapists? Name five disciplines that practice under this category.

CLIENT-CENTERED REASONING
ACTIVITIES FOR CHAPTER 4

1. This chapter presents six different issues regarding clients' rights. They are: whether or not or when to use ECT for depression, third-party reimbursers driving the length of stay and types of interventions, whether or not or when to force medication, whether or not or when to extend a hospital stay against someone's will, whether or not or when to send people for long-term intervention at a State hospital against their will, and how much freedom versus restriction is necessary to keep someone safe during a psychiatric hospitalization. You have already discussed the pros and cons of each issue as each issue relates to mental health. Now do the same for physical disabilities. Compare and contrast each issue as it relates to the practice areas of physical disabilities versus mental health. Are the rules the same or different? Why?

2. Set up a mock court trial for each of the scenarios below. Make it as real as possible, presenting all sides of the issue at hand using the different characters in the identified narratives.

   a. Someone play the part of Anne, the client in Laura Bella-Bryant's narrative, who wants to leave the hospital because she believes that her rights have been taken away.

Someone play the part of Anne's primary nurse, who escorted her to the shower, made her take off her clothes to give her an intramuscular injection against her will, and restricted her use of crafts. Someone play Anne's lawyer, who advocates for Anne's rights. Someone play Anne's doctor, by making up an appropriate script since Anne's doctor is not mentioned in the narrative. Someone play Anne's intern, who feels bad for Anne because of her loss of freedom but is also aware of her potential for violence. And finally, a jury of nine is needed to agree on the types and amounts of restrictions (if any) that would be necessary for Anne to get the most out of her hospital stay and whether or not she should be in the hospital at this time. The jury must explain their conclusions.

b. Someone play Meibel, the client in Liliana's narrative who may be discharged before she has a place to live that provides structure as well as a bed. Someone play the director of the residence that takes four months to process a referral and generate a bed. Someone play a staff member at the drop-in center that provides a place to sleep but no structured activities or therapeutic groups and is about to receive Anne unless she finds an alternative living arrangement. Someone play a representative of Meibel's managed care company, which is denying her payment of further hospitalization. Someone play Meibel's intern, as described in the narrative. Someone play Meibel's doctor, who is at odds with all managed care companies because of the restrictions they place on his ability to treat his clients the way he believes to be the most therapeutic. And finally, a jury of nine is to decide the best possible outcome based on the evidence provided.

c. Set up a trial about the use of psychotropic medication. Discuss the intricacies of when and how it should be used or not used, how much input people taking the medication and their family members have, if it is necessary to take the drug for life, and so forth. Present all sides of the issue by including the following people from the narratives in this chapter: Denise, Denise's doctor, Denise's student intern, Mr. Leavy, the anonymous author of "Medications: Pro," and Wesley Morrow. In addition, include made-up scripts for the family members and neighbors of Denise, Mr. Leavy, and the anonymous author of "Medications: Pro," and for the parole officer of Wesley Morrow.

3. The final narrative about the life of Theresa, written by intern Eileen Tierney, illustrates many of the practices mentioned earlier in this chapter. Space has been left for you to write your thoughts between the lines as you read.

THERESA

EILEEN TIERNEY

I first heard about Theresa on team rounds, when each morning, various staff members discuss clients and whatever progress they may have made. Theresa's description was given as follows: The client is a 38-year-old divorced white woman who lives with her current husband and two boys, ages 17 and 6; she has a history of bipolar disorder, currently in a manic episode, with multiple psychiatric hospitalizations. She left her home the day before Halloween to attend a party; and when she did not return home, her husband, Scott, filed a missing person's report. Theresa was soon found in Port Authority bus terminal walking around with no shoes on, claiming that they were stolen along with her pocketbook. The police brought her into the Psychiatric Emergency Room, where she was evaluated and described as, "extremely agitated, incoherent, yelling, and threatening staff." Theresa was given intramuscular medications and put in four-point restraints. She was a "danger to self and others" and would require hospitalization.

When Theresa came onto our unit, via a stretcher, she was still quite sedated from the medications. A few hours later she awoke and was very disoriented. She did not know where she was; she was yelling, screaming, and threatening to the staff. Theresa felt that she was here by mistake and should be released immediately. She continued to be loud, uncooperative, and threatening. Security was called, and Theresa was escorted to the special care section of our unit, where she remained under close observation. This section is set up with to provide special attention to those who need additional observation for either medical or psychological reasons. Again, she was given medication to calm her and help her to sleep. Theresa awoke the next day still very angry and with pressured speech. At this point, I still had not spoken to her because the nursing staff advised me that she was still too distraught. Generally, when a client whom I have not encountered is in special care, I approach the nurses for their advice on the person's aggressiveness or vulnerability. I try to orient clients to our unit on their first or second day, but in this instance, it was suggested that I wait until tomorrow for the client to calm down. However, even though I am not meeting with the client, I gather information from the team rounds and various progress notes in her chart. The information from Theresa's first two days is based on such reports.

On her second day, her husband came to visit her, and after his departure, an unopened pack of cigarettes was found in her possession. At this point, the staff penalized her, according to regulations, by administering visitor restrictions. A first-time offense mandates that a client be not allowed visitors for 24 hours. A second offense calls for a two-day visitor restriction; and after three offenses, the staff makes a therapeutic decision regarding a penalty. Theresa was having a difficult time adjusting to her stay on our unit because she was aggravated at having to be there in the first place. In addition, she was now being limited, in that her husband could not visit. Her distress was visible and further exacerbated as she was still displaying symptoms of mania; her speech was pressured, her thoughts were delusional, and she was very restless. She took her medications reluctantly and was seen trying to put her bed linens in the toilet. Theresa was not ready to attend any of the therapeutic groups. To make matters worse, early the next morning, Theresa somehow set off the fire alarms. Staff reacted by placing her in seclusion, whereby she was not even allowed to use the bathroom unattended. Seclusion rooms are used only under extreme circumstances, when people are in a danger of losing control. Unlike other rooms on the unit, those in seclusion are quite basic. The only thing in the room is a bed. There is no adjoining bathroom, to avoid clients hurting themselves. Theresa remained here for one day because she did not display any signs of responding to limits or maintaining control of herself.

At this point, I still had not actually spoken to Theresa; I had only seen her in the halls. She has long, strawberry blond hair combed straight; she is about five feet and six inches tall, and has a wide smile. During the first few days, Theresa did not smile much; in fact, her facial expressions were very constricted. Theresa was upset and so her emotional state was very volatile. I had seen her quickly pacing the halls and hanging around elevators that did not work, in an attempt to escape our locked unit. To be honest, I was a bit afraid to approach her because her mannerisms were almost menacing. She had a crazed look in her eyes, and she was so restless and angry that I felt she might lunge at me if she took the notion. I knew that she is manic and that irrational actions may occur spontaneously. I also knew that this is not her fault, because it is part of her illness; nonetheless, I was hesitant to approach.

In addition to what I observed, the tidbits about Theresa given in team rounds did not cause me to rush over to get personal with her. Twelve years ago, before her first episode, Theresa worked as a psychiatric nurse. She was knowledgeable about all the medications prescribed to her as well as how certain procedures should be carried out. A few of the nurses did not find this appealing; in fact, they found it irritating to have someone reminding them how to do their job. Also, one morning, I was in the nurses' station looking up a chart and Theresa came over to the door and was very angry. She told one of the nurses that she was upset with so many people knocking on her door to ask her so many questions and so she wanted to have a list of all the staff who were assigned to her. This deterred me even more, because I feared that if I did approach her and my name was not on her list for some reason, she would lose control. So here was Theresa, this boisterous ex-nurse who was loud, disruptive, and intimidating to those around her. I felt I was losing control of the situation, and I wanted to do something fast to regain my stature.

That afternoon I found her in the day room. I introduced myself and asked if I could speak to her. To my surprise, she smiled, her eyes lit up, and she said, "Absolutely." I was not expecting this response at all; I was anticipating her reaction to be dismissive. I then proceeded to go over our unit's orientation booklet with her, describing the various activities, schedules, rules, and staff members. She let me know immediately that she was once a psychiatric nurse and therefore was aware of most of what I told her. I also realized that she was having difficulty keeping her eyes open, and so I asked her if she was tired. She said that she was a little bit drowsy because of the medications. (I also attributed her serenity and lethargy to this fact.) I did not want to force her to talk, and so I said that I would either meet with her later that day or early the next morning, depending on how she felt. Theresa agreed and said she was very glad to have met me.

And so, there was our first encounter, just about the opposite of what I had preconceived in my mind. Based on all her previous actions, I expected her to be just as short-tempered with me as she was with most of the other staff. Theresa had almost immediately found a connection with me. I believe this is because she saw that I really cared about her and was willing to listen to whatever she had to say. She bonded with me that day and from thence forward, she considered me someone she could open up to about anything. It is amazing what one can learn from a simple encounter. In just 10 short minutes, I had witnessed behavior from this woman that contradicted much of what I had learned of her in rounds. I previously had fears that Theresa would be very agitated and irritable with me. I am not ignoring that she was delusional and slightly bizarre, but I began to see past that and look within her. There were underlying qualities and strengths that I could focus on and work with while Theresa was on our unit. I was not yet aware of them all, but at least I had recognized that they were there, although dormant.

Theresa attended a therapeutic group the next day, and I noticed that halfway through the group she fell asleep. When the group was over, she woke up and came over to me. She remembered who I was but had forgotten my name. I introduced myself again, and she asked me if I wanted to talk again. I sat down with her and she began to tell me how she ended up in the hospital. Her account did not coincide with what was reported in the chart; "This whole thing is a setup," she claimed. As she continued, it became evident that she was paranoid, delusional, and grandiose. She proceeded to tell me that she was a member of a research team that had found a cure for AIDS. This was Theresa's fourth day, and while her agitation and hostility had markedly decreased, her thoughts were still delusional and grandiose.

Theresa continued to tell me more of her life story. She told me that her mother had been diagnosed with unipolar depression, so she helped her father, who was a superintendent, raise seven children. They lived in a very diverse neighborhood in Staten Island, and Theresa says this is the reason she is able to get along with so many different types of people. Theresa, a middle child in her clan, said that she loved to do things for her younger siblings. She enjoyed taking them to the movies or buying them little gifts. To do this, Theresa said that she had to work at a candy shop when she was 12 years old. While she was at this job, she was sexually molested for the third time in her life. On the first two occasions, she states that her uncle committed the act when she was 8 years old. This time, however, the owner of the candy store acted out against her. Theresa said she quit the job that very day, and it changed her life in ways she still does not really understand.

Theresa began to experiment with the opposite sex at a young age. She met her first future husband, Matt, when she was 14 years old and quickly took on the lifestyle of sex, drugs, and rock-n-roll. Theresa said that she was trying to grow up too fast. Matt was the same age as she but he introduced her to an adult world that she wishes she never entered. She began taking many different drugs because he was taking them, and she loved being with him. Theresa and Matt hung out with an older crowd, who would help them get alcohol. Also, at this young age of 14, Theresa found herself spending many nights having sex with Matt in motels.

Theresa's hypersexual thoughts began to reveal themselves. Hypersexuality is a common symptom for manic people. Although I was aware of it and its existence in such clients, I had never witnessed the process of its unfolding during an interview. It caught me off guard because here I was getting a lot of relevant information from this client, but I had to keep redirecting the conversation. Theresa's focus would return to the topic at hand but only after much verbal prompting. Theresa was still experiencing manic symptoms at this point, as was evident in her pressured speech. She had so much to say and wanted to say it all in a short amount of time. I told her that she could take her time because I was available everyday to hear whatever she wanted to tell me.

In time, Theresa went back to talking about drugs and her early teenage years. She said that she began to smoke marijuana when she was 15. Within about a year, she began taking LSD, uppers, and downers. I asked her to explain some of these drugs and their effects, because, quite frankly, I have never heard of some of them. Theresa said that tripping on acid (LSD) was a horrible experience and she regrets ever doing it. It messed with her brain and distorted her reality. Not all trips were the same, but during some of them she felt that she would never come out of it, and she felt very scared. Uppers and downers each do what their name implies. Uppers made her feel so incredibly high and amazing, but, "the feeling does not last that long and when it is over, boy, do you feel like complete crap!" Downers "mellow you out and make you feel really relaxed," and when they wear off, they would just make her very tired. She said that she regrets taking all of these drugs because they just made her feel dirty inside. Although she has come to this realization only recently, she said that these days she gets all her highs from God. When asked why she did these drugs, she blamed Matt; she was so in love with him at the time and just wanted to spend time with him, even if most of that time was spent all drugged up.

Theresa continued living this way throughout her teenage years. The one thing that may have saved her life was her determination to become a nurse. Theresa said that, at a young age, she felt a premonition to go into a healing ministry whereby she would use her hands to help others. She finished high school at 17 and soon after had an LPN degree. She married Matt two years later, at the age of 19, but she continued to stay focused on her career. Theresa states that this was not an easy period in her life. While she was very much in love with Matt, he began to use heavier drugs, and he introduced her to these heavy drugs, too. Looking back, Theresa is not sure how she was able to attain her nursing degree because she spent so many nights all coked up. She did manage to become a registered nurse at the age of 21, within days of giving birth to her first child, Matt Junior. The drugging did not stop though; in fact, it got worse. Matt and Theresa began using heroin, but in between this time many accidents occurred.

One of their first accidents took place on New Year's Eve, before Matt Junior was born. Matt and Theresa were driving home from a party in Theresa's little red car; they had both done a considerable amount of cocaine before they left. That night, Matt somehow lost control of the car and it flipped over twice. Theresa says she does not ever remember being so scared, to awake upside down in a car, at night, and high as a bird is not something she wishes to think about often. They both survived the accident and continued on with their lives. Theresa bought another car, this time it was a van, and two years later they had another accident. Matt had been drinking in addition to taking downers and Theresa had been doing the same but in smaller quantities. Matt Junior was with the couple this time, so Theresa wanted to drive home, but Matt refused. Their van ended up colliding head on with another vehicle, and Theresa broke her wrist as a result. The accident was not terribly severe but it upset Theresa to talk about it. She did not wish to go into details of other accidents but she said that while she and Matt were married, there were seven more accidents.

These days Theresa has a lot of time to reflect on the past. She thinks back to those earlier days and does not know how she made it to this point alive. Again, she places a lot of faith in God, but it does not take away from the fact that she feels she is living, and has been, on borrowed time. Theresa says that she thinks her time should have been up a long time ago. She says that she has lived through so much and Theresa is not even an old woman; she is only 38. Theresa is tired, though, and finds it very difficult to find the inner strength to carry on. She says that her reservoir of inner strength has been dipped into so many times that she cannot understand how there is any strength left.

When Theresa was 26 years old she had her first manic experience. It occurred six months after Matt lost his job, and they were experiencing both financial and marital problems. She does not remember the day vividly; all she recalls is being at work one morning and trying to read papers. Her vision became blurred until she could not see anything. She retreated to her office and sat down until she felt a little bit better. She then drove home but does not remember this. Theresa had to take sick leave from her job due to this illness, and she has not returned to her former profession in over 12 years. Her marriage failed shortly after the outbreak of her illness. Theresa remembers doing a lot of cocaine the weekend before her manic symptoms revealed themselves, and she could not deal with the fact that Matt was still caught up in all the drugs. In addition, Matt had lost his job, and they were experiencing many financial problems.

Theresa fought this illness for 12 years, while going through about 16 psychiatric hospitalizations. Throughout each of these, she was prescribed different medications. On one occasion, after being married to her second husband, Scott, Theresa was hospitalized in a manic state. During this hospitalization she was given a mood stabilizer that she begged them not to give her. She was aware of the side effects and of the possibility that she may be pregnant. Theresa took a pregnancy test but the results were a false negative and she remained on her medication for two months before it was confirmed that she was pregnant. Needless to say Theresa was extremely upset because she had feared the worst. She was informed that a D and C, dilation and curettage, would have to be performed, where the lining of the uterus is cleaned after a fetus has been aborted. This procedure had to be done because the fetus had suffered deformations during Theresa's hospitalization. She began to cry at this point, and I really empathized for her. The pain she must have gone through and the torment at knowing that it could have been prevented is something that haunts her to this day. I tried to offer her some soothing words and eventually she calmed down, but it is difficult when your heart saddens over what another has lost.

Theresa described her mood stabilizer as the worst drug she has ever been medically treated with. She says it caused her to rock back and forth in addition to being teratogenic, or genetically deforming, to her fetus. Currently Theresa is on a mood stabilizer and an anticonvulsant. She says that she likes the mood stabilizer because it helps her get her thoughts back together. Theresa was not fond of these other medications because they made her hands tremble and gave her ataxic symptoms, stiffening her arms, legs, her entire gait, as well as making her drowsy. She was compliant with her medications at this point because she knew she had to take them to get better and return home. Toward the end of her 16-day stay, her mood stabilizer level was approaching its therapeutic point. It is important to increase the levels at small increments because it can be toxic. Theresa did experience some toxic symptoms, as she occasionally had diarrhea and vomiting. Theresa was able to contact nursing for assistance, and her doctor reduced her dosage.

Theresa had come a long way during her stay. On her tenth day, the staff recognized that she had been able to maintain control of herself; therefore, it was decided in rounds to change her status from special care to level one, whereby she was then allowed to wear her own clothes. This decision was reached during one of our team rounds, whereby I encouraged them to make this therapeutic decision. Theresa had gained insight into her illness. She was able to think back to her first few days and realize that she was not in control of herself. From the beginning, Theresa never had any problems socializing; and she was always eager to participate in our groups. Theresa could be loud and disruptive at first, but she responded well to redirection. Toward the end of her stay, she was quite helpful in our group meetings, because she was insightful and offered much advice to other peers.

One of her goals was to work on her frustration tolerance. In our group we went over tai chi, different relaxation techniques, and when to implement these techniques. On one occasion, Theresa became quite upset with nursing for not responding to one of her requests. I happened to be with her when she said she was going to the nursing station to "raise hell." I asked her to wait a minute, take a couple of deep breaths, and think about the consequences of these actions. I asked her, if she went down there angrily, would it solve her problems any faster? Theresa knew the answer, and so she continued taking deep breaths for another minute and then calmly approached the nurses' station. During our next encounter, I asked Theresa why she had difficulty using the relaxation techniques that she had learned. She said it was not that she had forgotten them, but rather she just did not think of them in the heat of the moment. Based on this information, I decided that it might be helpful if we went over stressors that may cause her to get upset and work from there. This proved to be effective when Theresa had a small altercation with Scott over the telephone. They were discussing their financial situation, which she had identified as a stressor, and she needed time to calm down, and so she asked Scott if he would call her back in a little while. I was very pleased and a bit proud of myself that the intervention we had worked on had actually worked effectively.

Theresa's concentration levels also improved, but it may have been secondary to her medications. I encouraged her to come to our skills development group, where we work on accomplishing different tasks. At first, Theresa made a beaded necklace, and she did not display any difficulty adhering to the task. It is a fairly basic task but the degrees of performance vary. What I looked for in Theresa's performance was how well she worked. Due to her mania, she could work quickly on tasks, but I wanted her to work efficiently and accurately. I observed the manner in which she beaded the necklace to see if there were any patterns. Theresa was capable of doing this; she coordinated the beads by color in alternating patterns. Due to this, at our next meeting, I encouraged her to try something a little bit more involved. Theresa simply declined, though; she wanted to make the necklaces because she wanted to give them out to people when she was discharged. After two more meetings, I convinced her to make an ashtray, a task that generally involves more cognitive skills. Theresa demonstrated little difficulty with this task as well. More steps are involved in this task and the directions are more intricate. I explained each step; then went through them with her one at a time. Theresa picked out the tiles that she wanted to use and proceeded to glue them to the tray. At this point her anxiety got in the way of her performance. She did not want to wait for the tiles to dry before adding the grout. I intervened and asked her what she thought would happen if she sped through the project. Theresa was able to admit that sometimes she just gets so restless that she needs to keep doing something. I offered her a smaller task (beaded necklaces) to do while she waited for the tiles to dry. Mixing the grout was also problematic for Theresa, as she had a tendency to add too much water. After the third trial, she got the hang of it and proceeded with her project. I was impressed when she resumed beading the necklace while waiting for the grout to dry. Breaking down the steps of the task greatly benefited Theresa and her work. Her ashtray came out very nice and she was quite proud of her work.

Another problem of Theresa's was smoking on the unit. She had been caught, numerous times, either smoking or with paraphernalia. I had spoken with her many times about this issue, and I had brought her pamphlets to try to increase her awareness about the damage to her health as well as to those around her. It was to no avail; she continued to smoke but did it discretely, so as not to lose her level one status. This was a bit upsetting to me, because I continued to pursue the cause and she showed no signs of attempting to better the situation. From this, I learned that it is extremely difficult to achieve all or even most of the goals set for clients, especially when hospitalizations are rather short. The best one can do is try to realistically figure what they can work on during a stay and try to achieve those goals.

Theresa was cooperative with making discharge follow-up plans, so a social worker, a psychologist, and I set up a family meeting for Theresa. My goal in the meeting was to assess the level of support Theresa would receive from her husband after her discharge, which is a difficult period for many people. My concern was that, after discharge, Theresa would stop taking her medications. She had been having manic episodes for over 10 years. What was to stop her from having another one next year? I wanted to increase her husband's awareness of the importance of taking her medications regularly and adhering to follow-up interventions. To facilitate this, prior to the meeting, Theresa and I created a schedule, detailing when her appointments were and when she would need to take her medications, as well as when to renew them. In addition, we had made a copy for Theresa's sister, because Theresa had cited her sister as someone who in the past had been involved with funding her prescription renewals at times. Theresa and Scott were given a list of numbers to call in case any questions should arise. The meeting went well. Theresa was calm and acted appropriately, and many details concerning her discharge were discussed. At this time it is still difficult to foresee if and when any problems may arise. I am not certain that everything will go as planned because she has had many problems with relapse in the past, but all I can do is hope for the best.

Theresa had a rough start in life; she began doing many of the wrong things at an early age. Theresa became involved with hard-core drugs at an age when most people are looking toward their future. In Theresa's case, her future was rapidly deteriorating. Theresa regretted the mistakes she had made; she felt that all those years of drugs and recklessness had rotted her brain and wore down her soul. Theresa said that her illness further exacerbated this, and she has lived a lot in the time that she has been on this Earth. She is mentally, emotionally, and physically tired of this way of life. Her mind is not as sharp as it once was and her body movements are not as quick as they once were. At times, Theresa says that she is just waiting for her existence to expire. She is not suicidal, she states, because she still has a lot to live for, particularly her son, who is only 6. Theresa is just finding it hard to have the strength it takes to make it all the way.

I learned a lot from this client. I believe that something can be learned from every client encountered, whether it is trivial or significant. I learned that I do attach certain prejudices or preconceived ideas about what a client may be like, and I learned that it is critical to overcome these notions because they are not always right and they interfere with intervention.

Client-Centered Reasoning Activities

1. Finish the narrative.
2. In addition to the ones given here, write your own client-centered reasoning questions and activities.
3. Write an occupational profile for Theresa.
4. Write a questionnaire.
5. List additional assessments you would use with this client.
6. Write an occupational performance analysis for Theresa.
7. Write an intervention plan for Theresa.
8. Readjust the intervention plan for Theresa if you were working with her in the following settings: a day treatment program, once-a-week family therapy, a 28-day drug/alcohol rehabilitation facility, a holistic healing center, and an outpatient clinic for bipolar mothers. Write an intervention plan for each setting.
9. Write two progress notes at two different points in her intervention. Compare her progress.
10. Write a discharge note.
11. Make referrals to other services.
12. Write a group protocol for a craft group that Theresa could participate in. State how this group would address her specific goals.
13. Identify the types of clinical reasoning you have applied in writing Theresa's assessment, occupational performance analysis, intervention plan, discharge plan, referrals, and group protocol.
14. What frame of reference or theory have you applied in creating Theresa's assessment, occupational performance analysis, intervention plan, discharge plan, referrals, and group protocol? Provide support for why this theory is appropriate for Theresa's needs. What other frame of reference might be appropriate and why?

5

Am I Mark When I Am Manic?

How do psychosocial issues affect personality? Most clients will say that they are totally different people when they are symptomatic or that the onset of their psychosocial issues has changed them into different people, people they and their family no longer recognize or understand. Over time, certain clients and families have expressed the following sentiments. "When I am manic I embarrass myself in front of others doing things that I would otherwise never do." "When I am manic I am not myself. People tell me that I did things that I do not remember doing." "I like to be hypomanic because I am more creative, have more energy, and can stay up all night. I adjust my medications so I can achieve this state of being all the time but it does not always work." "I am afraid of my son. I never know when he is going to go off. Last time he got sick, he physically hurt me." A more detailed description of how bipolar illness has affected the personalities of four clients is expressed in the following narratives.

SUNSHINE AND RAIN

THOMAS DANIEL

> Because of my illness I am not as outgoing as I used to be, I do not have as many friends. In fact, now, I do not have any friends. Because of my mood changes no one really wants to be around me much, because some days I am happy and want to play, and some days I am sad and feel the whole world is against me. Even my own wife does not want to be around me because I am so depressed. I always spoil the mood and say something to make everything all wrong. Because of my illness, a day that should have been the happiest day of my life turned out to be one of the worst days ever. The day I got married should have been really happy because I loved my wife a lot. But for some strange reason, after the wedding, I got really depressed and hid in the basement and played with my model cars. I felt that for some reason my family was not happy with the decision I made. I came to find out they were happy with the decision I made. It was just my illness

playing tricks on my mind once again. My illness turned a beautiful sunny day into a rainstorm of sadness.

HAPHAZARD

ANONYMOUS

I find that I am more emotional than most people. Maybe that is a personality change resulting from mental illness. I found that being more emotional helped me academically because whatever I read—a short story, a historical document, or a biography of a mathematician—I became totally and emotionally engrossed in it. Being emotional though had its drawbacks when I was in school. I was overly affected by what other people thought of me and I avoided taking risks, such as meeting new people, raising my hand in class, or trying out a new writing style. So, I grew up loving books, information, and solace. I also grew up terrified of people outside of my immediate circle of friends, usually Chinese American Christians from my church.

That was just me growing up, when I did not even know that I had a mental illness. When I look back, I do not see anything particularly strange. Maybe I was just more analytical, emotional, and withdrawn. Church, though, did not allow me to withdraw much. Going to church, and being deeply involved in it, forced me to normalize my behavior.

I did not realize that I had manic-depressive illness until the end of my high school career. When I went to Taiwan that summer, I had my first full-blown episode. It was similar to the one that landed me in the hospital from which I write today. I became paranoid (I am also psychotic to a certain degree). I thought the police, FBI, CIA, or authorities of some sort were following me, through bugs or undercover agents. I thought God and other people were talking to me. In one episode, God told me I was a prophet; and in the same episode, I thought God told me I was Jesus Christ. In another episode, I thought people were talking to me (extrasensory perception) and I could talk to others. In one episode, I cried uncontrollably because I thought I heard people talking about me and mocking me. In another episode, I cried uncontrollably for the suffering in the world.

All these episodes share some things in common: They happened in places that were foreign to me (Taiwan, freshman year in college, New York City) and they happened after a period of stress or little sleep. All together, I had about three severe episodes and three mild episodes. Those six episodes consisted of personality changes like overanalysis, paranoia, overemotionalism, and intense and false religiosity.

As I write, I realize that I have been given a haphazard explanation of how my personality changes because of manic-depression. I hope it helps to describe the thoughts that flashed through my mind, in an equally haphazard way.

THEY CALL ME CRAZY

STEPHEN DOMINA

I am comfortable with bipolar manic-depressive disorder but not everyone else is. It feels bad when people turn me down because of my illness. Some do not want to be my friend anymore, while others call me names and call me crazy. My family treats me better when I am on medication. When I am manic, things from the past come back to haunt me. I believe people set me up by telling me the world is going to end. I think the whole world is running together. I hear people talking about me. I have trouble making decisions and focusing.

DISORGANIZED AND DELUSIONAL

ELODIE MONTIVERO

In the following narrative, intern Elodie's clinical reasoning has already been identified and labeled in parentheses, as have the questions and activities at the end of her narrative. Write how each type of clinical reasoning identifies the text preceding it.

It was a regular morning on the unit and I was going about my normal routine of seeing my clients. I like to meet with my clients in the morning for intervention before I attend rounds. A team rounds is a meeting that consists of psychiatrists; occupational, recreational, art, and dance therapists; nurses; social workers; psychologists; aids; and interns. These meetings address each client's current psychosocial and health concerns, reactions to medication, psychiatric symptoms, functional capacities, unit management issues, and follow-up intervention plans (* diagnostic and content or knowledge). My morning interventions (* interactive) allow me to obtain more information about the clients I treat so that I may speak about them in subsequent team meetings. As I was walking the hallway, I passed a young man and greeted him, "Good morning." This client was tall and masculine, had broad shoulders and appeared to be Hispanic. Instead of replying back, he gave me a look that made me feel like he wished I was dead. His walk was heavy and sluggish as his hands formed tight clenched fists that hung at his sides. From his body language and expression I could tell that he did not want to be bothered (* inductive). I had not seen him before nor did I hear his case presented in team meeting. I thought to myself, *I hope he is not one of my clients*. I felt extremely uncomfortable when he gave me that look.

Unfortunately, when I attended rounds I found out that I was assigned to work with him. In rounds, the psychiatrist presented this client as having a serious anger management problem; he has a history of being abusive and destructive. The psychiatrist also mentioned that his diagnosis is bipolar affective disorder, currently in a manic episode. He has been placed in the special care section from the minute he was admitted to the unit due to his hostility. Special care is a section in the hospital for individuals who lash out and have poor impulse control. He would remain in this section throughout his entire hospitalization stay. After rounds, I reviewed his chart to get more information before I oriented him to the unit. I tend to review the chart first when clients are agitated and could be dangerous. I wanted to know what to expect so I would not be shocked (* content or knowledge).

Hector Riviera was his name, and due to the incident from the morning, I already knew that he was going to be difficult to handle (* inductive). I proceeded to knock on the door and enter the room with caution. Hector was lying on his back on top of the bed, staring blankly at the ceiling. I greeted him, giving my name and telling him I was an intern. Hector did not acknowledge my presence and proceeded to stare at nothing. I then asked him, "Is this a bad time, should I return at a better time for you?" Hector replied, "I do not want to be bothered so get out now." From his tone of voice and discussion in rounds, I knew not to push him too far. I decided to leave him for the time being (* inductive and predicative) and possibly return when he was less irritable (* interactive). That afternoon, I decided to be persistent and try another time. This was a successful effort, as he was more approachable. Because he was more approachable, I felt more comfortable and confident with myself and explained to him again who I was and how I could help him. He agreed to be oriented during this process. Hector maintained good eye contact throughout the orientation but did not seem to understand. He would just gaze at me, shaking his head, acting as if this really did not matter to him. When I finished the orientation I knew to leave him alone, because I sensed that he did not want to answer any questions (* inductive and conditional or predicative). I decided to wait a couple of days before evaluating him (* interactive). I left the room and went back to his chart to gather as much information as I could (* content or knowledge).

Hector was a 23-year-old living with his parents. He has been diagnosed with manic-depressive episodes since the age of 17. This was not Hector's first hospitalization; in fact, it is his fourteenth. The police brought him to the unit because he was found sleeping on the subways, appearing disorganized and delusional. On arriving, Hector displayed classic signs of mania: racing thoughts, agitation, obsessive exercise, decreased need for sleep, poor concentration, paranoia, and grandiosity. He had been involved in several arguments with neighbors as well as strangers. Hector was not only noncompliant with his mood stabilizing medication, he was also neglecting his insulin for diabetes.

A few days later after he had a chance to settle into the unit, I felt it was time to evaluate him (* inductive) so I could begin an intervention plan that would meet his needs and help him return to society. Hector was extremely guarded, due to his paranoia. I wanted to ask the correct questions (* procedural), so I had to be prepared. He would give me two- or three-word answers, appearing bothered and agitated until I brought up a topic that interested him—basketball (*conditional or predicative). Since he was exercising obsessively, Hector had great interest in many sports, but a particular one was basketball. I saw him brighten up when I mentioned this sport, which made me feel comfortable because I, too, am an avid athlete. Now we had something in common. Hector stated that "Basketball is a game that controls the mind and body and since nobody tells me differently, I have the power of the game." Hector felt that playing this game allowed him to have freedom and control of himself and other people. He has a serious anger management problem; when someone tells him to do something, Hector tends to get argumentative. This was a main reason as to why he did not take his medications on a daily basis. Hector stated, "I know that I am manic, but when someone tells me that I must take my medications, I will do the opposite." He had slight insight into his illness but could not pinpoint what triggers his episodes. Hector had great interest in weight lifting as well. He felt that he needed to become stronger so that nobody would hurt him (* interpretive and interactive).

Hector had been timid and isolative throughout his childhood years and rarely socialized with children from school. He was, however, able to befriend some children from his neighborhood. Hector's first episode occurred when he was attending high school, at age 17, when he flashed his private genital area at a girl. The girl got extremely upset and told her brother, who eventually wanted to fight him. Hector could not remember if he had really exposed himself and tried to back away from the situation. "I am not the type of person to fight; in fact, I try to talk my way out of those situations, but if I must defend myself, I will." Hector found this to be an extremely humiliating situation, especially because he also ran away from the fight. This incident led him to compensate by lifting weights and obsessively exercising two or three times a day. He would go to the library to find books about fitness and health, gathering as much information as possible. Hector dropped out of school after this incident occurred.

Unfortunately, this was not Hector's first time dropping out of school; it was his second. Hector had dropped out two years earlier because he felt that school was too difficult. He lost interest and could not comprehend the classwork. Hector was too embarrassed to ask for help and would lie to his parents about school. He would tell them that school was fine and he was doing well. He would skip school and hang out on the streets alone, riding the subway, going from place to place stating, "I love being outside and going places; it makes me feel free and I love watching the people on the streets." After a phone call from his school that he was not attending classes, his parents found out the truth. Hector was out for five months, but with the support of his parents went back the following year.

At this time, Hector began to display extreme changes in his personality that were noticed by his parents. He was sleeping less and staying out all hours of the night. His parents never knew where he was; and when they would speak to him, he would get irritable and abusive, throwing objects around in the house. At times, he would bring home strangers he had met from the streets, telling his parents that they just moved onto the block. Hector had a rapid loss of his appetite and would speak his mind, saying anything that came to his thoughts. He had been afraid to talk when he was young, because he thought that he would get beaten up, but now that he was stronger he felt could say anything, no matter what anyone told him. Hector's behavior was getting more bizarre. He began giving speeches in his neighborhood, preaching about God and how he knows better than anyone else does. His belief in God occurs dramatically when his manic episodes begin. Hector was never able to manage a real job, although he did walk his neighbors' dogs for money and helped one of his friends with an ice cream truck one summer. Hector's life was not normal. His parents found him emotionally draining and decided to seek help.

Before his first hospitalization, Hector explained that he was lonely, depressed, isolated, and felt bad about himself. He remembers the holidays very clearly because he never wanted to participate in the family reunions and would stay in his room watching television or sleeping. Hector stated that, when he was young, he was selfish and hated everyone. Everything was given to him and he never really worked for anything. When he got to his teenage years, Hector tried drugs but never pursued them. He stated, "God did not use drugs in His lifetime and I do not feel that I need to." Hector got into some mischief and was lucky enough to get out of these situations. When Hector hung out with his friends, they would write graffiti on stores and windows, steal from the Chinese vending stands, throw onions at cars, and break into and steal cars. He recalled, "The worst incident I remember is when I stole this car and crashed it, hurting innocent people." He had felt bad, especially because he ran away from the scene.

At 16, Hector experienced a major shift in his sexuality. He came to the realization that he was not only interested in girls but boys as well. I knew to keep this situation on a professional level and not to pressure him to speak about sexual identity issues if he did not want to (* ethical). Hector was very open and comfortable talking about his sexuality change and displayed great concern in being unsure of his role as a young man. Hector did not have any healthy male role models to look up to, since one of his brothers is in jail, his father suffers from bipolar illness and alcoholism, and his other brother is absent from the household, away in the German army. He was the third son in the family and was expected to maintain the house. Hector's parents never educated him about girls. As he spent more time with boys, he grew more interested in them. Hector stated, "I felt as if I did not know my self-identity. I was not sure if I was gay or not." Hector's anxiety eventually led him to experience dating both male and female partners to help him make up his mind. He admitted that he enjoyed being with both. He could not decide which gender he preferred, because he saw them as individuals (* interpretive, narrative, interactive, and collaborative).

As Hector and I built rapport, he began to trust me. I began to feel very comfortable with him and less afraid of what would happen if he became angry or agitated. I felt confident in myself and knew what needed to be done if the situation got out of hand. At times, when I proposed certain questions to him, he would give me a look with a determined stare and I would change my wording (* inductive and conditional or predicative). When he did not want to talk about certain things he would address me in a direct manner, stating, "These questions are bothering me today. Can we talk later?" He respected me, and I gave him that same respect back (* interactive). On the unit, Hector would participate in as many groups as he could tolerate. I began to work on his concentration skills, so that he could focus on one task at a time instead of jumping from one activity to another (* procedural). I recommended that he be involved with the anger management group because he wanted to improve the way he deals with anger (* procedural and collaborative). His manic symptoms started to subside, and he seemed more reality based and less grandiose.

I also worked with Hector individually. I enjoyed teaching him the skills he needed; it allowed me to realize how I helped him progress. Hector and I talked about his future plans and what he wanted to do upon discharge (* collaborative). Hector's parents are having financial problems and he wants to be able to help them. Hector feels that this might be one way that his parents would accept him back into their lives. He figured, "My parents have done as much as they could for me, it is time to start giving back." Hector and I talked about a possible job that he would be interested in (* collaborative and interactive). At first he talked about wanting to be a bike messenger. He liked the idea of traveling from one place to another. He then was talking about five other jobs he would be interested in. I made it clear to Hector that he has to do one thing at a time and not to take on so many tasks at once. Hector and I came to a realization that he wanted to get his general education diploma (GED) so that he could find a better job (* conditional or predicative). I thought this goal was quite impressive. Hector is very intelligent and when focused on one task accomplishes it. I explained to him how stressful studying for the GED could be. He understood but was still determined. I had brought this conversation to the attention of his social worker, who was an intern. The social work intern, Hector, and I sat together before he was discharged and came up with a couple of places that offer classes. Hector became more motivated as the intern and I worked with him toward this goal. He seemed very positive about this, and I think that he will eventually proceed with this goal. Hector and I accomplished a lot of goals (* collaborative). I was very pleased with the results. He and I talked about the importance of taking his medication and insulin on a daily basis. He now understands that, by taking his medications, he may avoid being hospitalized. Hector made an agreement with me (* conditional or predicative) that he would continue with follow-up interventions because he knows that he needs it.

Hector and I decided on an intervention plan that would help him organize his thought process (* procedural). The results were marked. Hector was hard to work with at first but once I gained his trust, he was easier to work with. I expected to be afraid to work with him. Hector taught me a lot about myself (* knowledge-reasoning integration) and gave me the confidence I needed to work here (* pragmatic). I now have a better understanding and realization that people are unique (* interactive).

Client-Centered Reasoning Questions

1. What precautions would you take with Hector and why (* procedural, conditional or predicative, and inductive)?
2. Hector is diabetic. It was noted in his chart that prior to admission that he had not been compliant with his insulin injections. What are the symptoms of diabetes when insulin is neglected (* content, procedural, categorization)? Compare these symptoms to the symptoms of a bipolar manic episode. How can you tell the difference (* content, procedural, categorization)?
3. Elodie states that Hector likes to control himself and other people, but often cannot control himself. Perform an activity analysis of basketball and weight lifting to identify all the ways each sport could be satisfying Hector's needs. In doing so, be sure to identify his needs. How is each of these sports therapeutic for him? How or when or did they become antitherapeutic for him and how can you tell (* content, procedural, interactive, narrative, conditional or predicative, inductive, categorization, pragmatic, knowledge-reasoning integration, interpretive)?
4. Elodie states that "Hector and I came to a realization that he wanted to get his GED so that he could find a better job." What is the danger in arriving at this realization during the same individual intervention session that Hector speaks about five different jobs he is interested in pursuing (* knowledge-reasoning integration, categorization, inductive, conditional or predicative, interactive, diagnostic, content)? Elodie also states that "Hector became more motivated as the intern and I worked with him toward this goal (obtaining his GED). He seemed very positive about this, and I think that he will eventually proceed with this goal." For someone that still might be hypomanic, does strong motivation necessarily correlate with achievement of goals? (Remember that Hector was motivated to pursue five different jobs.) If so, is it a positive or negative correlation (* content, conditional or predicative, deductive,

categorization, knowledge-reasoning integration)? Do you think that pursuing a GED is a good discharge goal for Hector? Why or why not (* pragmatic, conditional or predicative, knowledge-reasoning integration, interpretive, procedural, diagnostic, interactive, inductive, categorization)?

Client-Centered Reasoning Activities

1. Finish the narrative (* narrative).
2. Write an occupational profile (* interactive and interpretive).
3. Write a questionnaire that would help you gain additional information about Hector in order to treat him (* interpretive, procedural, interactive, and diagnostic).
4. What assessments would you use with Hector and why (* procedural and interactive)?
5. Write an occupational performance analysis for Hector (* interpretive, conditional or procedural, and diagnostic).
6. Write an intervention plan (* procedural, interactive, conditional or predicative, categorization, pragmatic, knowledge-reasoning integration, and interpretive).
7. Choose an appropriate intervention setting for Hector after his discharge. Readjust his intervention plan if you were to work with him in this setting (* narrative, programmatic, conditional or predicative, knowledge-reasoning integration, interpretive, and procedural).
8. Write two progress notes for Hector at two different points in his intervention (* procedural and diagnostic).
9. Write a discharge note (* procedural, diagnostic, interactive, conditional or predicative, categorization, programmatic, knowledge-reasoning integration, and interpretive).
10. Make referrals to other services (* interpretive, knowledge-reasoning integration, programmatic, conditional or predicative, categorization, interactive, diagnostic, and procedural).
11. Identify the types of clinical reasoning you have applied in writing Hector's assessment, occupational performance analysis, intervention plan, discharge plan, and referrals.
12. What frame of reference or theory have you applied in creating Hector's assessment, occupational performance analysis, intervention plan, discharge plan, and referrals? Provide support for why this theory is appropriate for Hector's needs. What other frame of reference might be appropriate and why?

CLIENT-CENTERED REASONING
ACTIVITIES FOR CHAPTER 5

1. Compare and contrast all the ways that Thomas, the anonymous author of "Haphazard," Stephen, and Hector changed once they became symptomatic with bipolar illness (* procedural, diagnostic, categorization, and interpretive). In Hector's

case, for each of Hector's actions, thoughts, wishes, and ideas, how do you know if they are symptoms of mania/hypomania or his personality (* diagnostic, content, interactive, inductive, categorization, pragmatic, knowledge-reasoning integration, interpretive)?

2. Answer the title of this chapter, is Mark still Mark when he is manic? Use quotes from the narratives in this chapter as supporting evidence. Use any other references or life experiences to justify your answer (* inductive, content or knowledge, procedural, diagnostic, narrative, interactive, teaching as reasoning, categorization, knowledge-reasoning integration, and interpretive).

6

I Feel Like I Am
200 Years Old

The first person to speak in my group said, in a hostile, bitter voice, "How can you help me? You have no idea what it is like, what I have to go through and how I feel." I asked, "How do you feel?" She responded, "I feel like I am 200 years old."

IT IS ALL IN THE MIND

Aviva Graber

Write between the lines.

There are two types of illnesses—mental and physical. As an intern, I observed behaviors, talked with clients, and learned (*) that most people with psychosocial issues suffer from both illnesses simultaneously. In talking with them, they describe to me their mental anguish as well as their physical aches and pains. Their lives are infested with demons of the mind and physical debilitation. To these clients, which is more debilitating? They cannot answer. Are these aches and pains real? Is it for us to decide?

Sharon Walker is a 45-year-old African American woman who was brought to the unit by the police because of a violent outburst caused by her refusal to take her medication. The police reported that they were summoned to resolve a physical altercation she was having with a neighbor. Sharon entered the hospital with a previous diagnosis of schizoaffective disorder. She is currently prescribed antipsychotic, antidepressant, and benzodiazepine medications.

Sharon is five feet, seven inches tall, an obese woman with short kinky black hair. Her bruised face bears the scars of her tragic life. The right side of her face droops and her cracked lips reveal a mouth filled with yellow, rotted teeth with her two front teeth missing. Her arms and legs have many scrapes and black and blue marks, evidence of the battery she had been exposed to. Her fingers are distorted and appear twisted and bent. She appears disheveled and unkempt, with a reeking odor emanating from her body.

As I walked into Sharon's room one day after her arrival, her expression was one of despondency. She was dressed in pajamas, sitting up on her bed, muttering to herself. I greeted her with a cheerful "Good morning," to which I received no response or eye contact. I sat down on a chair next to her bed and introduced myself as an intern who would be working with her. I told her that, to help her, I had to learn about her background. Sharon seemed suspicious and reluctant to talk to me. She told me that she was tired, since she had not slept well because of all the noise in the hallways. I told her that if she felt uncomfortable talking to me, I would not force her, and that I would come back later that day (*).

I then went to check Sharon's chart. Her chart revealed that she refused her medication and did not attend meals. She remained in bed in a depressed mood. I decided (*) to wait until the next day to talk with her. The next morning I went to her room but Sharon was not there. I found her roaming the hallways. This time, when I asked if we could speak, she agreed.

Sharon told me (*) that her mother was an unwed teenager when she gave birth to her. She put her in Angel Guardian Home, an orphanage for abandoned infants. At age 1, Sharon was placed in the foster care of an African American family, the Johnsons in Bridgeport, Connecticut. The Johnsons were a middle-class family who provided her with the basic necessities and lots of love. Suddenly, at the age of 6, her maternal grandmother filed for custody. The Johnsons had grown to love Sharon and were extremely upset. After a drawn-out custody battle, the grandparents were awarded custody of Sharon. Sharon then moved in with her maternal grandmother and step-grandfather at Utica Avenue, Brooklyn. Sharon missed the Johnsons and the security of the only family she knew. She lay in bed for nights crying, wishing she could return to the Johnsons. Her grandparents were strict disciplinarians and beat her with a strap when she disobeyed them. Her step-grandfather sexually abused her and won her silence by threatening her. She tried to soothe herself through food consumption, which caused her to become as obese as she presently is.

At this point during our interview, Sharon suddenly bent over screaming and holding her stomach. Sharon yelled, "The pain is so horrific—it is like gnawing, something chewing away inside of me." Sharon explained to me that she has a peptic ulcer. She described the pain as constant and vicious and compared it to a tug of war with people pulling in opposite directions. She said that the pain was so bad that she wanted to rip her stomach out and bang it against the table and walls.

The next day I went to check on Sharon, and she was anxious to continue telling me her life story (*). She told me that, at age 18, her grandmother passed away, at which point her grandfather forced her to pay rent to she could continue to live in the house. She got a job as a store clerk and lived there until she was 22. At age 22, Sharon moved into her own apartment, which she shared with a troubled female roommate who had two children. During this period of her life she began to drink, experiment with drugs, and experience psychotic episodes. She explained, "I began to hear voices that would command me to do evil and harmful things to others. The voices would keep on repeating the same things over and over again. They would not go away. I could not stop them. I would put pillows over my head and play loud music to block and muffle the voices, but they only continued."

Sharon also began experiencing visual hallucinations and delusions. She had vivid memories in the form of realistic flashbacks of the traumas of sexual abuse she had experienced as a child. She convinced herself that her step-grandfather was looking for her and wanted to kill her. Sharon began sleeping with a kitchen knife to defend herself. At this point, it became evident that Sharon needed help for her uncontrollable symptoms and thus began her journey of admissions to various psychiatric hospitals.

At the end of our conversation, Sharon returned to her room, claiming she was fatigued. She did not attend any groups and spent the remainder of the day in her room.

The next morning, I attended the team rounds. Sharon was the first client to be discussed. It was noted that her depression was worsening. A discussion on the various antidepressants ensued, and the attending psychiatrist changed her medication from a monoamine oxidase inhibitor (MAOI) to a selective serotonin reuptake inhibitor (SSRI) (*).

After team rounds, I went into Sharon's room. I found her sitting and staring at the walls. She had a blank look on her face and her eyes were red and swollen, revealing (*) that she had been crying for hours. She told me that she wanted to be left alone and asked me to leave. She said, "I do not want to do anything or see anybody." I asked her if she would attend our stress management group. After much reluctance and display of negativity, Sharon agreed. Sharon walked with me to the activity room where the group was being held. All the members introduced themselves, and we began our discussion. Five minutes later, Sharon ran out of the room.

After group was over, I went to Sharon's room to see what had happened (*). Sharon began telling me of her pain and frustration. "This is the fourth hospital I have been to in four years. No one seems to understand me or what my problems are all about." She told me that people are always angry with her because she has difficulty caring for herself. She admitted that there are periods of time when she did not brush her hair or teeth or shower for weeks. "They tell me I am lazy, and that I want to be a client and sick so that people will care for me." Sharon defended her behavior by describing her struggle to pull herself together, stop drinking, and get her life back on track. "People do not recognize my efforts and tell me to snap out of it. They have never been there, so they do not know what it is really like. They do not understand that, on some days, I feel so heavy I cannot manage to drag myself out of bed. I have been up a whole night with buckets of sweat soaking my body, heart palpitations, and destructive thoughts on how to end my intolerable pain. I feel so sad and lonely. I feel unimportant, useless, hopeless, unloved, and unwanted. If I were gone, no one would miss me or even notice that I had left. I feel like I have no purpose in life. I feel like a child and

I want someone to take care of me and to love me. I feel pain, dark, and total emptiness in a fuzzy fog, nothing penetrates. Nothing is any good nor is anybody, and I am troubled."

Sharon told me that her whole body physically aches when she feels depressed. She said that the pain is absolutely excruciating, totally debilitating, and every part of her body is consumed with pain. She compared her pain to that of a thousand knives being driven into her body at the same time. "My body feels heavy and paralyzed. I feel as if I have a bad case of the flu. My head feels like it will explode. I feel like someone has clamped a brake on my brain and thrown a thick gray blanket over me." She reported constantly having blinding, splitting headaches in the back of her head. She said, "My heart hurts; it feels like it will stop beating. My chest aches; it tightens up and feels constricted. I have difficulty breathing. At times, I feel nauseous and constipated. My back and limbs ache. I experience muscle spasms and heaviness in my limbs. My eyes ache and feel heavy. I feel tired and exhausted, I have no energy or drives of any kind whether sex, appetite, or work. I fluctuate between no appetite, starving, and binge eating. I experience no pleasure in the usual things that I used to enjoy. Everything seems to be difficult."

I explained to her that, although she felt that things could not get worse and that her life was falling apart, the medicine would eventually start to make her feel better. The medicine is not magical and would not make her problems disappear. She would have to play an active role in setting goals and work hard to improve her life. I encouraged her to begin participating in the therapeutic groups that would help her begin to put her life back together.

By the end of the week, Sharon was showing definite signs of improvement. Her medicine was starting to take effect. Sharon's appetite seemed to be returning; she was attending meals and eating. Although she was still withdrawn, she was spending more time out of her room. I told Sharon that, at times when she felt good, she might not realize the value of her medicine and might be tempted to stop taking it. I stressed the importance of her medication in helping to decrease her symptoms and warned her that she should not cease taking her medication without the doctor's approval.

On Friday, I saw Sharon in the dining room at breakfast, talking to the others at the table. I reminded her about the skills group that would take place at four o'clock. I suggested that she might enjoy socializing at the group and could make something useful. At this point, Sharon began to sob and said that she could not make anything, since her hands constantly shake and tremble and that she had a bad case of rheumatoid arthritis. She lifted her hand and said, "Look at my ugly crooked fingers. They look like witch's fingers." She then proceeded to tell me how she used to play the piano, knit, and string beads for jewelry. "I can no longer do these things. The arthritis has robbed me of all the pleasures in my life. The pain in my fingers is crippling and burns me like fire." She said that the arthritis was God's method of punishing her for the time in her life when she was on drugs and alcohol and was forced to steal to sustain her addiction. I calmed her down, and we worked together on a schedule of groups that she would like to attend during the following week (*).

On Monday afternoon, I was surprised to see Sharon waiting by the door for the mind/body movement group. She appeared neat, dressed in her street clothing with her hair brushed. She seemed to have energy and was even conversing with other clients. After doing the relaxation exercises, all the clients were asked their personal view on the effects of the relaxation techniques. When the question was posed to Sharon she answered, "It lifts my mood, clears my mind and calms me. It gives me something to focus on and distracts me so that I can take a break from thinking of my problems and all my aches and pains."

At the next day's team meeting, Sharon's evident progress was discussed. I proposed that Sharon was ready for supervised, therapeutic walks in the community with other clients, and that we could shoot for discharge in one week. The attending psychiatrist agreed and approved the proposal.

Sharon continued to make further progress the entire week. The following Monday morning, Sharon approached me to say, "Good-bye." She thanked me and hugged me. She told me that she was being discharged and would be attending an outpatient clinic in the neighborhood for follow-up intervention. I asked Sharon how she was feeling today. She replied, "I feel fine. It is all in the mind."

I had mixed emotions about Sharon's departure. Although she had made remarkable progress, Sharon's past history of relapse invoked within me feelings of hesitancy about her readiness for discharge (*). I was proud of her present accomplishments and hoped that she would continue on her long and tenuous road to recovery.

When reflecting on my experience with Sharon, I have come to the realization that all sicknesses have physical components as well as emotional components (*). One's mind and body are actually integrated parts of a whole being. It is impossible for one part of us to change without effecting change in another part. I have come to believe in the words of Dr. Graham (*) of the University of Wisconsin, "Psychological and physical refer to different ways of talking about the same event and not different events. The difference between mental and physical is not in the event observed but rather in the language in which it is discussed."

Analysis

The order in which people present information is important. The mind makes connections between events as in free association. These connections are often unconscious to the person making them and to people listening; however, clinicians can be trained to listen for such connections to understand their clients better. Here, Sharon talks about her step-grandfather's sexual abuse and her resultant increase in food consumption as a soothing mechanism for the abuse. Immediately after sharing this experience with her intern, Aviva, Sharon experiences "horrific" pain from her peptic ulcer. For Sharon, her peptic ulcer and resultant periodic pain may be directly related to the trauma of her sexual abuse (*). Sharon describes to Aviva the pain of her peptic ulcer, "She described the pain as constant and vicious and compared it to a tug of war with people pulling in opposite directions." But this also sounds like a possible description of Sharon's sexual abuse: "constant" and "vicious" like a "tug of war with people pulling in opposite directions."

Sharon then expresses anger by saying "she [Sharon] wanted to rip her stomach out and bang it against the table and walls." It may not be her stomach that she would like to "bang against the table and walls," but perhaps she wants to punish her step-grandfather for the physical and emotional pain he caused her. Instead of being able to express her anger directly toward her step-grandfather, she internalized her own anger into her stomach. Instead of talking about wanting to rip her step-grandfather off of her body and bang him against the table and walls, she substitutes her stomach. Her seeming inability to express anger toward her step-grandfather may be the etiology of her ulcer.

Sharon is aware that she used(s) food to soothe the trauma of her step-grandfather's sexual abuse, but she may not be aware of the connection between her sexual abuse and her peptic ulcer. This awareness and recollection of past memories may have been too much for Sharon to handle until now, so these unexpressed feelings and memories stay in her stomach and may be adding to her feelings of depression.

The following descriptions of Sharon's depression may be related to her sexual abuse, because they sound like they could be describing her feelings during an unwanted sexual act or attack: "'My head feels like it will explode. I feel like someone has . . . thrown a thick gray blanket over me. My heart hurts; it feels like it will stop beating. My chest aches; it tightens up and feels constricted. I have difficulty breathing. At times I feel nauseous . . . my back and limbs ache. I experience muscle spasms and heaviness in my limbs. I feel tired and exhausted, I have no energy or drives of any kind. . . ." Sharon also describes her feelings of depression to Aviva as feeling the pain "of a thousand knives being driven into her body at the same time."

Shortly after thus expressing herself, Sharon gets better for a day and then gets worse. A short immediate release of information may have given her some relief and motivation to discuss more, but after discussing more and going even deeper, Sharon becomes more depressed. This is a common occurrence. The medical model's solution as presented here is to give her antidepressant medication. By the end of the week, Sharon is eating again and is ready to attend a week of therapeutic activities, after which she is discharged. When asked how relaxation techniques helped Sharon, one of her replies was, "It . . . *distracts* me so that I can take a break from thinking of my problems and all my aches and pains." When asked how she was feeling on the day of her discharge she replied, "I feel fine. It is all in the mind." Aviva states, "I had mixed emotions about Sharon's departure. Although she had made remarkable progress, Sharon's past history of relapse invoked within me feelings of hesitancy about her readiness for discharge. I was proud of her present accomplishments and hoped that she would continue on her long and tenuous road to recovery." Were Sharon's underlying problems adequately addressed during this hospitalization? Is an inpatient psychiatric hospital the appropriate setting to address such issues? How would you address such issues so as not to push Sharon into a deeper depression? If these underlying issues are never addressed, what may happen?

Client-Centered Reasoning Questions

1. Answer the four questions at the end of the analysis.
2. What precautions would you take with Sharon and why?
3. What parts in the narrative give you clues that Sharon may be ready to begin to make a connection between her sexual abuse and her depression and somatizations?
4. Is it possible that Sharon's substance abuse may also be related to her past abandonment by her mother and sexual abuse? If so, how could you help her?

Client-Centered Reasoning Activities

1. Finish the narrative as if Sharon's underlying issues were never addressed. Then, finish the narrative as if Sharon's underlying issues will be addressed.
2. Write an occupational profile.
3. Write a questionnaire for Sharon that will help you obtain more information about her life that would help you treat her.
4. What additional assessments would you use with Sharon?
5. Write an occupational performance analysis.
6. Write an intervention plan.
7. Readjust the intervention plan for Sharon for your treatment of her in an outpatient clinic in the neighborhood where she is going after discharge.
8. Write two progress notes at different intervals of Sharon's intervention.
9. Make referrals to other services.

10. Identify the types of clinical reasoning you have applied in writing Sharon's assessment, occupational performance analysis, intervention plan, discharge plan, and referrals.

11. What frame of reference or theory have you applied in creating Sharon's assessment, occupational performance analysis, intervention plan, discharge plan, and referrals? Provide support for why this theory is appropriate for Sharon's needs. What other frame of reference might be appropriate and why?

12. Identify types of clinical reasoning used by Aviva. The asterisks mark some but not all examples of when Aviva used clinical reasoning. Find the rest (also look in the author's analysis, the questions, and the activities) and identify them.

13. Go back to preceding chapters and identify the types of clinical reasoning used by each of the following persons. Asterisks are not provided.

- "Gabrielle Miller," Chapter 2.
- Nancy Moritz-Farajun, Chapter 2.
- Keri Reilly, Chapter 3.
- Lilliana Mosquera, Chapter 3.

MY BRAIN HURTS

FRANCIA BRITO

During a team meeting, it was announced that there was a new client, a woman by the name of Ms. Day. Ms. Day was going to be part of my caseload; therefore, after the team meeting, I went to her room to introduce myself and orient her to the unit. As I knocked on her door, she did not allow me to speak. The first words that came out of her mouth were, "I do not feel like speaking!" This occurred for three days before she would speak to me. As I came to find out through speaking to others and reviewing her chart, she did not feel well enough to speak to any of the staff members. She refused all medications and treatment. On approach, if Ms. Day stated anything at all, she would say, "I do not feel well, do not want to say or do nothing."

She was very psychotic and constantly responding to internal stimuli. This did not stop me from attempting to make contact with her for the first couple of days. I constantly passed by her room to tell her "Good morning" and to announce any groups that we were having at the moment. I would sometimes ask her if there were anything at all she would like to talk about and let her know that I was available. I did not really bother her about medications, because other members of the team were focusing on that. I just needed to develop a trusting relationship with her, even if she did not respond. I did this so she would understand that there are people who do care about what she is going through and to develop rapport.

Ms. Day finally decided to take her medications a couple days after a team meeting we had with her stressing their importance. This was the starting point for Ms. Day's journey to wellness, and how I began to get to know her better. Ms. Day's life is as follows. Ms. Day is a single, unemployed, African American woman, with a long psychiatric and polysubstance abuse history. She had her first experience of psychosocial issues in her twenties. She began smoking marijuana in her teens and crack cocaine in her twenties, several years after the onset of her psychosocial issues. Ms. Day has spent a lot of her time in the jail system, having been arrested two or three times for possession and sale of narcotics. She has been raped. Ms. Day has two children and a granddaughter, whom she wishes to care for but cannot. It is ironic how just a few short sentences can say so much about a person's life and the great obstacles that they have needed to face.

When I first met Ms. Day, I remember her appearing very disheveled, untidy, and malodorous. Her hair was not done, and she refused to wear shoes. She was paranoid about showering and grooming, but she also stated that she did not feel well enough to do them. Once she began to take the medications, she began to speak more and, day by day, she began grooming. As she once stated, "I just need to take it one day at a time." As time went by, she began attending groups and opening up more and more to me. What is ironic is that she reported feeling so sad, but she was always laughing and smiling at something. She appeared to be responding to internal stimuli, but I later came to find out that she was just imagining how she wishes her life to be. She says that she was laughing at happy things. She did not know whether what she imagined was her life, but she still laughed. Behind that laugher, there is a lot of pain.

We began speaking about her life and the course it took, her desires and goals, and what she wishes out of life. The first thing she started to speak about was the voices. She stated that the voices make her feel bad and "bug out hard." Ms. Day stated, "I am in nightmares most of the day. Sometimes, I feel like not waking up and knowing what is going on in my life." Voices remind her of the pain of mental illness. "Without taking medications, my brain and head hurt, and I feel like I am going to explode. Everything hurts—my legs, arms, hands, head, and my heart. I would like to read and write but cannot. It is too hard to hold a pencil, because it causes a lot of pain in my hands."

Taking drugs as a way of making friends is an every day issue for Ms. Day. She was insightful, in that she knew that those are the friends that she really should not have, but said that she did it anyway. It hurts her to take drugs, but Ms. Day gets so depressed that she just needs them as a way to escape from reality. Drugs have only made her reality worse. "It hurts me to take drugs, because drugs have made so much hurt in my life. I have lost money, my apartment, my boyfriend, and my family. My family does not trust me, and friends do not look upon me for anything.

I do not have anyone beside me. Drugs have destroyed my whole entire life. I lost my life, as I see myself taking drugs and abused my body," Ms. Day stated.

According to Ms. Day, whatever chances at life she had were destroyed by her drug use and exacerbated by her psychosocial issues. Ms. Day would always say how she wished to be young again. To do all of the things she has never done before. How she wishes she could read and write, dance, and draw. She once stated that she never had a chance at life. "I never had a life to begin with. I hold it in God's hands, if this is what he wants. This is not a punishment for me, this is only a bother."

Client-Centered Reasoning Activities

1. Finish the narrative.
2. Compare and contrast Ms. Day with Sharon from the previous narrative in this chapter.
3. Identify the type of clinical reasoning used by Francia.
4. Write an occupational profile.
5. Write a questionnaire that you could use to gain more information about Ms. Day in order to provide intervention.
6. What additional assessments would you perform with her and why?
7. Write an occupational performance analysis for Ms. Day.
8. Write an intervention plan.
9. Readjust the intervention plan. Pick an appropriate setting of your choice.
10. Write a progress note.
11. Write a discharge note.
12. Make referrals to other services.
13. Identify the types of clinical reasoning you applied in writing Ms. Day's assessment, occupational performance analysis, intervention plan, discharge plan, and referrals.
14. What frame of reference or theory have you applied in creating Ms. Day's assessment, occupational performance analysis, intervention plan, discharge plan, and referrals? Provide support for why this theory is appropriate for Ms. Day's needs. What other frame of reference might be appropriate and why?

REFERENCE

Graham DT. Health, disease and the mind-body problem: Linguistic parallelism. *Psychosomatic Medicine* 1976;29:52.

Rock Bottom: The Lowest Point in My Life

7

Hitting "rock bottom" or the lowest point in someone's life means different things to different people. For most, it refers to a series of losses. For the next five people, it means the loss of a normal thought process. The following narratives are samples of what may go on in someone's mind during a psychotic episode. Answer the questions to see how you would intervene with these people. The final narrative of this chapter addresses the strength of a psychotic episode in causing someone who has worked as an assistant manager for 15 years to move out of her apartment of eight years onto the streets of New York City with only pens, tissues, and a pocketbook and how she begins to rebuild her life with the help of therapeutic intervention.

QUICK

WESLEY MORROW

> Well, well of falling, a deep pit in my stomach, falling out of my ass, staying at the bottom is safe and cool for a second, then you want to get up. Getting up is faster than coming down; you must be faster than a bullet. Air time when you hit the top of the trees and sunlight is bright but immediately you have to pop somebody to stay up or you will go down eternally, which would not be so bad if not for the faces you see going down that you are going to see again on your way up again then down. If you get off the up and down fall in the well, up on the street and trees you have to go home.

Client-Centered Reasoning Question

What do you think Wesley means by the word *pop*?

Client-Centered Reasoning Activities

1. Interpret this writing in as much detail as you can. What do you think Wesley is talking about? Read your interpretation to the class and listen to your classmates' interpretations. How many different interpretations did the class produce? Were any similar? If so, what elements were similar? What did you learn from this exercise?

2. In "Quick," Wesley describes the up and down fall in a well that starts inside his own body then is externalized to the outside with no differentiation between himself and his environment. Clinicians are trained to treat their clients in context with their environment, but how do you help someone whose definition and boundaries of self are blurred and undefined, as in Wesley's case?

3. How may the lack of "well"-defined boundaries affect occupational performance?

4. What would your first goal be with Wesley and why?

5. List three intervention methods you would implement to help him achieve the goal you just identified.

HOMELESSNESS

LURLENE WILLIAMS

Medicine has been the topic for years; especially after having teeth pulled. For one thing, it is hard to means reach after you have been cited as being or becoming a homeless person. I did not realize during times that people steal from someone as having or had become a homeless person, #1 result. It is absolutely cold in this month of September, and no one really notices you, but today I became fortunate because I have received a gift from God that will never ever let me down in other times of tumult. What is so sad about what I have written is it cannot be taken up or erased.

Client-Centered Reasoning Question

What are Lurlene's two strengths, as mentioned in her narrative? How would you use these to begin your interventions with her?

LIFE

ANONYMOUS

Today is similar to yesterday. The old me and the new me. Life has improved. Starting over is a yes/no: no/yes depending how it is phrased. No cigarettes. Yes life! Yes life! No smoking! No nicotine! Yes breathing. Yes breath! No cigarettes. Life movement is growing. My life has developed in a better way. Every breath is essential life!

GOOD DAYS BAD DAYS

JULIE TAYLOR (written material)

> Live is a bad day day or good in sad because my live momie a parry oceace folese day go by they I doneg they a bomy lovenag's a good day.

This is what Julie Taylor said when she read the preceding:

> Life is a bad day or a good day, but when it is a bad day, it is a sad day 'cause my life is dealing with schizophrenia. When it is a bad day it drags on and I feel so all alone, like no one else has a problem like me and there is no one to help me. I am lonely. When it is a good day, I am not so lonely and I have found peace.

Client-Centered Reasoning Question

What are some of the reasons for the discrepancy in Julie's written material and her spoken words? What did you learn from this and how would you incorporate what you learned into your intervention of clients in general?

MY ASSESSMENT

MARC WOLSKY

> My assessment is as follows. When I was younger I could not fully negotiate all the things, ideas, and beliefs that I had, but three years ago that all changed for me. My academic education had finally paid off and left me on a plateau. Life for me is simple when all is complex and the tides turn to peace. Though some of these metaphors seem to be just delusions, I know what they mean and maybe you might, too, to a certain extent.
>
> How many years must a white dove sail? A lot. I know that there is not eternity ahead for all living things to set their reward on.

Client-Centered Reasoning Question

Often clients in a psychotic state will fully understand the meaning of what they write, even if no one else can, as emphasized by Marc when he says, "I know what they [his metaphors] mean and maybe you might, too, to a certain extent." Some of these people may also have difficulty expressing their thoughts verbally. How would you communicate with them and foster their self-expression?

STARTING OVER

REBECCA PHILIP

> I knocked on the door of 43A; a soft voice welcomed me to enter. There she was, Janis Hayes, lying on her bed with the sheets

wrapped all around her from neck to feet. Janis picked her head up off her pillow to see who was waking her from her slumber this time. I started off with an apology for waking her and then with an introduction, "Hello, my name is Rebecca; I am your intern." Janis lifted herself into a sitting position with the sheets still wrapped tightly around her, "My name is Janis, Janis Hayes," and then she stared at me blankly as she brushed back her hair.

It was obvious that Janis is a tall slender woman, even though she was sitting down. She is six feet, one inch in length with broad shoulders, and she has a streak of white hair running through the middle of her short black hair. I told her I would be back later to talk with her when she was out of her bed. She said that would be good because she wants to go back to bed. Janis resumed her position on her bed, but this time the sheets were pulled over her head as if to say, *leave me alone.*

At this point I had not read Janis's chart. All I knew about Janis was what I had heard in team meeting. Janis quit her job of 15 years as assistant manager of an insurance firm and was found one month later in front of Fordham University. What had happened in Janis's life that could have caused her to leave her job and home? Before Janis was found on the streets, Janis was living in Central Park. When I read her chart, a great deal of information that I was looking for could not be found. I wanted to know more than her diagnosis and her medications. Janis was able to take care of herself, hold a job for 15 years, and live on her own.

The Janis that I had just met was a different person. She did not know why she was here, her hair was uncombed, and it looked as though she had not showered for days, which was probably true since she was living in the streets. All she could remember was that she was spending her nights and days on a bench in the park.

The next time I saw Janis, she was in the day room. The television was on and the program appeared to be a Spanish talk show. Janis was seated on the far right of the round table in the day room. Her head was down and her hands were folded on her lap. I approached her quietly. As I reached her, I called out her name. Janis slowly turned her head to look at me. I asked her if this would be a good time to speak with her. She consented and got up from her chair, proceeding to go to her room as I followed. As we walked, she kept her arms crossed, close to her chest, and would look nowhere but forward.

We entered her room; she pulled out a chair for me to sit as she sat down on her bed. She stared at me with the same blank look she gave me earlier. "How are you feeling today Janis?" I asked. "I am all right," she replied, stroking her hair methodically. "Do you know why you are here?" I waited for a response. Janis immediately stopped stroking her head. She took a deep breath and gave me a brief history of what had happened to her.

Janis lived alone in an apartment in the city. She had been living there for eight years, working full time as assistant manager for a firm. She would go to work, come back home, make dinner, and watch television. After taking a shower, she went to bed and started the same routine all over again. She was fine with her routine because she was too tired after work to do anything else.

But after eight years of living in this apartment, Janis could not live there anymore. She was having paranoid thoughts of her landlord trying to rape her. Janis felt that she had to do something to protect herself. She quit her job and left her apartment taking with her two pens, two boxes of tissues, and her pocketbook. She sat on a bench in the park. She cannot remember how she got there, but she was safe from her landlord. At the time, it seemed like the right decision to make. She did not realize then how irrational her decision really was.

One month later, the police brought her to the hospital. She had thought that she was being brought to the hospital because of her swollen feet. Janis was very upset and angry when she realized she was brought to the hospital for psychiatric reasons. Janis described herself that day as being out of control; she was yelling at the nurses, refusing to cooperate. Janis could not help it; she was angry not just at the nurse but at herself as well. She had a good job and her own apartment. She was more fortunate than most people. She gave it all up—for what? It has been weeks since she showered, slept on a bed, or even brushed her teeth. I comforted Janis as much as I could. Janis was so full of emotions and racing thoughts that she ended the conversation and asked me to leave.

The following days, Janis went through a state of social withdrawal. She spent her days and nights in her room. She occasionally would be found in the day room, sitting by herself, staring at her hands folded on her lap. I would try to engage her in a conversation, but she would stare at me blankly or walk away. My greeting would be ignored as I passed her in the hallway; however, I did not let this discourage me or take it personally.

Janis closed herself to everybody. She would be encouraged to attend groups, but each time she would refuse. "I do not want to be around too many people," Janis would say. Her reason was that she did not know whom to trust and did not want to be responsible for anything. Most of the groups required patients' participation in discussion and volunteering for tasks, both of which Janis wanted no part of.

Gradually Janis's behavior began to change. Janis was following her medication regimen, and she appeared slightly more related. She still kept to herself, but if you passed by her, she would greet you with a smile. Soon she was conversing with me again, this time about the types of groups we had on the unit. Even though she inquired about the groups, she would still refuse to attend any. She wanted to stay away from the groups; it was as if she knew that once she attended groups she would have to face the facts of why she was here, and that was something Janis felt she was not yet ready for.

Janis was looking better, but was she really better? A battle was going on inside her. Would she choose to separate herself from reality or would she find the courage to fight? I would soon find the answer to my question. I had just finished a group. And as the clients dispersed, Janis was waiting by the door. "Janis, you just missed group," I announced. "What kind of group was it?" she asked suspiciously. I went on to explain the purpose and content of the group. Janis brushed back her hair and said, "Well, maybe next time." "There is another group later in the afternoon, and you can still come to that, it is exercise group, and you exercise your body and mind," I said. "Oh no, I do not want to do anything that involves moving my body." She pointed to her feet. "I do not want to make them worse," she pleaded. "That is fine, Janis, but there are a lot of other groups you can attend that can help you. A calendar outside your room lists the day and times of each group. Take a look at them and let me know which groups you would be interested in," I stated.

I went on to say that these groups were more than just ways to pass time, they touched on areas that she might want to know more about. Janis was especially pleased when I mentioned one group, in which she could make things like wood projects, leather purses, and artwork. After my speech was over, Janis waved her hand and signaled to me that she was leaving. "I will think about what you have said, and I will let you know," she said. She walked away from me smiling and then disappeared to her room.

Janis's smile was still vivid in my mind. It was a sign that Janis wanted to get better and that she would fight. Janis is a rosebud refusing to bloom, she is afraid that she would not be able to make it on her own again. But what fate awaited her if she did blossom? Would she have control over her life? There was only one way to find out. Janis was determined to not let her illness destroy everything she worked for, even it meant starting over.

I could see this determination in her eyes the next day as she stopped me by the nursing station. "Rebecca, I know what I would like to do!" She said with a bright smile and glaring eyes. I detoured from my destination and walked with Janis to her room. She told me that, last evening, she went to a group in which she made a leather purse. She enjoyed it so much, and she was so happy that she could make it. It made her feel good. "I do not have to sit alone and do nothing; there are plenty of things that I could do," Janis said proudly. We stopped in front of the calendar and she pointed to the groups that she would be interested in. Janis assured me that she would come to these groups, and I had no doubt in my mind that she would.

Janis's attendance in groups became a topic of discussion during team meeting. The doctor laughed, "Janis came up to me today, and she told me that she loves going to groups and that she has been dreaming about one group in particular which has to do with crafts." "Janis is always the first at the door to get into groups," the nurse added. "How is she in groups, anyway?" the social worker joined in. All eyes were turned to me, and so I figured that this would be a good time to speak. "Janis," I said her name proudly, "is doing well. She enjoys skills group the most because she gets to make things, and she likes to keep herself busy. However, in discussion groups, Janis is very quiet and only speaks if she is called on." The staff responded with sounds of disappointment. True, Janis was not as active as we had hoped she would be, but she was improving. There was no instant remedy or cure-all group for Janis. Janis understood this. She knew what she had to do and that was to take small steps to reach her goal. And her goal was to get better and return to living on her own.

Soon there was talk of discharge for Janis in team meetings. I would ask myself, *Is Janis ready to be discharged?* Her performance in groups was still the same. She rarely spoke and would not volunteer to take on any responsibilities on the unit, such as watering the plants or taking care of the books in the day room. However, Janis had improved considerably from her initial admittance to the hospital. She was taking care of herself, taking her medication, and interacting with the other clients and staff. She sat with other clients in the day room rather than alone and would often be found working on a project, whether it was leatherwork or a puzzle.

Janis looked good on the outside, neatly dressed, well groomed, and well postured. She was often described by the social worker as an elegant woman. I would have to agree; she was very elegant and charming. I was curious to know what was going on inside of Janis. Her doctor and social worker must have talked to her about a discharge plan. How did she feel about it?

I had the opportunity to sit and talk with Janis on several occasions about her plans after discharge. "I want to have my own apartment again," Janis demanded. "But I have been told by my doctor that I will be transferred to the residence Season House, until I am ready to live on my own." Janis understood that the move to Season House would be good for her. It was a comfort to know she would not be completely on her own after she leaves the hospital.

A worried looked shone on Janis's face when I asked what she would do after Season House. There was something on her mind, something that was making her feel out of control. Janis was worried about where she was going to live and how would she be able to pay the rent after she left Season House. Janis had worked since the age of 16; now 54, Janis was tired of working. She wanted to start over. She wanted to march out of the hospital with her head up high. But she was afraid—What if she could not succeed? What if she had no money and was forced to live on the streets this time?

Starting over was not going to be easy, and Janis knew that life could not go back to the way it was before her hospitalization. Janis was no longer an assistant manager nor did she have a home. Janis would have to start from the bottom. Janis decided that she would not go back to work nor would she be idle and do nothing. Janis had a clear plan of what she wanted to do after discharge but lacked the confidence to do it.

Janis did not let her insecurities stop her. Janis prepared herself for her pending discharge. The only clothing that Janis had when she was brought to the hospital was jeans and a tee shirt. It was winter now, and jeans and a tee shirt would not suffice. Janis told the nurse about her dilemma. The nurse brought it to our attention during team meeting. Arrangements were made, and Janis was able to go down to the hospital thrift shop and pick out a coat, shoes, and some clothes. Janis walked proudly in the hallways wearing her new attire. Janis was aware they were used clothes, but it was better than having nothing and, most importantly, they were hers.

A list of things to do was kept near Janis's bedside. The list contained things that Janis hoped to engage in after discharge. Learning how to knit, volunteering in a nursing home, and attending church were the top three on her list. I asked her how would she go about learning how to knit. She mentioned that she had already thought about it, and she heard that some churches offer classes. She would look into it, as soon as she is discharged. It was clear that Janis had gained insight about her illness. She knew that to stay in control she would have to do more than just follow her medication regimen. She had to balance her life between taking care of herself and doing things she enjoyed.

The day of discharge came for Janis. I found Janis in her room; the sight reminded me of the first time I met her, only this time Janis was wrapped up in her long brown coat, ready for departure. Janis was packing her bag with paper and artwork. On noticing that I had entered the room, Janis took out her hand for me to shake, "I am leaving today Rebecca; it was nice knowing you." "It was nice knowing you too, Janis. How do you feel?" I responded. I waited with caution to hear Janis reply. I was afraid that Janis would give me her worried look and tell me she was unsure. Janis looked straight into my eyes and smiled, "I feel confident that I will be able to put my life back together as much as possible, and I know I do not have to do it alone."

Janis drew closer to me and said almost in a whisper, "I know now what got me here in the first place; I stopped taking my medication, so then I started having these thoughts about my landlord that I know were not true." Janis raised her right hand as if she was taking an oath, "I learned my lesson, I will never stop taking my medication, and I will not be afraid to ask for help when I need it." Janis stared at me, not blankly as she often did, but this time with hope in her eyes. It was as if they were telling me, *Yes, I will make it!*

Janis, to me, was and is a remarkable woman who found the courage to overcome her circumstances. Her illness led her to lose all that she had, but her illness could not maim her spirit or preclude her from fighting. Janis helped me to understand that among the bedsheets lay great fears that wrap around us, forcing us to give up. But we have the choice to either let those fears take complete control of our lives or take back what is ours. Janis did exactly that; she took back her life and started over.

Client-Centered Reasoning Questions

1. Rebecca wonders whether Janis would "choose to separate herself from reality" or "find the courage to fight." Is this really a choice in Janis's case? Why or why not?
2. What precautions would you take with Janis and why?

Client-Centered Reasoning Activities

1. Finish the narrative.
2. Write an occupational profile.
3. Write a questionnaire.
4. What additional assessments would you use and why?
5. Write an occupational performance analysis.
6. Write an intervention plan for Janis.
7. Readjust the intervention plan for your work with Janis in a vocational program.
8. Write two progress notes at different periods of time during Janis's intervention.
9. Write a discharge note.
10. Make referrals to other services.
11. Write a group protocol that would address most of Janis's issues.
12. Identify the types of clinical reasoning you applied in writing Janis's assessment, occupational performance analysis, intervention plan, discharge plan, and referrals.
13. What frame of reference or theory have you applied in creating Janis's assessment, occupational performance analysis, intervention plan, discharge plan, and referrals? Provide support for why this theory is appropriate for Janis's needs. What other frame of reference might be appropriate and why?

There Is Nothing Wrong with Me: Denial and Defenses

8

As practitioners we focus the majority of our intervention efforts on functioning. However, people living with or overcoming barriers to occupational performance must deal with the painful reality that they are not functioning and possibly will not function the same way they used to. To deal with this painful realization, many people use defense mechanisms. Defense mechanisms, while they provide temporary relief of uncomfortable feelings, often affect people's ability to realistically understand how their barriers affect their occupational performance. Some people minimize their difficulties or completely deny having an illness. This chapter gives examples of people using different defenses and how interns have had to work through some of these defenses to maximize occupational performance and safety.

This first narrative addresses the defense mechanism of denial.

DENIAL AT ITS BEST

Marsha Eiserman

> Denial is used to avoid awareness of painful reality by abolishing external reality (Kaplan and Sadock, 1998). It is an unconscious defense mechanism used to disown or refuse to accept the truth. Often denial is one of the symptoms of a psychosocial problem. Everyone has used it at least once as protection from a harsh reality. Denial, however, becomes a dangerous tool when used extensively. Its existence may prevent a person from finding solutions to the problem. Not only does it prolong the psychosocial issue, it intensifies the issue.
>
> When a person is informed of a serious medical problem, such as cancer, it is natural to deny its existence as part of a shock reaction. So too with a psychosocial problem. When Betty was first informed of her diagnosis, bipolar II disorder, she denied it. Within months after being stabilized, she felt better and stopped taking medication. If one is not sick, one does not need medication. The

illness struck during the prime years of Betty's life. She was attending college at the time, becoming increasingly more independent of her parents. She thought she had her life mapped out, at least for the next four to six years, until illness hit. As Betty confided, accepting the diagnosis would mean accepting the fact that her life would never be the same again. This is Betty's second psychiatric hospitalization. She acknowledged the benefits of adhering to a medication routine. Presently, Betty views hospitalization as a bigger disruption of her life than helping her through medication and therapeutic intervention. With the aid of medication and therapy, she can function independently in the community.

Other clients, such as Linda and Juanita, who have a diagnosis of bipolar II disorder and major depression with psychotic features, respectively, are able to hide some of the psychosocial issues. Linda presents with a logical and coherent thought process when evaluated verbally. She is able to list her impairments, such as a relative decrease in concentration, and how she compensates for them. It is not until one observes her pacing in a corner of the hallway, responding to internal stimuli, that one can clearly see her symptoms at their worst.

Juanita was brought to the hospital after walking into a police station, asking for help. For four days prior to her hospitalization, she wandered the streets with her 5-year-old son in tow. She explained that she was standing on a subway platform with her son when teenagers, belonging to the well-known Manhattan gangs Crips and Bloods, blew rings of cigarette smoke and jeered at her as they passed by. Additionally, Juanita claims an old [boy]friend related to the gang is spreading gossip about some friend being the father of her son. As a result of the confrontation with the gang and the slander regarding the boy's father, Juanita is scared to return to her apartment, fearful people will find her there and hurt her. Juanita is also afraid people are continuously following her while she roams the streets.

During the initial evaluation she was observed vacillating between inappropriate laughter and tearfulness as she told her story. Although she offers explanations for living in the streets, she is anxious and guarded. Physically, she is weak and fatigued. On completion of her initial evaluation, Juanita became selectively mute, refusing to speak with staff members. When approached by the staff, she is extremely irritable and agitated. She appears to be preoccupied with feelings of hopelessness. Juanita continued with this behavior until she was forced under court order to take medicine intramuscularly.

Juanita was brought to court because she was noncompliant with medication. Juanita could give a strong presentation during her court appearance. Juanita was almost able to present a convincing, logical explanation for all questionable behavior. In her defense, Juanita told the judge that it is quite possible the teenagers do not belong to the Crips and Bloods. However, she went on to say, "Since they are wearing the colors blue and red, the colors belonging to the two gangs, I assume they are gang members. If you, the doctors and judge, tell me they are not gang members, so they are not. Is it not reasonable to assume they belong to these gangs based on their color clothing and the fact the neighborhood is gang infested? Is it not reasonable for a female, standing alone on a subway platform with a group of rowdy boys, to become frightened? Why should my running be considered paranoia and neglect of my son?"

Her story went on. When questioned about her four-day stay on the streets, Juanita explained that she could not return to the apartment, since some of the gang members know her address. When asked if she recognized any of the gang members, she said she did not. (The implication is, if she does not know them, they most probably do not know her. Therefore, the members of the gang would not know her address either.) When asked to explain why she did not go to the police immediately, she responded that it took her four days to organize her thoughts and ask for help. She defended her actions by saying that she fed her child all four days, managing to find shelter every night except the fourth. The churches were closed by the time she started looking for a place to sleep. Therefore, she came to the police to ask them for help in finding a shelter.

When asked about the rumor regarding her son's father, she denied the story. Juanita eventually denied a connection between the gang and allegations of her son's supposed father. Furthermore, she denied she is paranoid, although she confesses she is not comfortable in the hospital since it is a coed ward filled with really sick people. She refused to speak with staff since her arrival on the ward.

She was able to defend herself very well at court; however, because of the loopholes in her story, the judge agreed with the doctors to retain her in the hospital and administer medication against her will. It should also be mentioned that, after the judge ordered Juanita be retained by the hospital to receive medication, Juanita decompensated. She exited the courtroom in tears. Her crying escalated in the hallway, necessitating a speedy removal with the aid of the security guards and attending nurse. This was done to prevent the eruption of extreme emotional responses and chaos among other clients in the courthouse. Once Juanita was brought to the vestibule, she tried to escape the building, stating she would rather end her life than return to the hospital.

Initially following the court case, Juanita commented how she would not know if she were paranoid until she walked the streets of Manhattan. Eventually, she adamantly stated she is not paranoid, a stand she maintained throughout the rest of the hospitalization. However, she refused to return to her apartment. Instead, she plans to speak with her landlord concerning moving to a different apartment in the same building.

Since her denial is so strong and her ability to articulate the reasoning behind the actions is so good, Juanita initially was unable to gain any insight into her psychosocial issues. Not until she was on medication for two or more weeks was she able to recognize her symptoms as they began to lift. Juanita remained socially isolated as well; she did not interact with any clients. Juanita continued to maintain a very superficial relationship with staff members, never discussing any real issues except her desire to get discharged immediately.

George takes denial to a different level. He admits himself to the hospital due to suicidal ideation and delusions, such as that his organs are dying. Initially, George seemed to have some insight and judgment, since he was able to identify anhedonia, insomnia, and loss of energy as symptoms. George accepted suggestions and began attending scheduled group activities during the week and client-run activities over the weekends. After weeks of hospitalization, though, very little improvement was seen. He was no longer suicidal, but he started spending more and more time in bed. He complained of paranoia preventing him from leaving his room, as well as some psychosomatic symptoms, such as that his feet are too weak to hold him up. The closer he came to discharge, the more his symptoms increased. As a result of this behavior, George received more attention from staff. Although George denied it, he was acting out because he did not want to become independent. In fact, he liked the attention and assistance he received from the staff.

Denial with a delusional disorder is very difficult to treat. Al was infuriated. He offered rational answers for everything, except that his symptoms are so overt that nobody is fooled. He spends the day pacing the hallways, verbalizing his anger by screaming profanities at staff who try to set limits with him. Police brought him in because he was found swimming in a pond in Central Park. Whenever confronted with this behavior, he responds, "I started a new business and made twelve dollars profit on my first day. What is wrong with taking a congratulatory swim?" When told his place of residence does not want to take him back because he started a fire in his room, he would say, "The fire was caused by faulty wiring. I had nothing to do with it. They [the people at the residence] are just looking to blame someone."

Al is given a one-day pass twice to clean up his apartment. Photos taken prior to his visit display wall-to-wall piles of papers, magazines, household gadgets, and broken furniture. The residence agrees to take him back on the condition he cleans up the apartment, since it is a fire hazard. Al did not confess it is cluttered, even though he can barely open the front door to the apartment, but he agreed to clean it up, since it will enable him to be discharged.

Al returned in an extremely agitated state after each one-day visit to his apartment. Again, he was in denial. He blamed his agitation on being forced to return to the hospital, when in reality it is the opposite. Despite resisting help from the hospital staff, he really acclimated to the environment and likes the attention he receives. Cleaning up his apartment means he will be discharged soon, requiring independent living, without a 24-hour support system to hear his problems and profanities.

Al is in denial of his illness and all its ramifications, even at discharge. Since he perceives himself as being well and the rest of the world as abnormal, it is only going to be a matter of days before he stops taking his medication. I, therefore, expect him to return to the hospital within a short period of time.

Josephine is very psychotic. She arrived in New York on a Greyhound bus from Philadelphia. An emergency medical squad found her walking along the West Side Highway, carrying her luggage, in total disregard of oncoming traffic. On admission, she explained she was walking to Connecticut. She refuses to speak to the staff, since she was brought in against her will. She was verbally abusive, muttering profanities under her breath as she paced the hallway. She, too, refused to take medication since she felt she is not sick.

As a mental health professional, it is important to recognize and handle denial. Sometimes, clients are able to mask their symptoms and their denial, like Juanita. With experience, one is able to interpret clients' observable behavior much more accurately. For some clients, once the medicine takes effect, the symptoms, including denial, decrease, enabling them to deal with their psychosocial issues. In others, the denial is so strong a component, it causes the therapist to treat details of occupational performance without eradicating the denial. In some instances, a client has built so many walls and barriers, strengthening denial to such a point, the client is unable to discern reality from illusion.

Client-Centered Reasoning Questions

1. Marsha accurately defines denial, but then states that it is often a "symptom" of a psychosocial problem. Is denial a defense against or a symptom of psychosocial problems? Why do you think Marsha considers it a symptom?

2. Marsha writes, "Everyone has used it [denial] at least once as protection from a harsh reality." Describe an instance when you were in denial. What was the difficult experience that caused you to unconsciously use this defense? How did your denial affect your behavior and your ability to accomplish necessary tasks? How did you first become aware of the reality of your situation? What helped you see your situation as it truly was? How long did your denial last? Have you ever seen denial in other people? Describe these situations. Were the people aware of their denial? How did it affect their daily functioning? Did you try to help them? What did you do? How were your attempts successful or unsuccessful in helping them see the reality of their situation? Why?

Client-Centered Reasoning Activities

1. Sometimes people with mental health issues are in touch with their changes in functioning but their families are not. Denial can be just as strong in family members. There are many well-intentioned instances of family members pushing their loved ones to work or to complete college when they may be unable to perform in these roles at the particular time. Some family members mistake symptoms of depression, fatigue from medication, or negative symptoms of schizophrenia for laziness—if they just pushed them harder. . . . Sometimes people cannot understand why the person does not "just snap out of it," but one cannot just snap out of a psychiatric disability. Some days are better, some days are worse, some years are better, some years are worse, some people fully recover from a depression, but they never just snap out of it. Families as well as clients deserve to be educated about mental health. Your job as a practitioner includes families and other support groups. Set up, on paper, a program for family members in denial. How would you encourage attendance?

2. Marsha presents six different people (Betty, Linda, Juanita, George, Al, and Josephine) with different levels of denial in her narrative. For these people, describe what each of them is denying and how their denial affects their behavior and occupational performance. Marsha states, "Not only does it [denial] prolong the psychosocial issue, it intensifies the psychosocial issue." For these people, describe how their denial prolongs their psychosocial issues and how it intensifies their psychosocial issues. If the answers to these questions cannot be found in the narrative, write your own questions to each person to generate the information required. For each person, write a plan for intervention and how you would administer it. Include additional techniques not mentioned in the narrative that you could use to lessen some of their denial.

3. When people are in denial and do not want to hear what you have to offer, it usually helps to relate to them using their own words. For this, you must listen carefully. Here, the words are permanently written. After reading the following example, go back to the text and, for each person, pick out key words or phrases that could be used to form a stronger working relationship. Then, expand on their words by asking related questions that gently probe deeper. For example, Betty confides to Marsha that "accepting the diagnosis would mean accepting the fact that her [Betty's] life would never be the same again." Although it may be obvious that Betty's life will not be the same with bipolar illness, what having bipolar illness means to her may be different than what it means to you. So, find out what having bipolar illness means to Betty. What are the important aspects of her life that she feels will change? How will they change? Is this change realistic, based on what you know about bipolar illness? If not, help her with psycho-education.

If they are realistic, how can you help her manage these changes? Now do the same for the five other people.

NOT A CLUE

LILIANA MOSQUERA

I met a client, G, who is in denial about his situation. He has been here several days. Even after various individuals from the unit have spoken with him about the reason for his hospitalization, he is still unaware of why he is here. He was hospitalized after his girlfriend called the police because he was being physically aggressive toward her and would not leave the house when she asked. She was afraid he would hurt her, and she believed he was talking to himself. He thinks his admission was due to playing a video game. His insight and judgment are so poor at this time, he believes he did nothing out of the ordinary or bizarre to be placed in the special care area of an inpatient psychiatric unit. I will see him later this week to assess any other behavioral problems and work on his goals, especially his impulse control. The team has agreed to continue to leave him in the special care area because of his tendency toward violence.

Client-Centered Reasoning Questions

1. Some people do not actually remember a psychotic episode. Yet, sometimes, seeing someone from outside the hospital that they were with just before admission can help them recall how they were behaving. Here, G's girlfriend could be brought in for a family session when she felt comfortable being with G again and after G regained control over his behavior. Role-play such a family session with you as the leader and classmates for G and G's girlfriend.
2. List other ways that you could help G work through his denial.
3. What precautions would you take with G and why?

UNREACHABLE

KATE HARRINGTON

Maggie, a client who was transferred from the geriatric-psychiatric unit, continues to be unreachable. She has many delusions about the unit, how she got here, and what is waiting for her on the outside. She seems to think I am capable of getting her discharged, that I somehow have connections. I am able to see how she may think this, as I do work on the unit, but many other professionals work on the unit with me. Unfortunately, doctors from the geriatric-psychiatric unit are still seeing her, and on this unit she is being seen only by me and the nursing staff. She does not seem to understand my role. I have tried to explain to her, in more ways than one, that I am an occupational therapy intern and I can help her with various tasks related to improving her functioning. She, unfortunately, wants nothing to do with this, as she feels she is in perfect health and being kept here against her will. I am not sure how I am to intervene at this point. Every time I talk to her, try to help her, she becomes tearful and states that she does not belong here with all these "mentally retarded people." I have discussed this client with the occupational therapy, recreational therapy, and creative arts therapy staff on the geriatric-psychiatric unit, but they have not seen her since two weeks prior to her admission on this unit. They were able to give me some tips that they used to engage the client, but unfortunately these tips have not worked for me. I will continue to try to find my "in," as I am convinced everyone has one.

Client-Centered Reasoning Questions

1. What would you do to find your "in" with Maggie?
2. What precautions would you take with her and why?

Analysis

The idea of using clients' own words to work through their denial with them was illustrated in the client-centered reasoning questions of this chapter's first narrative. Kate's narrative above contains three clues that may help engage Maggie: "She [Maggie] seems to think I am capable of getting her discharged, that I somehow have connections." "She [Maggie] does not seem to understand my role." And, "She [Maggie] does not belong here with all these 'mentally retarded people.'" From the narrative, one can infer that Maggie would like to leave the hospital, since she thinks that she is being held against her will and nothing is wrong with her. You can use this assumption with the first clue, "She seems to think I am capable of getting her discharged, that I somehow have connections," as incentive for her to speak more with you. Since only Kate and the nursing staff are treating her, what she says in team meetings about Maggie's functioning will be heavily weighted. You can tell Maggie this. She may be interested in what you have to say and how you could get her out of the hospital. You then can tell Maggie that you need to see how she can function without any problems, so you can make a recommendation to the team. But, to do that, Maggie would have to show you, not just tell you. Maggie may now be more inclined to complete a functional evaluation with you. As she completes each section of the evaluation, you can ask her how she thought she did on that section. If she cannot point out her difficulties, you can give her feedback on her problem areas in a nonconfrontational manner.

With regards to the second clue, "She [Maggie] does not seem to understand my role," Maggie may not want to understand Kate's role. Maggie may be more interested in her own role. You could ask Maggie what her roles are, then try to help her with whatever she tells you in order to start to build a rapport with her.

To further strengthen the relationship between yourself and Maggie, agree with the third clue, "She [Maggie] does not belong here with all of these 'mentally retarded people.'" Tell Maggie that she is correct; she is not mentally retarded. Suggest that she disregard the other clients in the facility so she can focus on her work with you in order to expedite her discharge.

Denial can lift in a split second of insight, it can take years to slowly peel away, it can leave and then return again, or it could stay forever depending on the person and the situation. The next two narratives are written by the same anonymous person, F.T., who managed to gain remarkable insight through the help of her intervention team in a span of two weeks.

BEFORE

F.T.

> Being told that you have a mental illness can be devastating, especially when traumas of the past have left you with emotional scars. It is not fair that I am the one locked up here while the perpetrator of my abuse goes free to live his life. It is a gross injustice. Because I went to the doctor upon my father's request and not my own better and good judgment, because I was misdiagnosed 10 years ago and started on a mood stabilizing medication, my life has been devoid of the normal things people do.

> I do not think this is fair. I feel that, since I have taken the medication for 10 years, my body is addicted to it. I still maintain that I do not have a mental illness, only a need for love and affection from people, especially those in positions of authority, like my pastor and my doctors. This love heals me and restores to me my sense of dignity, self-respect, and self-esteem. Needless to say—needless to say—being in the hospital is very hard to deal with. Everything within cries out—this is not fair!

> I have tremendous joys and pleasures in life. Keeping me locked up and not free to pursue my interests (my four-mile-a-day run and my daily work) deprives me of my pursuit of happiness. I love life and I have a lot to live for. I have my pastor, my surrogate father, who has taken me into his arms and cared for me; my roommate, who is so genuinely fond of me; my sister, who told my mother not to call the cops on me; a grandfather, who loved me dearly even thought he is not here on this earth now; a grandmother, who cannot see or perhaps she does see why I am here withdrawing from my mood stabilizer.

> I started to take the mood stabilizer out of fear that something bad would happen to my beloved grandmother, not because I felt ill and needed medication, and not because my friends and relatives felt I needed it.

> I have the right to fight for what is rightfully mine—to fight for my right to be a happy individual. This is my life and I want and will be happy and fulfilled, as God is my witness. And I have the best friend and all the love I would ever need—God.

Client-Centered Reasoning Questions

1. At least five different examples of denial are found in this narrative. What are they?
2. Compare this anonymous narrative to the next narrative written by the same person, F.T., two weeks later by reading, then answering the questions at the end of the next narrative.

AFTER

F.T.

I do not like to admit that I have manic-depressive illness. I dislike it so much that I do not even let myself have any opinion about it. I tell myself that it is just a part of me, just another part of life. I mean, hey, life brings good and bad for both the "good" and "bad." Why get so bent out of shape over a natural part of life? Why fight it? Let the medication come, let the labels come. . . .

The first time I was hospitalized, 10 years ago, I did not really mind being hospitalized. Within a month, I was medicated, diagnosed, and discharged. It was a piece of cake. I finished out my college academic year and eventually completed college in four years with no other disruption. I was like any other human. I did not think too much about mental illness.

Like I said, that was 10 years ago.

Now, I am in the hospital again. I am writing from a hospital, and I am not as accepting of being here as I was 10 years ago. It could be that this hospital stay is not as pleasant as the one 10 years ago, or it could be that I am older now and I have to confront my illness. I know for sure that I am anxious being here in the hospital because my job awaits me outside these walls. I am a teacher and I miss my kids so much. I also am struggling with guilt, the guilt of letting my kids down, my kids' parents down, my principal and my school down. But this is something I have to deal with. This perfectionist inability to say "no" is what landed me in here. I accepted too much responsibility at work.

True, this hospital stay is more unpleasant than the previous one. Ten years ago, my peers were detoxification clients, mostly male and two other females. The hospital was smaller and there was more one-on-one attention. Now, I have to put up with conversations that do not make sense, with other patients, and slow nurse service. There are about 30 clients here.

And true, as an older adult, I do have to confront my illness. Not only am I kept away from my real-world job but I am also forced to accept that yes, indeed, I do have a mental illness. A second hospitalization proves it. I have to think about what caused me to become ill again. I cannot deny it. Here I am, an adult who can converse with other clients (not all of them are nonsensical) about medication and symptoms. Here, I am an adult who finally understands why she had to take medication 10 years ago. I am reluctantly coming to terms with the reality of having manic-depression tinged with psychosis.

I could write about how it takes two days to find someone to watch me shave my legs (since clients cannot use razors unsupervised). I could go on and on about how I dislike being in this hospital, about how inconvenient it is. (Do not get me wrong. I know there are positive aspects of hospital life, one of which is writing this piece.) But I would rather speak of something else. I prefer to speak about what manic-depressive illness means to me.

Initially, what comes to mind is that having manic-depressive illness means I cannot work myself into utter fatigue. It means that I need to eat regularly, sleep regularly, and learn to say "no" to responsibilities that people (like my principal or pastor) ask me to take. But it means more. It means I must *feel* something about it. I must have some sort of emotion about it, just an initial emotion is fine. Something that tells me I know my mental illness. It should be like the emotion I feel when I smell a bouquet of flowers or when I watch a gymnast executing a routine perfectly on the uneven bars. What kind of emotion should accepting a mental illness elicit? What is appropriate? What is not appropriate, but nevertheless expected? What is my emotion?

My first response is sadness. I am sad because I am not like most people. I know that anyone who has a physical defect probably feels different, so why should I feel sad? I know that every person is unique. But it is almost as if I have a defect that I cannot understand. Doctors do not know why lithium carbonate treats manic-depression successfully. I cannot explain why I have delusions that cause me to embarrass myself in front of the people of Manhattan. The episode that drove me to this hospital made me into one of those lunatics you encounter while you are eating at an outdoor café.

I am sad because I embarrassed myself. I am sad because I have been committed to mental hospitals. I am sad because I have an illness I will never completely understand. I am sad because I am like Vincent Van Gogh and Sylvia Plath. I used to think it was an honor to be like them—so sensitive, so emotional, loving life but being scared of life. I like that we love life—the beauty and beauties of life. Is it really true that manic-depressives are extremely creative? I know they are more sensitive than the average person is. Just wondering. But now . . . now, I see their lives and my life as just plain sad.

So now I am sad and glad about manic-depressive illness in my life. I used to think I was superior because I had this illness. It was my way of dealing with it. Now, I do not feel so superior. I feel sad, ashamed, and inconvenienced. I do not like being in this hospital. At the same time, I have learned. I have learned that I actually do have a mental illness. I have learned that I cannot be a workaholic; I need balance in my life. I have learned that I have to get proper rest (less responsibility) to avoid having another episode.

I guess I feel sobered. I still do not completely understand my illness. But, at least this time around, I will give it proper regard. If not for my health, then for the kids I teach—hopefully, both.

Do I believe my illness is real? Yes, and now that I know it is real, I will live a more balanced life. It will not come naturally for someone as extreme as me, but I will have to do it.

I cannot wait to get out of here. I have this itch to get back into life. I want to tweeze my own eyebrows, call friends without quarters, and socialize with people. (I do not socialize here—I need to focus on me. I get too involved emotionally with people— something else to work on.) So I long to live life again, and this time around, I live it along with my illness. No denial.

Client-Centered Reasoning Question

F.T. has worked through a lot of denial in just a few weeks; however, there is still one example of F.T.'s denial in this story. What is it?

Client-Centered Reasoning Activities

1. Finish the narrative.
2. Now that F.T. is more aware of her illness, write an intervention plan for one more week of individual and group intervention. What frames of reference would you use for each goal and why? What is your rationale for prioritizing her intervention this way?
3. Write an occupational profile.
4. Write a questionnaire.
5. List additional assessments you would use with this client.
6. Write an occupational performance analysis.
7. Write a two-week progress note for this client, using material from both narratives.
8. Readjust the intervention plan, as if you were treating F.T. in the employee assistance program once a week at her work site after her return.
9. Identify the types of clinical reasoning you applied in writing F.T.'s assessment, occupational performance analysis, intervention plan, discharge plan, and referrals.
10. What frame of reference or theory have you applied in creating F.T.'s assessment, occupational performance analysis, discharge plan, and referrals? Provide support for why this theory is appropriate for F.T.'s needs. What other frame of reference might be appropriate and why?

The following anonymous narrative has been included to demonstrate an absence of denial.

INSIGHT: MY THOUGHTS ON HOW I GOT HERE

ANONYMOUS

It all started approximately two years ago. I noticed that things around me had changed. I went through a divorce that I still, as of today, feel sad about. However, I must tell myself that life goes on and that I have to look forward to the future and what it has in store for me.

My therapist is a very important person in my life. She helps me through difficult times, tells me that there is a life out there and that I must fight for what is mine. She also tells me that I am an intelligent and fascinating woman of many talents. I also see a doctor who also treats me with much respect and devotes his time to see that I get the best help possible. Approximately two weeks ago, I was thinking of committing suicide because I could not face another day. I was very sad, so my doctor suggested that I admit myself into the hospital where they would help me with that kind of situation.

So, I decided to admit myself into the hospital. I arrived at the hospital and, with the help of my doctor, was placed in an institution for mental disorders. I was given medication to help me with my disorder so that, later on in life, I could deal with my emotional and sad moments.

Client-Centered Reasoning Questions

1. This narrator seems to respond positively to five things that her therapist and doctor provide. What are they?
2. What precautions would you take with this client and why?

Denial is just one type of defense. There are many more. They all serve the same purpose of avoiding painful realities, but attempt to achieve this goal in different ways. Some people use one type of defense throughout their lives, but most use several different types of defenses. The next two narratives may be seen as examples of two defenses that author Marc Wolsky uses: intellectualization and externalization.

INTELLECTUALIZATION AND EXTERNALIZATION

MARC WOLSKY

Mental health seems to be in vogue. Mental health professionals claim that they are helping their clients, but I do not feel that the treatment I have received here has helped me. I feel more like a prisoner of war whose captors are blinded by their own states' propaganda machine. What makes it even worse is that the people attracted to work in the mental health field appear ideally suited to separating the chaff from the wheat (not the other way around).

To me, the complexity of all this psychiatry is no longer all that mystifying. The real reason psychiatry is such a primitive science is that, by definition and nature, it asks fundamental questions of the mind and heart: who are we, where are we going, and how futuristic will tomorrow be? This is a complex project for anyone.

For me, the stigma of mental illness and its treatment are gone because I have won my own personal battle for a sane mind and a sane tomorrow.

God bless you, and may you reach all the stars in the sky and all the dimensions in the universe you will need to get you through the day after tomorrow.

And this is Marc's second narrative:

For much of my life, the mental health institution has left a scar on my memory and a stigma in my heart. I have, however, prevailed and now, instead of having a fatalist outlook on life, I feel privileged to know that my many years of supporting myself through progressive ideas instead of just supporting the status quo have brought me to a place with a real future, instead of just another day of watching the axis of the world turn.

I say this in prelude to my stay at this psychiatric unit, because now that I feel this way, I can really appreciate the quality of care given by your unit. It is not utopia, I do not believe in that way of life anyway. Thanks for putting up with my long-winded speech and inability to compromise, but I would like to add I hope you got as much out of my getting here as I got from both staff and patients.

Client-Centered Reasoning Questions

1. Write your own definition of the two defenses, intellectualization and externalization, based on Marc's two narratives.
2. Do you feel that you know Marc after reading his narratives? Why or why not? Did you feel that you knew F.T. after reading either of her narratives? Besides length, what is the difference between how these two people present themselves?
3. How do these defenses help Marc to avoid painful feelings?
4. Research and list other defenses and their definitions. Where did you obtain this information?
5. Besides denial, what other defenses have you used in your life? Give an example for each defense and state how that defense helped you avoid painful issues in each situation. Were you aware of your defense at the time?
6. Think of your acquaintances who have prominent defenses. What are they? How do they affect your interactions with them? Are they aware of the defenses? Do they affect their functioning? How?

Client-Centered Reasoning Activity

In both narratives underline examples of externalization with one color pen; then with a different colored pen underline examples of intellectualization. What is the difference between these two defenses? In what ways are they similar?

REFERENCE

Kaplan HI, Sadock BJ. *Synopsis of Psychiatry: Behavioral Sciences, Clinical Psychiatry*, 8th ed. Baltimore: Williams and Wilkins, 1998.

You Can Make It on Broken Pieces: The Experience of Psychosocial Distress

Despite well-defined symptoms characteristic of well-defined diagnoses, everyone experiences psychosocial issues in different ways. It is not enough to know that people are delusional without knowing the specifics of their delusions and how these delusions affect their lives. These few narratives are only a step into the journey of understanding how people experience psychosocial distress.

BATTERED AND BROKEN

Hellis Joyce Chatman

I was a battered woman for eight years. My children were battered also. My family told me to leave, but I did not listen. I am very stubborn. It was my fault because I should have left the first time he hit me. He lied, cheated, and slandered my name, so that my peace, my joy, my pride, and my dignity are now gone. I am on a psychiatric ward for all the anger that I have inside from his mental and emotional abuse. I felt suicidal.

I wanted to kill him, but today I have hope and a little strength. In the short time that I have been in the psychiatric hospital, I have gotten stronger. The voices, depression, and paranoia are not there as much as before. Today, I feel that I can make it without him, just my kids and me. I can do all things through Christ, who strengthens me.

I lost my kids because of my drug use. I have three. My oldest two are with my Mom and one is with their father. I do not call my son because I fear him [her husband, who batters her] putting me down and breaking my spirit. So now, I live in the solution one day at a time. I will grow. Pray for me. No more drugs. One day I will get my kids back. I will take them out of New York City.

I went into detoxification, where I called my son the last time. My husband's new girlfriend answered. I asked her to make my son some muffins to eat. She yelled at me and told me never to call and bother them. All this time, it has haunted me. I was in a big rage. He used my son to hurt me, but he does not realize he is hurting his son. He will lose his son if he does not change.

The groups have helped by letting me talk and get feedback from my peers, who gave me advice and held and hugged me on days when I felt down and needed help. I began reading my Bible again.

I miss my 7-year-old son, too. He is sad. He has no more clothes or bright smile, and he misses me very much. He does not want to stay with his father because his father still hits him. I should not allow my fear of my son's father to stop me from calling my son. I have to learn how to separate the good and the bad.

He told me I was fat and ugly, and I believed him. He said I would never find anyone else like him, so I would have to stay. I believed this, too. I would like to send a message to whomever out there is a victim of domestic violence. Get out of it. If you are on drugs, you do not have to use. It is all right to put your kids on the back burner so you can focus on your recovery. You can make it on broken pieces.

Client-Centered Reasoning Questions

1. How prevalent is domestic violence?
2. What are your legal obligations as a therapist if you suspect domestic violence has happened to your client, by your client, or to any child? What are your legal obligations as a layperson?
3. Where did you obtain the information to answer questions 1 and 2?

Client-Centered Reasoning Activities

1. Finish the narrative.
2. Rewrite this narrative four times, each time from a different person's perspective: the husband's, the husband's new girlfriend, Joyce's 7-year-old son, and Joyce's mother.
3. Write an intervention plan for Joyce, one for her 7-year-old son, and one for the intervention of her husband, as if you were the therapist of each individual. What would your countertransference issues be in each case? How could you prevent these feelings from interfering with your intervention with each person?
4. Write a discharge note for Joyce.
5. Identify the types of clinical reasoning you applied in writing Joyce's, Joyce's husband's, and Joyce's 7-year-old's intervention plans. Identify the types of clinical reasoning you applied in writing Joyce's discharge plan.
6. What frame of reference or theory have you applied in creating Joyce's, Joyce's husband's, and Joyce's 7-year-old's intervention plans? What frame of reference have you applied in creating Joyce's discharge plan? Provide support for why this theory is appropriate for these people's needs. What other frames of reference might be appropriate and why?

I AM A SABATA

LAURA BELLA BRYANT

Write between the lines.

Since the very beginning of my fieldwork experience, I remember a man whom I will call Melvin. Melvin is a 42-year-old, extremely slender, African American man who has a history of schizophrenia and AIDS. Melvin has been in and out of psychosocial institutions for years. Melvin is aware of his barriers and extremely expressive about his thoughts and feelings at times. Melvin is a friendly man, who always makes an effort to say "hello" while he paces the halls throughout the day. When Melvin smiles, everyone around him wants to smile, but when he is angry or upset, you could cry.

For the first few weeks of my internship, Melvin had his ups and downs, but he was basically well tempered. Even though he appears to be happy, he could break at any minute. Everyday, Melvin asks to go home, but everyone tells him that he is not quite better yet; therefore, he gets extremely frustrated with the staff at times and thinks that no one cares about him.

I have had therapeutic conversations with Melvin on a daily basis. Melvin has expressed his feelings to me about his illness, family, and life outside of the hospital. Melvin told me that his Mother abandoned him and his sister at a very young age; therefore, a foster mother and father raised them. He expressed the love he has for his foster parents and how much he has missed them since their deaths. Melvin told me that he has no one else in his life: "They were the only people that loved me. I have no family. I have AIDS. My aunts do not want anything to do with me. Many people have told me that I have no roots and I am nothing." He told me that he once spent five years in Kings County Hospital, and when released, he went to his aunt's house, but she did not even answer the door because she knew that it was he.

Melvin told me that he completed high school only through the ninth grade because he was stupid and had no interest in school. He said that the other kids were more advanced than he was and he would never be able to finish high school. He said that his mental illness began when he was very young, probably around the age of 18. He began hearing voices and doing things that he normally would not do. He would not go into detail. He said, "I have a space ship in my head and a transmitter in my cheek. The transmitter was created from semen." The voices say, "If you die, I will suffer. If I die, you will suffer." He expressed to me how horrifying these voices are and how he prays for them to go away. He also said that they have become part of his life and that, if they were not there, he would not know what to do. "Some days they are better but some days they can be worse." He paused and then said, "they tell me to do terrible things. They tell me that I am a Sabata. A Sabata is a spy that eats feces and cuts throats. I do not know what to do when they tell me to do these things, but I know that I am not a Sabata. Sometimes I get so upset, I am unorganized, I am stupid, and my mind is messed up! Will you just laugh at me, Laura?"

Melvin has also told me about his life outside of the hospital. He told me that he lives in a residence called the Sunrise Hotel, which he enjoys very much. He has his own room, where he is left alone. He told me that he always pays his rent on time and he is going to return there after he is discharged. He said that it can be lonely at times, but when he is there he is free.

Melvin's life is one that could make anyone sad. He has been in the hospital for over two months now and his freedom has been taken away. His clothes were taken and he now wears a hospital gown. He has AIDS and schizophrenia, the latter for over 20 years. He paces the halls daily and sleeps on occasion. During this hospitalization, Melvin has been placed in seclusion, he looks despondent while he stands by the window for hours looking out. Melvin wants to be on the outside with everyone else.

Today Melvin is being discharged from the hospital. He has been waiting for this day ever since his admission. He has had his ups and downs over the past three months, but now he is rapidly improving. When he came to the hospital, all of his clothes were taken away and from time to time he was placed in special care. Occasionally, he had the privilege of going on walks, which he always enjoyed.

I knew that it was going to be difficult to say goodbye to Melvin, but I never imagined it to be this hard. He was the client

I looked forward to seeing every day. He always made me smile. Since I worked with Melvin on a daily basis, I wanted him to use the skills we worked on. Before he left, Melvin showered, shaved, brushed his teeth, his clothes were clean, his bags were packed, and he was ready to go. The ambulette was not coming to pick him up until 3:00 in the afternoon, but he was pacing the halls in high spirits. He was looking forward to going back to his residence he loved so much due to the freedom it offered him. He told me that he was looking forward to the home-cooked meal he was going to receive that following night from the shelter next door, which he always went to on Saturday nights. He asked me about the new movies in the theaters. He was so excited to hear that one of his favorite movies was back on screen. He told me that he had so many plans, but he was too excited to talk about them. The most important thing was to be free.

Before Melvin left, I knew that I wanted to discuss medication compliance with him because he had a history of being non-compliant with medication. When I started talking to him about the importance of his medication, he said, "Do not worry, Miss Laura, I never want to be back here again or anywhere else so I am going to take my medication. It keeps me out of the hospital you know." I told him that he looked great. I was very proud to see him so well.

At 3:00 this afternoon, the ambulette finally came to pick up Melvin. Melvin was so excited that he did not know what to do. Before he sat in the wheelchair, Melvin decided to give me a huge bearhug goodbye. He told me that he was going to take his medication, bathe every day, and make sure to brush his teeth daily. As he said goodbye, I almost began to cry. He asked for his bags and then jumped in the wheelchair. I have never seen someone that excited to sit in a wheelchair before. I wished him lots of luck and told him to take care of himself. When he was being wheeled down the hall, I felt the tears approaching my eyes. Somehow, I held them back. I knew that Melvin was better. He was going to a place where he would be much happier, where he would have his freedom. All I could remember when he was being wheeled away was the one time I heard him say, "I want to be free!"

Client-Centered Reasoning Activity

Write your own client-centered reasoning questions and activities.

ABOUT MY SECOND ILLNESS

ANONYMOUS

I was scared all my life about mental illness due to my mother having it. It has not been easy dealing with mental illness. To open up old fears and secrets is very painful. I want to die because of my life's circumstances. I did attempt suicide at 13 and a few more times until I went into therapy and learned to talk out my thoughts to a psychiatrist. I started to heal. My struggle has been long and hard, and I will continue to struggle until I die. I have bipolar illness, posttraumatic stress disorder, and borderline personality disorder. I believe if I take my medicines on time, go to therapy, know my symptoms, and talk to my doctor when they occur, I can live a productive life. I believe I will end up in mental hospitals for life.

Client-Centered Reasoning Questions

1. If this client wrote her narrative in your intervention group, which sentence would you be most concerned about? What would you do about it and why?
2. What do you think about this author's last two sentences? Why do you think she wrote both?
3. What would your intervention priorities be with her and why?

Client-Centered Reasoning Activity

Often therapists will work with suicidal clients to create contractual partnerships that state that the clients will notify the therapist when they feel like hurting themselves before doing so, in order to get help and for the therapist to feel comfortable working with people who are suicidal. Work in dyads to create a contractual partnership for suicide prevention. One person acts as the therapist and the other acts as a client. Set up a contractual partnership together that you both sign before you can proceed with further intervention. Suicide is not the only way that clients try to hurt themselves. In your contract, include a list of all risky or self-destructive behaviors that are relevant to the client [played by a student].

CHANGES OF MY SEASON

KATHRYN FAZIO

Sometimes I crawl up into a shell
Stuffed up like a snail.
A bunch of escargot going nowhere.
Afraid of the chief warrior consuming me with forked tongues.
I am so withdrawn, and I feel dead.
It has not always been this way.
There have been songs for me,
Bird songs.
Liquid green and fuchsia parrots,
Riots of laughter,
The gauze of the sacred heart
Cured and protected.
So some days I am fine,
But let us not be asses.
It is not that one I feel well and another I feel ill.
Instead, it occurs in time spans.
It is like the winter of content
Or the winter or spring of not content.
And let us not be asses.
It is not some affective disorder either
But just times I feel the throng of discontent,
The ring of glimmering day disappearing.
Some periods of time the light does shine.
And so I shine. Jumping out of bed without thorns.
I listen to the flute of noodle songs from Chang Wang's Chinese
   restaurant,
And I am truly happy.
But let us not be asses.
Sometimes the noodles are each the twisted cock of the devil
Scaring the urine out of me making me run like a dead person.
Pleading, I beg for my medicine.

Client-Centered Reasoning Activity

Paraphrase Kathryn's poem.

10

Depression: Losses, Loneliness, and Interventions

Hopeless, helpless, desperate, lonely, sad, fearful, guilty, obsessing, worthless, perseverant, somatic, anguished, heartbroken, hurt, future-less, suicidal, anxious, angry, tired, despondent, anhedonic, isolated, withdrawn, sleep disturbed, loss of appetite, psychomotor retardation, poor concentration, poor hygiene, intrusive thoughts, unmotivated, dependent, needy, tearful—all possible characteristics of depression. How do you improve someone's occupational performance if they do not want to improve it, believe they cannot improve it, believe it is not worth improving, are afraid to fail, are afraid to succeed, or are too tired, angry, lonely, or unmotivated to work with you? The answers will come by studying specific examples of people struggling through their depression. This chapter presents eight such examples and begins with intern Kate Harrington's initial experience with a depressed person.

WHAT IS MY ROLE?

KATE HARRINGTON

> Depression sets in, at least for one client. I had the chance to sit in on a case study today. It was an interesting as well as a saddening experience. The case was presented to a team of residents and interns, followed by an interview with the client that was conducted by an attending physician. We were not only able to hear an in-depth history of the client; we were also able to hear first-hand from the client what he had been feeling and thinking. During the case study presentation and the interview, I asked myself various questions. How would I help this person? What could I offer? He had such strong feelings of hopelessness and despair and informed us that he wanted to be admitted to a state facility. He could not see any possibility of getting better. I acknowledged that he is acutely ill and proper medication will probably help him with the depression. In the meantime, what is my role?

After the meeting I had a chance to visit the client in his room. He was in bed, unshowered and seemed asleep. I actually had to speak to his roommate, too, and upon doing so, I saw him open his eyes. I introduced myself and asked him how he was doing. He said, "Not well." I had a calendar for him and asked him if he would like to put it on the wall. He declined. I put the calendar up for him and told him I would be back later or the next day. How far do you push a person before backing off? What are the parameters? These are questions I hope to be able to answer soon.

I admit, I do feel more confident and secure on the unit; however, there is so much I have yet to learn. For instance, how do I respond to clients who act inappropriately, say they do not want to be here or speak of hopelessness and despair? Sometimes, I feel as if clients are searching for answers and guidance, and I want to be able to help them. I am, however, not confidant that I am saying the right things. What if I contradict another professional or say the wrong thing? Unless I am 100 percent sure, I will refer the client to someone else, or find the answer first, and then return to the client. I do not mind doing this, as I realize it is more important to be correct, rather than to save face, although I do look forward to the day when I need not second-guess myself.

Client-Centered Reasoning Activity

Respond to Kate's seven questions.

DEATH

Anonymous

When I get depressed I usually do not eat or sleep and I get lonely. I take my medication every day. The first time I got depressed is when I lost my grandmother. My grandmother raised me like a mother. When she died, I stopped eating and grooming. I also stopped talking to all my family members. My family took me to the hospital for help because of my deep depression. When I lost my grandmother it was like losing my best friend, because she took care of me since my birth. She told me about the birds and the bees. When my mother became sick, I had to take care of her. My mother went to the hospital on January 5, 1995, because of her asthma. On January 30, 1995, my mother died. My best friend died of a heart attack in December 1995. She died in her home with her mother and brother and sisters. It took me a long time to get over her death. My step-grandmother died of cancer on August 19, 1995. It must be because she was there for me when my mother died. I became so depressed that I stopped eating for three days. I could not sleep.

Client-Centered Reasoning Questions

1. What are this person's symptoms of depression, and how do they affect her functioning?

2. List everything you know about this person from her narrative.
3. What kind of intervention would you provide this person to help her get over her grief?

A DEPRESSED DREAM

THOMAS DANIEL

I have no friends because of my depression. I am lonely and afraid to make friends. I am afraid that I will lose them like everyone else I loved. Sometimes, I wish I could have a friend. I feel that if they find out about the things I have been through (I was raped and molested), they would not be my friends anymore. I feel I have no life and no future. Most of the time I am so depressed that I wish I were dead. I hope that, if I go to sleep and not wake up, all the pain would go away and I could be with all the people I love and that people would love me. Sometimes, I think it is just a dream and I am going to wake up soon. One day, I hope I will wake up, but for now I will just sleep. I pray that when I wake up it will all have just been a dream.

Client-Centered Reasoning Questions

1. Thomas uses the image of a dream to express his wish to be free of depression. What kinds of creative exercises could you have him participate in, using the dream theme, to help him bridge the gap between a depressing dream and a life without depression?
2. What are Thomas's symptoms of depression and how do they affect his occupational performance?

Client-Centered Reasoning Activity

Write an intervention plan for Thomas for each of the following intervention settings: a welfare to work program, an inpatient psychiatric unit, a psychiatric day treatment program, a psychiatric day hospital, a residential community program, and an ongoing once-a-week session in your private practice. Explain your rationale. How does the intervention vary as the setting changes?

TINY LITTLE PEA—SMALL, SHINY, AND FREE

VLADIMIR RAMIREZ

I was born normal. Then at the age of 19, I started to have symptoms. They brought me to the hospital five times. I just cannot believe that I have the sickness known as depression. It is really messing up my life. How do I go about establishing a normal life? I believe that my depression is always there, that I am always blue. Blue is the color that describes sadness; it encumbers all angles of my life. Melancholy and infinite sadness are all that surround me. I was born sad and I will die sad.

Client-Centered Reasoning Questions

1. In speaking with Vladimir, how would you answer his question, "How do I go about establishing a normal life?"
2. You have to meet and interview Vladimir. You know that depression may cause psychomotor retardation and paucity of speech, so you choose your questions carefully, knowing that you may not have enough time to complete the interview nor may he be able to tolerate too many questions at any one time. What five questions would you ask him in order of priority? Why did you choose these questions in that particular sequence?
3. What are Vladimir's symptoms of depression?

Client-Centered Reasoning Activity

How can depression change one's perception? How may Vladimir's depression be affecting his perception? Write a narrative, in quotes of a dialogue between Vladimir and his therapist (you), describing how you would help him see that he may not always feel so depressed and how depression changes people's perception about life. What clue from his narrative suggests that Vladimir may not always envision himself in a depressed state?

DEPRESSION/DELUSIONS

KATHRYN FAZIO

Depression is the dark hole you fall through that makes you sad all the time. Delusions can come with depression. Delusions follow me as if they are the truth. I get afraid of how I let God, my family, and friends down. Depression makes me lie in my bed and not take a shower. How depression affects me is that I cannot escape the big foot that follows me everywhere.

With delusions, I think things are true. Delusions and depression can sure make it feel like it is the end of the world. For me, it is like I am bereft of spirit. I only wish I could shake loose the feelings, or rather thoughts, I have, but every time I try, something else happens to point to the depression and delusions being real. I do not deal with delusions because they are so powerful. It is like Popeye pouncing on Sweet Pea, but I do try to tell myself that delusions are just that—delusions—and that they have no reality base to them. I try to do this but the delusions are strong, like a big wave taking away all of life's goodies from me.

Client-Centered Reasoning Questions

1. What is the definition of a *delusion*?
2. In what other diagnoses besides depression could delusions be present? How can you tell the difference? Where did you get this information?

3. What are Kathryn's symptoms of depression and how do they affect her occupational performance?
4. What further questions would you like to ask Kathryn in order to work with her and why?
5. How could you (or could you) help Kathryn identify her delusions as delusions when she is in a delusional state? Describe five approaches to solving this problem.

CHILDHOOD TRAUMA

Mark Jules

Some people say every disappointment is a blessing, others may say that there is a light at the end of every dark tunnel. I may agree with the second saying, but I am not really too sure about the first. When I look back at my life, I see that there were many disappointments where my feelings were concerned. At the age of 10, I had the biggest disappointment of my life; I got separated from my mom and dad. They were the only two people that could really be there for me when I needed somebody to talk to. After I lost my parents, I stopped trusting everybody else. No one else could understand me the way my parents had. I felt really hurt inside. I kept my feelings to myself. I never wanted to ask anybody for help because of the lack of trust in others. There were many other disappointments where my parents were concerned, but I never got the courage to tell anybody else. The lack of building trust in others stays with me, I guess, all of my life.

ISOLATED

Anonymous

My illness makes me feel depressed because I am not normal like everyone else. My experience on this psychiatric ward makes me feel kind of good because I am among friends and everyone is like me. I have met a couple of friends here. It has been a good experience for me here, one I will not forget.

LOSING SOMEONE SPECIAL

Corey Simmelkjaer

Once upon a time there was a teenage boy who grew up in the Abraham Lincoln Projects. He was the only child, and his mother was a single parent. The boy lost his father when he was around 10 years old. The loss of this father caused him a great deal of depression because his father always took him and his friends to the park to play sports.

Anthony always felt lonely and sad about his father's death. He always thinks to himself about how his life would be if his father were still alive. Every year around August, the month when Anthony's father passed, he gets real depressed.

ON ONIONS AND DEPRESSION

KATHRYN FAZIO

How many onions are there in this day I live in?
Unfortunately there is no other day than this one that I can
   depend.
I feel the flood of secretions in the moon of the onion.

I am not cooking.
So why are there so many onions on palm trees?

Even the birds that sing merrily with flute
music against their ears are aware of
the onions on the beach of the shore.

I wonder why they fly so quickly across oceans.

I cannot even contain a telephone call that
will hold me up from this depression by the
seat of my pants—by the seat of telephone wires.

I am grateful I get to hear others who are
sound of mood and spirit when I speak on the phone.

The tombs in Egypt open and the spell
shatters the silence of spirit and brings solitude.
I could say there was hope.
But will I say hope in the face of this
miserable world with everyone fighting.

Mostly control issues surround me. I do not even
have the option to sit and pray as I please.
I seem to have forgotten how to pray.
But I remember the trees and the smell and burn of onions.

Today and tomorrow I desire my heart to lift up to music
And to ignore the stench of onions. Yes, let me taste the sweet oils,
taste onions when they do not tear me apart.

Perhaps a Sunday dinner with my family will do it.
I know I need so much now. I just hope the onion truck goes
   around another
corner tomorrow bypassing the supermarket I shop in so that I
   could go to a
small quaint store and enjoy the loneliness of the one I peel on
   that day.

Perhaps an onion soup. Perhaps an onion tough with character.
I need to be left alone by onions galore. The smuggle of onions
   into my
Dreams. The themes of wasted time. I have done so poorly at
   ignoring onions.
Perhaps there is a 12-step program: Onions Anonymous.
Let me breathe again without the choke and gag of sorrow or burn.

Client-Centered Reasoning Question

What are Kathryn's symptoms of depression?

CLIENT-CENTERED REASONING
ACTIVITIES FOR CHAPTER 10

1. Compare and contrast the different symptoms of depression and how they affect the occupational performance of the anonymous author of "Death," Thomas, Vladimir, Kathryn, Mark, the anonymous author of "Isolated," and Cory.
2. Compare and contrast the causes of depression for each of these people. What are other causes of depression? Is there ever depression without an environmental etiology?
3. Anger is usually closely associated with depression. In some instances, depression is anger turned inward. Go through the clients' narratives and record in quotes hints of anger. Are there many? What could you do to help these individuals get more in touch with their anger? How would getting in touch with anger be helpful to a depressed person?
4. You are conducting a therapeutic intervention group with the anonymous author of "Death," Thomas, Vladimir, Kathryn, Mark, the anonymous author of "Isolated," and Cory as members. You have six sessions to complete the intervention. Write a group protocol. Include specific exercises you would use and the areas you would cover in each of the six sessions and why. What types of clinical reasoning did you use? What frame of reference or theory did you apply when writing this group protocol? Provide support for why this theory is appropriate for these group members' needs. What additional frame of reference might be appropriate and why?

11

Substance Abuse: Triggers, Recovery, and Relapse

It is so weird because when the drug is sitting on the table it has no power. But, when I pick it up and put it inside my body, it causes me to lie, cheat, steal, kill, and become homeless. (Clifton Winston)

The following are a series of narratives written by 11 people with various addictions, followed by three written by interns and finally an intern's log, all depicting what it is like to have a substance abuse addiction and how to help people that do.

THE COURSE OF MY ADDICTION

ANONYMOUS

Everything started when I was a freshman in high school. I would go to all the parties and just want to fit in. I started drinking beer and smoking cigarettes with some friends. In the beginning, I felt sick. I would be nauseous and vomit. But I continued to drink and smoke because, even though it made me sick, it was still cool. I eventually started liking the use of alcohol. My friends and I started hanging out more and doing these things more often. At first it was once every three weeks, then once a week, then every day. Smoking was becoming good, so I started drinking alcohol along with the cigarettes. Any kind of alcohol would do.

Years went by and none of the students knew what they were doing with their lives. They were only in school because their parents made them be there. For some reason, I was placed in a music class, and I learned how to play the violin. When music entered into my life, my life changed. The "in" thing for me was not drinking and smoking anymore. Things started slowing down for me, and that is when I mastered the guitar. I then went crazy. All I did all day was play the guitar. I did not care about anything except music.

One day, I got hired as a musician and started playing in an amateur band. I was good enough to make money, and I started having easy access to drugs. Cocaine was always a part of the scene. Maybe there were one or two people not using drugs, but they would be drinking everything in sight. So I kept playing these small gigs in these types of settings. I was playing Latin music, and at this point I was getting not only caught up in the music but with the drugs as well.

I then ran into a Latin band that traveled all over the world for a long time. They auditioned me and offered me a part in the band. They made thousands of dollars and got whatever they wanted. To me, they had the most exciting lifestyle. I knew they were successful. They always had girlfriends, money, and all the drugs they wanted. I always felt like a celebrity. I started making thousands of dollars, and I felt like I could take any drug that I wanted. I started sitting in the VIP sections at all the clubs. I was able to do anything I wanted to do. I was surrounded by beautiful girls that would do anything for me just so they could be seen with me. I loved this feeling. I felt so powerful and high.

This went on for many years, and my use of drugs became more and more frequent. We no longer would use drugs to wind down, but we always needed drugs to feel up. Before a gig, we all had to use. The addiction kept getting worse. I became very dependent on drugs. I felt like I could not play or do anything without getting high. I started losing interest in girls because I wanted to get high with some friends and not with some random girls.

The addiction was becoming stronger and stronger. I did not realize it at the time, but I was deteriorating inside and out. My band mates and my career were going down hill. There were nights that I could not show up to gigs. This was a big deal because people were coming to see me perform. If I did not show up, I would be letting everyone down. I was one of the four main guys in the group, and everybody counted on me to be there. I started letting everyone down, and I realized that drugs were destroying my life. Drugs were messing up my responsibilities. I knew that I needed time out. Drugs were fun in school and fun when I first started taking them, but now they were just messing up my life and the lives of people around me. I started feeling irresponsible and decided that this lifestyle was not good for me anymore. I kept thinking. I did not tell anyone that I came to detoxification. I knew that I had to either come in here or just stay out there and rot. I knew what I had to do. I lose money while I am in here, but I was going crazy out there. Coming to detoxification was right for me even though people out there in the world may think that I am weak. The reason why I could not tell anyone was because they would judge me. I have to do this for myself, by myself.

It is hard. You cannot just quit on your own, but I know that since I decided to do this it will mean more to me. I decided to go for a detoxification because I want to see the difference in myself and my life. I already stopped smoking. Some people have the willpower to just stop. Even though I know what this addiction does to me, for some reason I keep going back to the drugs. I need help. It is like when something bad happens to you on a street, a person will do anything to avoid that block so they do not have to deal with the painful memories. It is the same with drugs. You have to take a different route to reach the same destination. I know that I should be going the same way and not down the same path, but I keep going back to get beaten up or something worse.

To get to this point right now, it took a lot of thinking. I had a crackhead brother, and he got to his lowest point while using drugs. He would sleep in the gutter and not take a shower or brush his teeth for days. One day he woke up and said, "no more." He now preaches the words of God. It was an inspiration to me to know that he did this by himself. I know that I could follow his footsteps and do the same thing.

Last night, I considered leaving the detoxification unit because of temptation to use again. I am at the beginning of my treatment and chances are that I will be tempted again. I have to remain strong and motivated.

Addicts are so stupid. Once we get to a point that we can be on drugs and still lead our lives, we are not happy with this and we want more. I could never stop. At first, I was able to function normally. Sometimes my lips would twitch, I would not stop talking, I would have nervous movements, and I could not find a posture that was comfortable. There is no level of drug that is safe to consume. It is written all over your face. There is no way to hide it. My mother always asked me, "Who do you think you are fooling?" I would be sweating even if it were 30 degrees outside. I was messed up. I would ask myself: How did I get to this point? How did this happen? Why can I not just stop?

I have had my share of excitement and fun. I have made unbelievable friends and connections. I put money into suites, champagne, limousines, girls, coke, and whatever the people I was a friend to at the time wanted. It was a great feeling in the beginning, but I know these feelings will not last forever.

Right now, I want to go back to school and maybe make a solo album. I never thought that I would end up in detoxification. This all shows me that there is still hope for me, and I am just beginning a new life for myself. I just have to remain focused and keep on being strong. I cannot fall into the peer pressure or situations around me anymore. I have to live life for myself the way I am proud and happy to live. I am excited for this chance at a new beginning.

DRUGS CHANGED MY LIFE

Anonymous

At the age of 14, I lived with my uncle who gave me two beers for my birthday. I started drinking with friends in junior high school on the weekends. In high school, I started drinking every day due to peer pressure. I had low self-esteem, and alcohol gave me false courage. When I went to college, I drank even more with my friends. I was surrounded by people who always drank. In high school and college I was involved in music groups. My drinking increased as a musician. After college I felt bored, so I started drinking even more. I went to the Navy and drank in the Navy. I met a girl in the Navy in 1982. She gave up her medical school training to marry me. (I feel really guilty about that now.) I cut down on my drinking. In 1986, I married her. I got a job at the Department of Corrections. This job was very stressful for me, so I started sniffing cocaine with other staff members at the job during work. Throughout the time period of 1986 to 1990, I drank and sniffed cocaine. In 1990, my family made me go for detoxification and rehabilitation treatment. It was hard for me to go because it meant that I could not work. I did not really want to stop working because I had no money and bad credit. I went anyway. I stayed sober for six years, the best six years of my life. During this time, I completed general electrician training, became closer with my family, and stopped hanging out with the bad crowd. In 1996, my wife was murdered. I started to drink heavily, so I came back to detoxification treatment. I began drinking as soon as I got out, so I went to rehabilitation treatment in Albany for 28 days. This time I stayed sober for 10 months. In 1997, I began to drink again until today when I am currently in detoxification treatment writing this story of my life as part of my treatment to become drug free. Writing this helped me see my past the way it really was.

IT JUST GETS WORSE

MANDY FERNANDEZ

When I first relapsed, two weeks ago, after being sober for six months, I felt really bad. I went out on Thursday and did not come home until Saturday morning. I caught myself. This time I did not want to do it again, so I came for detoxification.

Now that I am here, I feel a little better. I was scared when I was taking drugs for the third straight day. How can I go back to this way of life? It just gets worse. Never better. I cannot do this anymore. I always feel it will go a different way, but it is always the same thing; it just gets worse. This time I caught it early.

I was getting high for years before I lost everything. I had no work and was not on public assistance. I was out on the street selling drugs and doing awful things. My kids are not with me because of what I did. This time I was so close to getting them back. I figured that I would catch it early so I would get my kids back, because they mean so much to me, and I have to keep trying to change, not only for myself, but for them, too.

I was in the Bronx Lebanon Hospital in a drug psychiatric facility for parents. They have groups on women's relapse prevention and GED classes. I just completed my orientation for the GED.

I had the certificate in my hands to go on. I was so disappointed that I was messing up again. I knew I was messing up when I started missing my appointments. My counselor confronted me about missing some classes, so I relapsed because of the stress. I felt like she did not care about my problems but cared about the fact that I was missing the class. So, I stopped going all together. I went back to using drugs. I now want to continue where I was and go back to the program because there is no other way for me to stay drug free. Now, I can go back to the program because I went to detoxification, and I am dedicated to fix this problem.

I started doing everything when I was young. I had my first beer at 2 years old. I really started smoking marijuana regrettably at age 13. My aunt gave me a joint, so my family introduced me to drugs. At age 16, I sniffed cocaine and started drinking liquor. I took dust, acid, and popping pills. At age 21, I started smoking crack and it became a big problem. I kept going for years and years until I went to detoxification in 1999. In Jacobi Hospital, I realized I had to fix a problem that was a problem for my whole family. I stayed clean for six months and started using again. After that, I decided to go for detoxification at the Bronx Lebanon Hospital. I went straight to a rehabilitation facility when I came out. After that, I went to an outpatient program. I just relapsed a few days ago. From here, I want to go back to the Bronx Lebanon facility to fix this problem for the last time.

Right now I feel better than I did a few days ago. I am going to put my foot down and stay on the right track this time. I realize there is a life out there, and it is beautiful, and I can experience it. I have to stay away from people, places, and things related to drugs; go to meetings; and do what I have to do. This is for me. I learned that drugs are not for me. Nothing ever changes with drugs. It just gets worse, and eventually you die if you do not take the chances you are given to get better.

I STARTED DRINKING AT THE AGE OF 8

JEROME E. BOWENS

I started drinking at the age of 8. Mom and Dad partied. There was always liquor in the house. In third grade, I went to school drunk. I was buzzed, so my teacher hit me with a stick. I hit the teacher back with a pencil. I was punished and sent to a home for boys for nine months. That is when I started hating the white people because they hit me. So, at 8 years old, I started drinking and fighting. At the age of 8, I became an alcoholic.

My mom used to be a nurse. Her job was to help perform abortions. She used to make me throw away the bloody stuff. My father left when I was 4 years old. My mom was an alcoholic.

At the age of 10, I started selling drugs, and at age 15, started using drugs. At age 12, I started having sex with older women who were drinkers. I did not like women. I used them for sex. I used to hurt women emotionally because I enjoyed it. At age 15, I went to the county jail for the first time for fighting. At age 16, I burnt down a store and went to prison for 9 to 10 months in New Jersey. I abused drugs and alcohol throughout high school but graduated anyway.

After graduation, I went into the service, the Green Beret Special Forces. I used drugs and alcohol in the service. In the service, I got caught selling guns and drugs. I was sent to federal prison in Kansas for three years. I went back to the service for one and a half years, 1979 to 1981, then left with an honorable discharge.

In North Carolina, I was arrested for murder but was found not guilty.

My father had a lot of children. I have twin sisters that I keep in touch with. I never had a close family. I keep in touch with my younger brother and older sister, Sarah.

After coming back from North Carolina, I got married, then moved to Washington, D.C. I met a woman, Bracerla, in Washington, D.C., at work but did not want to get close to her. She was persistent and I started trusting her, and we married a year later. I continued to drink throughout my marriage, but my wife supported me and tried to help me. I have two daughters and one granddaughter. I was never close to my daughters because I was out drinking all the time. My wife left me a couple of times, but I would always go and get her back.

This is the first time I have been away from my wife for such a long period of time (30 days). She brought me for detoxification and rehabilitation so that I could get help. She is very supportive of me.

I wanted to stop drinking after I got married, but I could not because of this addiction. I am tired of the lifestyle and want to stop fighting and selling guns and drugs. I want to turn my life around. I feel like I lost control over myself. I feel confident that I will get my life straight by seeking help from detoxification and rehabilitation. I got tired of all of the blackouts.

I REALLY MESSED UP THIS TIME

JOY CHATMAN

I really messed up this time. Two of my children stay with my mother but my son stays with his dad. My son is very, very unhappy and very sad because of me. He used to have a beautiful and bright look on his face, a gorgeous look. Now, all I see is a very unhappy 7½ year old. Lord, forgive me for all my sins and wash me white as snow, especially my kids. I love them too much. I cannot handle looking them in the face. I failed as a mother. My children are hurting and so am I. I am struggling to stay off drugs. I must find out the reason that I keep getting bad breaks. All I know is that I do not want to hurt my kids, my mom, or myself. It is time to say "no" and mean it. My life has been like a roller coaster. I have come a long way. I have been beaten and raped by my man, not once but twice, hard. I give you all the glory and the prayer because you are walking of the Pnozs. One day at a time, a mind at a time, and everything will fall into place. I am grateful for being clean and sober $2\frac{1}{2}$ weeks. I do not want to go back to drugs.

RELAPSE

CLIFTON WINSTON

I was married for five years but I am now separated for six months. I lost a beautiful coop, job, wife, daughter, friends, and numerous bank accounts. Now, my credit is very bad. I gave away most of my material things so I could use drugs, especially crack. I picked up drugs to cover the pain in my relationship instead of communicating and getting help. The drugs would always mess everything up. While using, I would stay out three or four days, and then I would detoxify in the house and just lie around and do nothing. It got to a point where I needed the drugs so badly that I began stealing things from my house. I was lying to everyone.

As long as my wife was with me, I knew that everything would be all right and that I could get help, but as I learned later, she could not do anything for me, I had to do it all by myself. So, she left me. I could not believe that she had left me because I was afraid of being alone and abandoned. Thoughts came back of my childhood, and I became scared. When my wife left me, the pain would not go away, so the only way that I could solve it was by using crack. I became worse. I kept calling my wife and making her life hell. It eventually reached a point where I was emotionally and spiritually bankrupt. I had thoughts of suicide but no thoughts of helping myself. I felt no hope. I called my wife one last time, and she told me that I could be drug free if I wanted to, so I listened and I signed myself into a 28-day rehabilitation program.

After I completed the rehabilitation program, they told me that I was going to Long Island, where I was going to be out in the middle of nowhere. Before I went, I was able to catch a train and take it to my apartment so I could collect my stuff. When I was in the apartment I got depressed because there used to be such life and now the apartment was desolate. When I went to Long Island, I was very upset. When I arrived they informed me that, because I arrived on Friday, no one would meet with me until Tuesday. I felt alone and detached from society. I kept wondering if I would ever get back together with my wife. I felt it was not fair because my wife left me because of my disease. This disease robbed me of my life, and it took away everything.

I did not stay with the program in Long Island because I needed to want to be there and I did not want to be there. I also needed to internalize what had happened in my life thus far and reflect in order to get better and I did not want to do this either. I was not content with a roof over my head and food to eat as the Long Island program provided. Instead, I wanted to be productive and make things happen. But, as you will see, everything went wrong.

I came to New York on Sunday. I was debating in my head whether to pick up again or not. All of a sudden the need to pick up got very intense. The disease was cunning and baffling. It was the disease's fault that I picked up again. I decided to put clean urine in a bottle so I could pick up one or two, and nobody would know, because when I got back to my rehabilitation site and they tested me to see if I was clean, I would just swap the urine. Time kept passing and I stayed out all night, got high and used all the money I had. I came to a detoxification program the next day and they gave me a bed.

Coming back here was like déjà vu. Here I am, and I have to do it all again. The pain was still there, the pain that caused me to relapse. I felt like nothing would ever change and my life would never go back to normal. I felt alone and abandoned. It is a feeling of hopelessness. When you go through something again and again, you feel it will never be different.

The intake counselor told me that I used the pain of my wife leaving me as an excuse to use. I believe this because my addiction cost me all my possessions and my life. I always knew if I saw the sun come up one day I would come back to detoxification. Now I want to go to a religious sober house. I know I need to attend meetings so I do not have to run the streets. I lost the ability to speak up because I felt that I was not worth listening to.

Before I picked up drugs again, I was holding my head up high. I was happy. I learned lessons along the way. I learned that things would not fall into my lap. I just want to get my life back together. I know that I do not have a family anymore, and this is something that I have to deal with.

This disease can only hurt you if you use it; and if you do not use it, then you are miserable. Your thoughts and feelings turn into your actions. I have irrational thoughts. I go from feeling to action. I need to take time to think. The feeling of wanting to get high is sometimes stronger than other feelings.

My wife asked me to please let her go. She knew this was the key to my sobriety. As long as I held on to her I would continue to relapse. She knew what I had to do. I was holding on to my wife and the pain, and I was feeling like I wanted to share my life with her. The disease did this. I sometimes feel like it was not me that made a mess of my life but it was my disease. I usually try to take the focus off me and put it on the drug, but my family had to leave because I could not do anything. Now I accepted the fact that she had to go live her life. Now I have to find myself so I can live a drug-free life. The only way is to let go. The problem is that I was stubborn and I did not want to let go. At the core of my disease is self-centeredness. It is like I am a baby. Nobody takes care of grown men, so I have to deal with the consequences. This is the insane part. I look at the consequences and the pain and know that I have to remove the pain. Now that I am becoming clean again, the pain is back, even though I did not feel it at the time. I feel the pain now.

I feel like I lost everything except my life. I feel like Job in the Bible. They took everything from me. The disease puts a wall between my higher power and me because I feel ashamed. I know God has the answers and I have to keep feeling motivated. It is scary because you do not know what this disease will pull next. Drugs used me and I got nothing. Now I realize that I have the faith but I have to now combine it with hard work in order to succeed.

This disease has never told me the truth. Whatever it can do to get me to take the first one it will. If I take just one I will do anything to not stop. It is so weird because when the drug is sitting on the table it has no power. But, when I pick it up and put it inside my body, it causes me to lie, cheat, steal, kill, and become homeless. When the drug is done with you and it got you to lose control, it leaves you and goes into the next person. You can end up in jail, dead, or if you are lucky in rehabilitation. The drug leaves you miserable, dead, or suffering. If I keep up this behavior, I will die. I have been in jail and in institutions, so the next thing left for me is death. So I turn to a higher power, I know I have to take what I can.

It is my fault for picking up the crack. I was wrong to take crack. I have never felt such strong loneliness or abandonment before. I use my drug so I do not have to feel. I took the cowardly way out. I will not give up this time. I do not like feeling pain. I hate emotional pain. I have to stop using excuses and stop punishing myself.

After detoxification, I must live with someone else in his or her house, not in my own by myself. I have to take all this pain with me. The only thing that I can take is the recovery. It is about time for me to live and take care of my health so I can be happy, joyous, and free. All I want is closure and to let go of my past. I have surrendered. I am going to do whatever it takes to stay clean. I am going to do the best I can.

HOMELESS AT 60

CARL JAMES

I was born in 1941. My mom was in prison in New Jersey when she delivered me. They took me away from her. She was only 17. They put me in a foster home in Philadelphia, where I was raised. As I got older, I went to jail at a state prison in New Jersey. I was young and stupid. I have never seen my mother or father. I was in jail for 10 years. I became interested in music because they put me to work in the kitchen, where there was a band. I would always watch this one man play the piano. He was amazing. He was missing his pinkie and half of his ring finger. I was not supposed to be there listening, so I kept getting locked in the hole (solitary confinement). After being in the hole 9–10 times, an officer told me,

"I am tired of putting you in the hole, and I see you love music," so he said he would take me out of the kitchen and put me in the auditorium as a porter. I took the job. I would do anything just to be around music.

They put me in the band. This one person used to show me stuff on the piano. One day he said, 'There is something over there for you," and he brought me a keyboard. He said, "This is what you have to practice on." So, I kept the keyboard the whole time. People would go to the yard and lift weights, but I would just stay and learn from him. He taught me how to read, write, and play music on the keyboard. I got so good that, when the person who was in charge of the band went home, they put me in charge. I asked the man why he did so much for me. He said, "Because you pay attention."

The parole people told me, "You have come a long way, so you will be allowed a visitor." One day the prison guard told me I had a visitor. There was a woman waiting for me. I had never had a visitor before. A man called me and told me my mom was there. She was sitting waiting with apples and candy. I had never met my mother or father. When I walked in the visitors' room, I did not know who I was looking at. There was this short woman standing up. It was my mom. It was a funny feeling for me. She started crying, and I felt nothing. I was now 25, and I felt I was looking at a stranger. She explained to me what happened. She was a chronic alcoholic. I would not call her Mom. I just kept thinking of all the years I missed. I kept saying to myself that maybe she did not want me.

It came time for me to get paroled, November 22, 1963, the same day John F. Kennedy was assassinated. I will never forget this date. They asked me what I would do if they let me go. My mother arranged something with them to have me come to New York. So, I came to New York. My mom brought me clothes and everything. I was never in New York before. I did not know how to get anywhere.

I was not comfortable in New York living with my mom. She was a church person. She cooked food for me and did everything. It was new to me. I looked in the corner and saw a piano, so I stayed there a few days.

One day, I got up and just played the piano. My mother was listening to me, and she told me I played very well. There was a club around the corner. One day I saw a sign that said "guitarist wanted." My mother knew the man in the club. So, my mother convinced me to go down there and audition. He hired me. There was a guy in there practicing. He could play the board but not the pedals, so I auditioned. I stayed there for three years. I got offered drinks all the time. One day a man came in and closed the place down because they were selling drinks without a license. Everyone there liked me because I was nice to everyone.

After that, I moved to another club. Everyone in this club was on dope. I kept drinking to socialize, and drinking became a habit. I stayed there for a year and a half. I moved uptown. I started making money, but I started blowing it as fast as I could make it. I had money in the bank.

One night while I was on the bandstand, they told me I had a phone call. I had gotten married in Philadelphia. My wife always stayed with me. She became sick. She had leukemia. The call said, "Come to Metropolitan Hospital; your wife is in bad shape." The disease went through her body and she passed away.

It destroyed me because I loved that girl. Before she got ill, she used to work so I could stay home and practice. Her death took a lot out of me. She was gone, and there was nothing I could do about it. I started drinking more progressively out of sorrow and pity. Then things started going downhill. I got to the point where there was nothing to live for because she was all I had lived for.

I had two sons. About a month after my wife died, one of my sons was found dead in a hallway. He overdosed. The needle was still in his arm. My other son is doing life in prison. I started hanging out and drinking. Nothing really mattered anymore. I would use my money in the bank to drink.

Then I went to jail in New York. There I lost my cabaret card (like a union card). The card is needed to play where liquor is sold. It is hard to play in New York without that card. I started spending money like it grew on trees. I spent all of the money I had in the bank. I could not play anymore without the card. I knew things were going down. I did not have the desire to get back up. I had nothing else. My wife was dead, my son dead, and my other son in jail.

I wound up on the Bowery paying $10 a night for a room. I used to have a big pretty apartment, and now I am here. I was drinking heavily. One night I was in a club (not playing) and I met a musician named Miles Davis. He told me that he heard that I played the piano. We waited until intermission and he asked me to play one of his songs. So I did play. He then asked me if I had a suit. I said, "No." He asked me if I had a cabaret card. I said, "No." At that time, there were a lot of pawnshops. He put $700 up for me, and he got me a cabaret card. So he told me that he wanted me to play with him. (I told him about the man I met in prison.) About a week later, I was in Germany with him. We played all over Switzerland. He paid top dollar.

We all came back to the states. I met Louis Armstrong. He called me because he knew I knew Miles. Sometimes music can be depressing. Things went on for a few years, and I went down. I figured I had nothing to live for but myself. I gave up on hope, life, and a lot of things.

My story is not unique from anyone else's. Things happen. A lot of people I associated with and the stars I met used drugs. I used to buy dope from the stars. People used to give me big sums of money because they liked me. But things happened, and the drinking progressed out of boredom and loneliness. Everyone ends up on the Bowery or Skid Row. It happens time and time again. Whatever you do excessively is never good.

My drinking got so bad. One night I went out to the subway train on Second Avenue. I leaned over the track drunk; I did not even see the train coming. Why it did not kill me, I will never know. It has been downhill for me.

I have had good breaks and good times also. I met a lot of nice and good people.

Things happen. I asked Miles one day why he took me to so many places. He told me I was a likable person. He said, "People like you."

Alcohol got the best of me. Everybody's life cannot be peaches and cream. Now, I am on in age. Life has passed me by. The other day someone on the street called me Pops. I told him that the trick is not being old, the trick is getting old and that I was lucky enough to get here.

I went to detoxification treatment because I was not working. I could not hold a job because I drank too much. I got a job as a porter, but got fired because of drinking.

Life is a dream. It is what you make of it. I see a lot of young fellows messing up—people who had opportunities look at things differently, people do not know how fortunate they really are.

Maybe this was my destiny. You never know what will happen in life. Who knows? I once said to a young boy, "You look at me like I am old. I may outlive you. You never know."

I wound up a drunk. I was not always a drunk, but this is what happened. I think about this a lot and what I would have done different. I reached a certain age, and now I feel it is too late for me. Alcohol took me to a point where you would no longer recognize me. Things change. The world has changed. People change, everything changes. You never know what destiny will hold.

I cannot bring it back. What happened? You cannot cry over spilled milk. My life has spilled.

It is not the idea that I am bitter because I have wasted my life. I did it. It is no one else's fault. I had a lot of breaks. Sometimes you can have breaks and not know how to use them. Life keeps passing you by.

I have never been homeless until now, 60 years old.

RECOVERY: THE DREAM AND THE LIFE OF A FOOL

CARL JAMES

My life has been in shambles. Drinking alcohol and fast living have made my life so miserable. I have done horrible things to myself. Anyone who wants to live the life I have lived is a fool. All you are doing is fooling yourself. When you are young you think you have all the answers, but you do not. I would advise you change your life and your ways because one day it will catch up with you. Life is a dream.

BUMBLEBEE

JULIE TAYLOR AND ANONYMOUS

> Beneath the ocean, under the sea
> Lives a giant spider named Bumblebee.
> He laughs, he smiles, he wonders, he grins,
> When he looks at me he then becomes free.
> How in the world you might ask
> Did a spider get such a mask?
> How could this bee be under the sea?
> Did he fly, did he crawl, did he swim or flee
> From above the earth to buzz under the sea?
> How in the world you might ask
> Did he get to be such a drunken ass?
> Come back up you silly fool
> Up to the place where you once knew.

TRIGGERS AND CRAVINGS

KATE HARRINGTON

Cheryl, one of my first clients, had been using crack cocaine since her late teens. She is currently 27 years of age. She ran away from home and moved to New York City when she was 17 years old. Cheryl stated that she could not live at home any longer; there was nothing left for her there. When she moved to New York City she was able to get a single room in a hotel-style building. To make money, Cheryl would prostitute herself and use the money to buy drugs. She began prostituting when she started using drugs. This battle with drugs began a war that she continues to fight daily.

Cheryl was initially hospitalized because she had wanted to commit suicide. Prior to admission, she had been on a four- or five-day crack binge and had been gang raped after trying to prostitute herself in a crack house. Cheryl went to the emergency room and told the staff that she was going to kill herself. On evaluation, the doctors in the emergency room admitted her and transferred her to this psychiatric inpatient hospital. She initially slept most of the day, appeared irritable on approach, and wanted nothing to do with me or the hospital. When I administered my evaluation, I was able to learn about Cheryl's past history of drug and alcohol abuse. She told me stories of how she obtained money for the drugs (prostitution), how long she had been using (10 years), and how detoxification and rehabilitation programs never worked for her. Cheryl said being in detoxification and rehabilitation programs were fine when she was there; she was able to comply with the intervention, and almost always felt she had rid herself for good from drugs and alcohol. Once she got back to the streets, however; feeling good and in control, she thought she could handle using drugs again. I wanted to ask her more questions about the drug use, but she said, "All this talk about drugs makes me want them more." It was obvious, or at least I thought it was, that it was too much for her to be talking about her past, and current, drug use. I also had not been able to build a rapport with her, as of yet, and did not want to push her beyond her limits. I would wait until another time to discuss the trigger and cravings of her drug and alcohol abuse.

A few days later, in discharge issues group, I was able to learn more about Cheryl's urge to use drugs and alcohol. She had mentioned to the group that she was nervous about being discharged because she knew she would want to use again. She was asked to describe what her cravings were like. She said she knew she wanted to use crack when she started to crave meat. The reason she knew this was because, when she is not using crack, her drug of choice, she is a vegetarian. I was fascinated by what she was saying and wanted to ask her more questions about the cravings she had and the experiences that go along with these cravings and triggers. We were able to talk a little more about the specific craving for meat and the relationship between this craving and Cheryl's drug use; for example, what to do when she felt this craving coming and what actions to take to try to avoid using drugs. This discussion was limited, however, because there were other people in the group and other issues to discuss; but I planned on discussing this further at another point in time.

Cheryl had a lot of difficulties adhering to limits set in groups, as she would often display attention-seeking behavior. When she would see me on the unit, she would always come up to me, asking me to come to her room to talk about something or showing me projects she had worked on in the skills development group. I had established a rapport with her and felt comfortable talking about her past drug use, including how the substance abuse started.

Cheryl stated that she did not use crack when she lived at home in upstate New York. She had watched her mom take drugs and prostitute herself but did not engage in these activities when she lived at home, before moving to New York City. As stated earlier, Cheryl moved to New York City when she was 17 years old. She had had a few jobs, including working in a retail clothing store and working as a waitress. She lived in a single room in a hotel-style building. She said she loved living there and having her own place. Cheryl stated she did not meet many people when she first moved to New York City. Cheryl's sister also lived in New York City; therefore, many of the people Cheryl met were through her sister. Cheryl's sister had been using crack regularly, even before Cheryl got involved with the drug. Cheryl stated she started using marijuana and drinking when she was about 15 years old but stayed away from crack. When Cheryl would hang out with her sister, she would smoke marijuana and drink beer but would stay away from using other drugs. Eventually, though, the temptation to use crack grew too strong for Cheryl to resist, and she started using it. She stated she thought she would be able to control the drug use, but before she knew it, her life had escalated out of control.

Not long after Cheryl began using crack, she started prostituting. Her crack habit was expensive, and she needed quick and easy money. Cheryl prostituted for an escort service, making enough money to support her habit and herself. Sometimes, she would go on binges and use the drug for three or four days straight; and other times she said she could use the drug intermittently. Usually, though, she would start out using intermittently and end up spiraling out of control.

We discussed what made her crave the drugs. What about the drugs was so enticing? First, she stated that using crack was like no other feeling she had ever experienced. She said she had no worries when she was high; it was like flying. She said she would often start out drinking beer or hard liquor, depending on what kind of mood she was in, then smoke a joint, and then use crack. This was the usual progression. She said the alcohol and marijuana often made her crave crack.

Another trigger was the people she associated with. Her sister and the friends she met through her sister were all involved with drugs and alcohol. There was a lot of environmental influence to use. She says it also seemed like "no big deal," since everyone else was using. She said she knew it was not the best thing to be getting involved in, but the feeling she felt when she used ("invincible") and the people she hung around with made it extremely difficult for her to stop.

Another trigger that Cheryl often battles is the trigger of feeling in control. She says that, when she has money, a place to live, and a feeling that her life is in order, she can use drugs and alcohol; she can control her substance use. This is the reason she thinks that detoxification and rehabilitation programs do not work for her. She thinks she can control her substance use. She said, however, that she realizes now that she cannot control the use.

As stated earlier, she has been using crack for about 10 years and alcohol and marijuana for slightly longer. She said she has gone through cycles of having housing and a job to having nothing. She said she goes from being in control of her life to being completely in a "vacuum of drugs, sex, and craziness." On top of everything, Cheryl is also fighting the battle of AIDS. She thinks she got AIDS from an ex-boyfriend, but nonetheless it is another battle she fights. She said there are times when she uses substances because she has the mindset that it does not matter what happens, since she is destined to die anyway, to times when she feels empowered and wants to kick the habit for good, then help other people who suffer from addiction.

Cheryl stated there are many different triggers and cravings, everything ranging from emotions, to environmental circumstances, to thinking she can casually handle intermittent drug use, to life stressors. She said, again, she is ready to receive help and kick her substance abuse problems for good. She wants to attend a combination program, one that specializes in persons who have AIDS and substance abuse problems. She thinks this time will be different; she is ready for a permanent change. Cheryl has expressed that she knows there will always be triggers and cravings, that it is just a matter of identifying them and finding another way to cope, other than the drug use. She knows it will be a tough road ahead, but one that she has traveled down before, one that she is ready to travel down again, for the last time.

PREGNANT AND ADDICTED

KELLY MORALES

When I first encountered Jacklynn, many emotions arose that I was not quite sure how to handle. I had worked with many clients before on the detoxification unit, but she was different. Jacklynn was the first detoxification client I met who was pregnant, and very pregnant at that. Jacklynn was in her seventh month and had been using drugs throughout her entire pregnancy.

Knowing that the protocol for a pregnant woman allows for a longer stay than the average detoxification stay, which is three to five days, I was aware that Jacklynn was going to be on the detoxification unit for just over two weeks.

I wondered, *Why was she admitted now? And why did it take so long into this pregnancy for her to come for help?* As a mother myself, I was very scared for this unborn child. The adverse effects of the drugs that Jacklynn had used on this baby throughout an important time in the development of this unborn child were something I could not help thinking about.

Throughout the duration of Jacklynn's stay, she and I spoke every day. She always found her way down to the activity room, and we would talk endlessly. She loved talking and having someone to open up to and share her past. I quickly became at ease with Jacklynn. There was a level of comfort between us, as if we had known each other for years, and I was there to listen.

Jacklynn grew up in Harlem. Her family was broken up; between her mother and father, she had 14 brothers and 4 sisters in all. There was no family structure or authority in Jacklynn's life. Jacklynn was her own responsibility; she came and went when she wanted and did as she pleased. Having no parental structure, Jacklynn dropped out of school in the 10th grade. Her life then had no direction. Jacklynn hung out on the street until all hours of the night. At this point in Jacklynn's life, she occasionally drank alcohol and smoked marijuana; this lifestyle led to a downward spiral in Jacklynn's life, starting with teenage pregnancy.

Jacklynn became pregnant with her first child at age 16 and her second child when she was 20. Shortly after her second child was born, Jacklynn began to use crack. Over the next five years, Jacklynn had two more children. Somehow, Jacklynn always managed to clean herself up during the last three to four months of her pregnancy, so her children were not born addicted to drugs and removed from her care. Jacklynn was now 26 years old with four children, living in the ghetto, supported by welfare, and addicted to drugs. Jacklynn's life was out of control; she soon began using heroin and was addicted now to both crack and heroin.

At age 28, Jacklynn became pregnant with child number five, but this time things changed. Jacklynn's baby came early and was addicted to drugs. Jacklynn was unable to take this baby home. Her child was taken away from her, and her four other children were placed into the foster care system. Jacklynn said that having her baby taken away from her after being in labor for 15 hours was something she would never forget. Her life was filled with a pain she could never explain. Jacklynn remembers the last time she saw her baby before he was taken away, he was only three days old, but he seemed so small because the hospital diaper was so large compared to his fragile little body.

After this, Jacklynn went back out on the street, with no children, and was now using crack and heroin more than she ever had before. Her addiction was taking over everything. She began prostitution to support her habit. Sounding disgusted with herself, Jacklynn said, "You would not believe the things an addict would do for drugs; it is insanity." She remembers standing on the street corners in Harlem and the Bronx, fornicating with anyone and giving sexual pleasure to anyone who could pay her with money or drugs. Jacklynn recalled providing her services anywhere available, sometimes in the person's home or her own apartment, a cheap motel (usually known as a crackhead hangout), in the customer's car, or even right there on the street.

Jacklynn, now 37 years old, has continued this lifestyle of abusing drugs, prostitution, and never regaining custody of her children. Jacklynn, sounding upset with herself, trying to talk through the lump in her throat, said, "I never even attempted to clean my life up after my children were taken away from me."

Jacklynn has been prostituting herself now for nine years after she lost her children; she had never used protection and had never become pregnant. Jacklynn did not think she could get pregnant anymore. To her surprise, at the age of 37, Jacklynn became pregnant with her sixth child. This pregnancy stirred up a lot of painful thoughts and memories. Jacklynn was struggling inside. Unfortunately, she was not ready to take the steps she needed to take to clean up her life. Jacklynn continued prostitution and drug use throughout the first two trimesters of her pregnancy.

As her stomach began to show, Jacklynn would wear black to hide her pregnancy. She did this so she could continue selling her body. This was her only source of income. She said it was hard to support her habit, because some men refused her services once they noticed her condition. Because of her pregnancy, she was performing more fellatio than intercourse, which did not pay as much.

Jacklynn recalls seeing many women on the streets just like her—pregnant and prostituting themselves. Jacklynn recalled seeing one of these women sitting on the steps in front of a building as the baby came out of her body into her sweatpants, but this woman would not leave to go to the hospital until the "dope man" came. This sight frightened Jacklynn and brought up her own painful memories. She knew this child would be addicted to drugs and taken away, if it even lived at all.

For the first time in her life, Jacklynn decided it was time to get help. She decided she wanted to be off drugs; she could not bear the pain of the thought of having this child taken from her, as her last baby was. She thought for a moment and said, "It is so sad. I could pass my baby today on the street. I would never know that that was my child, nor would it know I was its real mother." She has memories of what her other children looked like, but so many years have passed she is afraid that they might not even be recognizable to her if she could see them. She figured, if she cleaned herself up, that this could be her chance to make up for her past mistakes and finally be a real parent. This is what led Jacklynn to the detoxification unit and her present situation.

Because it was her first time in any detoxification unit, she did not know what to expect. She was surprised that not all individuals who are in detoxification want to get clean (drug free). Jacklynn imagined a detoxification unit like some magical place that detoxifies you, and the people who go to detoxification are dedicated and have seen the error of their ways and want to change.

During Jacklynn's first couple of days on the unit, she was approached by an individual who was supposedly trying to clean up her life, too; this client managed to sneak contraband onto the unit in her hair and propositioned Jacklynn. Jacklynn was now faced with the option of using, which she very much wanted to be able to do, or staying drug free. She told the client that she was interested in buying from her, and Jacklynn went to her room to get some money.

When Jacklynn got to her room she began a fight with herself and broke down. Jacklynn wanted to take the drugs, but she did not. She thought about the consequences before she acted and decided it was not worth it. If she got high, chances were it would not end there. She would be discharged from the detoxification unit, with no where else to go but back to the streets and continue this vicious cycle, which would eventually end in the loss of this baby she wanted to keep. The thought of having this option available to her on the unit was something she knew she could not fight for long, so she informed hospital staff and the temptation was removed.

I performed an assessment on Jacklynn in order to identify facilitators and barriers that could be used to help overcome some of these obstacles. Jacklynn decided she needed to work on stress management. Jacklynn has used drugs to mange her stress in the past, and she was unaware of healthy ways by which she could deal with stressful situations. We talked about the groups that were offered on the unit and which would be beneficial for her to attend.

Jacklynn put a valiant effort into her recovery. She always attended intervention groups. She would preach to other clients about the benefit of coming to the activity room for groups. She would always manage to talk other clients into attending therapeutic groups. I stopped in Jacklynn's room one day. She had been in detoxification for so long and had always kept herself occupied with some activity or craft that she obtained from the activity room that her room looked like none other. She had her room decorated with pictures and crafts she had made. There was such color and character to her room that, for a moment, it did not seem like a hospital room.

Jacklynn learned she had a strong interest in arts and crafts. She discovered that while engaged in crafts she felt calm and at ease. Being occupied with crafts was a constructive way for her to utilize her time in a stress-reducing manner.

Jacklynn loved the feeling of the activity room. To her, the room felt safe and warm, like a home. For the first time in years, Jacklynn felt a sense of stability and structure in her life. She was sleeping and eating regularly, her time was occupied constructively, and she had a room of her own (something a lot of us take for granted). Jacklynn was finally receiving prenatal care, which she had never received before.

Her life was changing. She spoke adamantly about the baby she was carrying and how her life was changing because of her pregnancy. She was finally getting on the right track. She said it was God's way of giving her another chance. She would sit in the activity room and make things for her baby, saying things like, "This will look nice over the baby's crib," and "I will always cherish this as a reminder of where I was, to keep me strong and moving in the right direction."

Although I felt Jacklynn had a strong will to remain sober, I know what struggles and stress come along with taking care of a baby. The responsibilities are immense and could easily become overwhelming, especially for a single parent who is trying to get her life together. We spoke about these issues regularly, and occasionally I would bring her parenting magazines for her to read and educate herself on her own time. We sometimes would talk about the stress and struggles I endured as a parent. I was trying to open her eyes to the fact that dealing with parenting is hard, even for those who do not have other issues, such as addiction, to overcome.

Knowing how important it is to have a support network, I looked into various programs available for pregnant women as well as women who have children. I was telling Jacklynn about programs available for mothers and expecting mothers. She quickly became interested, and coincidentally, a representative from a program came to our unit to speak about what is offered at their facility the very next day.

I sat and listened as the representative spoke about her program and watched Jacklynn as her eyes lit while the speaker spoke about the program for mothers and children. Jacklynn was alert and interested. She asked so many questions. Jacklynn wanted to know how to apply for this program, and what steps she needed to take to become enrolled. Soon after the meeting ended, Jacklynn set up an appointment to speak with her counselor. She wanted to discuss her aftercare plans. She felt she now had a plan and needed help putting it into action.

A long road lies ahead for Jacklynn. She had been doing three to four bags of heroin a day for 10 years and about $30 worth of crack per day for 16 years. Jacklynn had never been tested for AIDS, a disease to which she was possibly exposed with the lifestyle she had led, and Jacklynn had no home of her own to raise a child. Although Jacklynn has a lot of things going against her, she still seemed positive and had a lot of hope for her future. She spoke about eventually trying to regain some type of relationship with her other children, once she was sober and had a life she is proud of.

So how many detoxifications does it take? Unfortunately, there is no definite answer. For everyone it is different. This was Jacklynn's first detoxification, after using drugs for most of her life, and I hope it will be her last. Jacklynn said she would call us in the activity room when she had the baby. I hope to hear that call from her and run into her someday in the future, hoping that she is still clean and that for her it only took one detoxification.

UNDER THE RAINBOW

CHRISTINE WEISS

"Growing up, there are two absolutes in life, truth and lies." This is the first sentence that Luke told me upon entering his hospital room. I continued by introducing myself and then asked him what he meant by this statement. Luke stated that his first memories of his parents were of their instilling in him the utmost importance of always telling and indeed living the truth. In contrast, lies were the telltale sign that a person was not merely bad but outright evil. This, he said, is the philosophy of life and religion in his family's Christian home.

As an intern, it is my job to orient and evaluate clients on my team. Before I meet a client, I always read the chart, so I know if the client is dangerous or easily agitated. From the chart, I learned the details of Luke's suicide attempts, his drug addictions, and his HIV-positive status. I knew about his male companions and his severe depression. Therefore, I had a picture in my head of this horrible-looking drug addict. I expected him to be overweight, bearded, and completely disheveled. I did not expect what was to follow.

When I first walked into his room, I saw him lying on the bed with the blanket covering his entire body, including his head. I introduced myself as his intern and asked him if it was all right for me to ask him a few questions. He replied with a very stern "no," then he uncovered his face and had a big smile and said, "Ha ha, just kidding." I then noticed his striking good looks, blond hair, and blue eyes. He looks about 28 years old, is about 5' 10", and weighs approximately 170 lbs. When he spoke, it was obvious to me that he is an intelligent individual. He maintains good eye contact and is able to communicate well.

All I could think about was, What could have possibly happened to this man, with his looks and intelligence, to get him to this point in his life? I asked Luke if I could interview him and then write up his story, the story of a man who has struggled throughout his life to hold inside how he really felt and be a model son to his wealthy, religious Virginia family.

He sat across the table from me, slouched over, waiting for my first question. I began to ask him some very simple questions, such as where he works, where he lives, and if he talks to his family often. Luke is the kind of person who, if he begins to speak, cannot stop talking; he loves to tell his story. He even offered to write the story on paper, but I asked him just to speak to me.

Luke currently lives in a one-bedroom apartment and works in pharmaceutical advertising. He is an only child. His father used to own a company that sells large farm equipment, so Luke thinks. His mother held a few small jobs to fill up some time, but she was socializing with friends most of the time. Luke never said anything nice or warm about his mother. The family has been in Virginia for several generations. As the only child, it was Luke's job to carry on the family name. It was a constant joke in the family that Luke would have at least five sons, since he was the only male child in the entire family with the family name.

Luke stated that, as a young child, he was afraid of blowing his nose the wrong way. Any transgression against the wills and laws of God would result in a certain and swift punishment from above. At the age of 7, Luke began to question the church's and his family's belief system. Of course, his parents were not happy with this and punished him when he asked any questions about his religion. One time, he asked his parents why he had to go to Sunday school while his friends played outside. His parents locked him in his room every day after school for a week. They thought that this would stop him from questioning his faith. This began to make him furious over the whole situation and further question his faith.

Luke was an excellent student in school, receiving mostly As and Bs in order to please his parents. To him, schoolwork was an escape; he immersed himself in his work and was the model student. When he was in fifth grade, he received an award at graduation for having the highest average in the school.

During the interview, I began to imagine how proud his parents must have been when he received the award or when he received high grades in school. Except for the time he questioned his faith, everything in his life seemed perfect. He had everything that money could buy, nice clothes and the best looking cars. He was raised by a nanny and always had servants at his disposal. From an outsider's point of view, it looked as if Luke had the perfect life.

Luke began to tell me how his father was never around to talk to, always working, selling farm equipment, "so I think." His mother was too busy socializing with the neighbors. He stated that, "She cared too much about what the neighbors thought." His mother wanted neighbors and friends to think that the family was close and well to do. As a child, he was alone the majority of the time. He had to entertain himself or find friends in the neighborhood to play with. Luke, at the age of 9, began to play with Jason, a boy who lived two blocks away. Jason's parents were around most of the time, and Luke enjoyed talking to them. Luke and Jason had a special friendship; they were always together, playing ball or studying for an exam. Luke always envied the relationship that Jason had with his parents. Luke wanted his parents to be loving and caring like Jason's.

I then realized that maybe Luke's life was not so perfect. He was just a boy that was trying very hard to please his parents to get some kind of verbal approval from them. His parents praised him only for his good grades; they never showed any other attention toward him. He wanted someone to show affection toward him. He said that neither his mom nor his dad ever hugged or kissed him when he was a child. He was neglected, and although it is not considered child abuse, it really should be. His father was never home. He suspects that his father was having an affair but there was no proof.

Luke's parents fought a lot while he was in high school and finally divorced by the time he was 18 years old. This did not surprise Luke, because of the constant screaming and yelling in the house. Luke would visit his dad on weekends, but at 19 years old, he went away to college and that stopped any of the weekend visitations. Luke attended an Ivy League school that made his parents proud. He still visited his mother on the holidays but stopped going to church with her.

Luke started to tell me about another issue, his homosexuality. "I am gay," a fact that he had known since he was very young. He has referred to homosexuality as, "the love that dare not speak its name." Indeed, in his hometown, the word was never mentioned at all except during the preacher's every other year sermon about man not laying next to man, for this was an abomination. As a 7-year-old, the first time Luke remembers hearing this sermon, he did not have a clue what the preacher was talking about. He did notice that this sermon made most of the men squirm in their seats and say, "Amen," more often than any other sermon.

Luke did not actually have the term or explanation of gay until he was in third grade, when he learned that the word *gay* means that the individual is associated somehow with the devil and is damned for the rest of his life. Luke did not realize he was gay until he was in high school and did not understand why he was attracted to the same sex. Luke, knowing that being gay meant that you were damned, kept his feelings to himself. He felt that he should pretend that he was someone else. He did not think that family and friends would accept him unless he pretended to be something that he is not, a straight man. He continued to bury himself and his true emotions in his schoolwork.

As he grew older, this pattern of burying himself and his emotions in his schoolwork grew more pronounced. Luke started law school at the age of 21. In addition, Luke also discovered that drugs and alcohol were ways of numbing his emotional conflicts. He could never be himself. He was trying desperately to fit in with societal norms and be the good son that his parents wanted him to be. But he could no longer pretend to be a religious heterosexual man. This led him to "come out of the closet." At the age of 21, he told his family that he is gay.

Luke's parents disowned him and he lost his inheritance. He said, "I can no longer live the lie that I have been living my entire life." Luke said, "I had a choice to make, either to live truthfully or to live a life of deceit." Although Luke was happy about the choice he made to tell his family, he became depressed and turned to drugs and alcohol to numb his feelings of losing his family.

Luke continued to drink alcohol on a daily basis and dropped out of law school, becoming easily depressed about his family's rejection of him. He would try to talk to his family on a regular basis, by either calling or stopping by the house. His family would not speak to him and asked him never to come home. Luke would drink every night to forget about his family's rejection.

At this point, Luke asked me what I thought about his coming out of the closet. I told him that, if he felt that he had to tell his family and stop living the lie, then that was the correct thing to do. I thought about how he needed to tell his family what he really felt inside in order to make himself happy. He could no longer live the lie that his parents wanted him to live. I feel that if your family loves you, then they will support you in anything that you decide to do. For some reason, I did not tell this to Luke. I think that I was afraid of rubbing in how loving and caring my family is. Instead, I just said, "It must have been difficult to tell your family that you are gay, especially since they have been telling you for years that you must carry on the family's name." He replied by stating that it took him several years to get the courage to tell his parents because he knew that they would not approve of this lifestyle. I kept thinking how hard it must have been for him to tell his parents how he really felt inside, just to be ostracized from them. Even though he was never very close to his parents, they were still his family.

Luke's first relationship with a man was with Jason, the boy he grew up with. They lived together for about six years. They both were addicted to drugs and alcohol. Somehow they were able to get good jobs to support themselves, although being out sick a lot was normal for them. Luke and Jason broke up when Luke was 27 years old. Luke took the breakup hard and became depressed. He had a plan to commit suicide by jumping in front of a train and left a note for Jason. Jason found the note before Luke was able to complete the act of killing himself. Jason called the police and they found Luke, crying in the subway station by his apartment. The police took him to the hospital where they gave him some antidepressants and kept him overnight. In the morning, they let him go. He went back to the apartment to live for three months, when Jason asked him to leave. Luke took his things and moved into an apartment by himself. Luke had never been alone before. He no longer had his boyfriend or his family.

Luke spent several nights at bars picking up several different men, just so he would not have to spend another night in bed alone. He would drink alcohol on a daily basis and do cocaine and heroin at least three times a week. Meanwhile, Luke's job in advertising was suffering from his all-night endeavors to bars and his excessive drinking to numb his emotions. He somehow managed not to be fired. He is in pharmaceutical advertising. This job requires a lot of creativity and intelligence.

Luke wanted to take more antidepressants, so he had three primary care physicians. In a suit and tie, he looks professional, and he would ask the doctors for a prescription. The doctors would not think that there was any kind of foul play. Each would write him prescriptions for antidepressant drugs. Therefore, he always had a large supply.

Luke, in the last few months, has continued to sleep with anyone that would stay over with him. He admitted to losing all self-esteem. Luke volunteered to be involved in an HIV study in which he was tested weekly; the tests were negative until just last week, when one of the tests came back positive. Luke became severely depressed and once again tried to commit suicide. This time he took several antidepressant medications at once with as much alcohol as he could swallow. Luke then tied a plastic bag over his head. Luke had been in the apartment for 10 hours with a bag over his head before he was found. He had left his suicide note on the apartment door. His neighbor found it and called the police. Luke is currently in the hospital's inpatient psychiatric unit trying to piece his life back together.

I remember learning in school that men are more likely to actually succeed at a suicide attempt than women. Men usually commit suicide violently, jumping off a building or in front of a train. Luke in his first attempt to commit suicide left a note in the apartment for a long time. In his second suicide attempt, he sat in his apartment for 10 hours with a bag over his head. This leads me to believe that Luke did not want to kill himself; he just wanted some attention from Jason or from his family. It reminds me of what he said earlier, that he would immerse himself in his schoolwork, have a high GPA, and receive attention from his parents.

In the hospital, Luke attends all the group therapy sessions that are given. He is cooperative and easygoing; I guess that is why I decided to write about him. Luke spends the majority of his day pacing the hallways, telling me that "I am climbing the walls." This could be part of his drug addiction coming out. Luke stated that he feels like a caged animal locked away for doing something wrong.

He made me think about how I would feel, being locked on this unit. I consider myself to be somewhat bright and articulate. The unit does not have a lot of activities that stimulate thinking. I thought about how bored he must be, spending the majority of his day watching the television. I started bringing Luke a copy of the *New York Times* after I was finished reading it. I did this for the three days prior to his discharge.

As an intern, I lead group therapy sessions in areas such as self-awareness, goals, grooming, and current events. When I attend rounds, I am asked about the patients assigned to me. Yesterday, the physician asked me about how Luke was doing in groups and if he was attending. At first, I felt that I was put on the spot and everyone was staring at me, waiting for an answer. I then said that he comes to every group and fully participates. He is eager to leave and wants to get well. Luke is functional; he showers daily, brushes his hair, and makes his bed. The only thing he does not do is wear street clothes. He wears hospital attire daily. I knew that Luke would not be at the hospital for more than a week. In rounds on Friday, we talked about discharging Luke to his apartment and an outpatient drug rehabilitation program on Monday.

Luke said that he will no longer do drugs. Something tells me that Luke is telling the truth and does want to get better. He has a long road of drug rehabilitation in front of him, considering that he used drugs on a daily basis prior to hospitalization. Luke has a good job in advertising and an apartment to return to. He has some very supportive friends, who come every day to visit him in the hospital. Part of me says that he will go to rehabilitation and get well.

My biggest fear is that he may not go to drug rehabilitation and will go back to his lonely apartment, with no support from his family or friends. Luke could end up in the same hospital with another suicide attempt. This time, however, the bag will accidentally be too tight and he may die. I think that Luke tries to commit suicide to get some attention from his ex-boyfriend Jason or even from his parents. He really does not want to kill himself.

Luke's mom does not know that he has been hospitalized; his father knows but refuses to come and see him. In addition, his parents do not know that he is HIV positive. He said that he does not want them to know that he is sick and that he no longer is speaking to them. I believe that, if his parents knew that he was HIV positive, they would come to New York and spend some time with him. It is hard for me to believe that deep down his parents do not still care for him and want him to be healthy and have a good career.

After I completed the interview, I realized that Luke was just like you and me. Growing up, he played with his friends went to parties and had dreams for the future. Luke just wants to be accepted for who he is, not the man he was pretending to be. He stated, "I do not want to continue to live the life of deceit and lies, I am happy with the choice that I have made." His family would not accept him for who he is, and as a result his family disowned him. I sometimes wonder what I would do if my family disapproved of my life. I am not sure that I would have the courage to tell my family something that they did not want to hear like Luke did.

CLIENT-CENTERED REASONING QUESTIONS FOR THE NARRATIVES IN CHAPTER 11

You just read about the lives of 11 people with addictions: Julie, two anonymous writers, Mandy, Jerome, Joy, Clifton, Carl, Cheryl, Jacklynn, and Luke. Answer the following questions based on their stories, using quotes and supporting material whenever possible:

1. Make a list of all the things these people have in common. Make another list of all the ways that they are different from one another.
2. Identify the reasons each person started to use drugs for the first time. What are some additional reasons people may try drugs for the first time? Have you ever tried drugs? What led you to try them?
3. List the triggers that caused each of these people to use drugs after the first time. What are some other triggers not mentioned in these narratives that often cause people to relapse?
4. Identify the things that helped each of these people stay clean (refrain from using drugs). What other things often help people stay clean?
5. How do you know the difference between abuse, dependency, and recreational drug use? Define each. Pinpoint the time at which each of these main characters made the transition from recreational substance use to abuse to dependency.
6. What is polysubstance abuse? Which of these people would you consider polysubstance abusers and which not? Why or why not?
7. What effect (positive and negative) did each of the families have on these people's recoveries from substance abuse?
8. Identify what you find to be the most disturbing issue in each narrative. Why is it so disturbing to you? How would you solve the problems around each to provide effective intervention?
9. Which areas of life do addictions affect (be specific—i.e., finances, children)? Describe how the addiction affects each area and why the addiction has this effect.

10. List the losses each person incurred because of addiction. Include physical, emotional, spiritual, and material losses.
11. Identify each person's facilitators and barriers.
12. What precautions would you take with this population and why?

LOGS FROM A DETOXIFICATION UNIT

PHILIP MACRI

3/23—We started the day with a staff meeting, where I realized that detoxification was a business like any other. I found out that there is a real competition between hospitals with detoxification wards for so-called bodies. Detoxification is a real moneymaker for hospitals, and they like to keep the place as full as possible.

Sara, the OTA of the department, and I ran an assessment group in the afternoon. One person in the group was here for alcohol detoxification. Sarah immediately picked up on this, based on the redness of his face and the tremor in his hand. All new clients need to be assessed. The assessment asks questions about work history, skills, stress and time management, and hygiene. It is an excellent tool to help clients look inside themselves and let them become aware of how their substance abuse has affected all areas of their lives. After the assessment, we talked about what they wrote down and ways in which they could improve themselves in these areas. One client who was detoxifying from heroin was very agitated and really did not want to be in the group. He spoke as if he had all the answers but did not know how to follow through. He was yelling and cursing at Sara, not showing her any respect. She was able to redirect the conversation and have other clients speak about their problems. She did not let herself get angry, like I think the client wanted her to. Sara is very good at dealing with difficult personalities and has an understanding of clients. What clients say is not always how they truly feel. They often have a lot of built-up anger toward themselves and society. They say that society views them as second-class citizens and they need to voice how they feel in ways that are different than others would. Detoxification is a difficult part of recovery. Compassion can be a strong therapeutic tool.

3/24—I attended a group on the detoxification ward that discussed an outpatient program available to clients once they finished detoxification. It is a program where clients could go to get continued counseling and support. When looking around the room during the group, I could get an idea of who was really interested in continuing their recovery program and who was just going through the motions. Clients that said they were going home after detoxification probably will not stay drug free. Detoxification is not rehabilitation; it is only a stepping-stone to a long road of recovery.

3/25—Some people in detoxification have many questions about how they got here. During a group today a woman asked, "Why me?" Before Sara answered, she asked if anyone in the group would like to answer her question. One gentleman in the group raised his hand and answered with, "Why not you?" I was awestruck by an answer so simple yet so powerful. As the gentleman went on, he said to the woman, "We are the ones that pick up the bottle to drink. We are the ones who put the pipe to our mouths. We are the ones who put that needle in our arms." Detoxification is a place where past decisions can be changed. It is a place for reflection and a place where people can clear their heads so that new, more positive decisions can be made.

3/26—I sat in on a mandatory client meeting run by a counselor named Don. Don is a recovering addict and has been for 29 years. He knows what clients have been through and what they are going through. Don does not let clients fool themselves or others. His group was very powerful. He was confrontational and truthful with them.

When sitting in on the group and observing clients, I realize that I cannot figure out which ones will go on to rehabilitation and recover, but I can tell which ones may not. The ones I feel will not are the ones looking out the window or not paying attention. I hung on to every word Don said, and I am not someone looking to get clean. A lot of what counselors say fall on deaf ears. I have come to realize that this is all right. If people are not ready to recover, there is nothing you can say to change that. I hear stories of family members of clients who have begged, bribed, and pleaded with them to stop using. If clients are not willing to listen to people that love and care for them, they probably will not listen to others. Counselors understand this and do not let this discourage them. They know that they need to try to help everyone here. Ultimately, it is up to the clients to use the help or not.

3/27—Today we played therapeutic bingo with 23 people. Each person received a prize before the game started, so even if they did not win at bingo, they went away with something. The game can get out of control. It is important to lay the ground rules from the beginning. Someone who wins needs to publicly answer a question pertaining to recovery before receiving a prize. It is important for clients to have fun while they work their recovery. Learning how to have fun through an activity that is drug free is part of recovery. It is important for clients to be involved in therapeutic groups during detoxification, not only to benefit from the contents of the group but also to avoid the negative talk that occurs with clients who do not attend groups but stay in the solarium and talk to each other. Some people that are on the detoxification ward are not there to recover but rather for rest or food. These people plan to leave the hospital and go back on the street to do what they were doing before they came here. They talk about getting high when they leave and where they are going to go to get their drugs. It is good to get the clients who are serious about their recovery out of that negative environment and into a more positive one like the activity room where we run groups. The groups we run vary from crafts to stress management to goal setting. A lot of clients lack social skills, caused by isolation and depression brought on by drugs and alcohol. Self-disclosure is a good way to help people get to understand themselves better so they can interact with others in a more positive way. They need to learn acceptance of themselves before they can accept others.

3/29—We did a craft activity today that involved woodworking. Being a carpenter for 10 years, I felt comfortable with this task and could foresee some of the benefits it may have for the clients. Most clients never do crafts except when they are in the hospital, but crafts are an excellent way to stay occupied when they are not in the hospital. Staying involved in activities that are void of drugs and alcohol is one of the best ways to keep from relapsing.

3/30—Self-awareness is a very important part of detoxification and recovery. It is very helpful for clients to write down why they came here, where they are going, and how they are going to succeed in their recovery. The reason it is important to write it down is because it can be easily referred to rather than possibly forgotten due to consistent use of drugs and alcohol. I have found it extremely helpful to keep a daily log since I have been here. It forces me to look inside myself and think about what I have really gained from the day's experience. I find that I learn something every day, and I am a better person and therapist for it. A client told me today that I have helped him more than anyone on the ward to find what his reasons for relapse were and how he can avoid them in the future. I found great satisfaction in his thanks, and it made me even more eager to help others who want to recover from their addictions.

3/31—Today, I was speaking to a client who was being discharged tomorrow. We sat down in the activity room and talked about his plans for discharge and what he wanted to do in the future. As we were speaking, other clients walked by and wanted to know if we were having a group. I told them we were just sitting here talking, and if they wanted to come in and join us, they could. Before I knew it, eight clients were sitting around the table talking about what they wanted to do after discharge and what their goals for the future were. I realized this was my first unsupervised and unplanned group.

4/5—Today a new student, Joan, started on the detoxification unit. We went over what goes on in the detoxification unit, and I introduced her to various staff members. I was able to answer any questions she had. I find it comforting to know that, after two weeks of working here, I was able to do all this and feel comfortable with it.

4/6—Some people do not want to attend groups. They have often been betrayed in their lives and sometimes do not know whom to trust. Some have never had anyone take an interest in them and cannot understand that there are people who actually want to help them.

I once thought that, if clients attended groups from the start of their recovery and engaged in positive conversation, they were serious about their recovery. I find this not to be so, based on people I have met here that have done all this and then discharge themselves early. I am constantly learning that you cannot categorize people into the ones that will make it and the ones that will not.

4/7—When listening to people's stories I realize that the problems I complain about in my life are nothing compared to the things that have happened in their lives. They often tell me about their parents, who were both unemployed, addicted to drugs or alcohol, and living with many children in the house. There are stories of sexual abuse by family members, such as uncles and stepfathers. One client told me that he started to drink alcohol at age 7, when his uncle gave him liquor because he enjoyed watching him get drunk and stumble around. Some clients have never left the block they were born on, let alone their neighborhood. When people grow up in an environment where things like these go on, they do not know another way of life.

In the afternoon, Joan and I ran a crafts group. Working on craft projects gives clients a feeling that they can control some aspects of their lives. Clients get great satisfaction out of creating something they can keep and show or give to others. One client told me that this was the first thing she had ever completed.

4/8—Therapeutic groups are mandatory because they offer clients a forum to speak about problems or concerns they may have. They also help clients understand their options about where they can go once they leave the hospital. The hospital has people come in and talk about the dangers of consistent drug and alcohol abuse and give them information about HIV prevention and nutrition.

I am learning to do assessments more efficiently. Some clients are very needy because they have no one to speak to about the problems they face in their lives or the feelings they have. If you let them, some clients will talk forever, so I need to use my professional experience to decipher what is important information and then help them understand why it is something we should work on. Time is very limited and I am learning to divide it equally among the tasks that need to be done during the day.

4/9—The spirituality group is very important to some clients, who benefit from it greatly. There is a real sense of comfort in the group. When speaking to clients afterward, they tell me it really helped them look inside themselves and helps them determine what they need to do when they leave the hospital.

4/12—I ran a group today that I developed, called the process of making changes group. We went through the various stages people need to go through in order to make changes in their lives. The clients were very receptive and verbal during the group. One client, who had been in detoxification eight times, had a lot of information for the other group members. Clients answered questions at the bottom of the handout, such as what important changes are you currently working on, what stage in the process are you at, and who can assist you to move forward in the process? We discussed their answers at the end of the group.

4/13—A client told me a story that helped me understand how a drug addiction can control every aspect of a person's life, especially their mind. He explained how, one day, he walked into a shooting gallery. Not the type of shooting gallery where people go to shoot guns, although I am sure there were guns there. No, this is the type of shooting gallery where addicts go to shoot heroin to get high. The client told me about a beautiful woman that walked into this shooting gallery to get her fix. She sat down with her works, which is what addicts call the equipment they use to get high with. This would include a syringe, lighter, water, and spoon to melt the heroin in and a string or belt to tie off with, so that they can find a vein more easily. The woman wore a pair of pants that came up to her knees. She rolled one of her pant legs toward her thigh. She removed a bandage on her leg. She then took a pair of tweezers and started to remove maggots from the open sore on her leg and place them on the table in front of her. She then prepared her fix and injected it into an exposed vein in her wound. When she finished, she placed the bugs back into her leg, put the bandage back on, and rolled her pant leg back down. The client who told me this story asked her, "Why do you not go to the hospital and get that taken care of?" The woman said that, if she went to the hospital, they would take her leg and she would not be able to get high for a while. The maggots that she was keeping in her leg were eating the gangrene that had developed in the wound and was slowing the infection down.

When the client told me this I remember being in shock. I thought to myself, this is what a drug addiction can make you do and think. To neglect your body and risk your life, just for the sake of getting high. The client later told me that, when he saw this, he then realized he needed to get help before he started to act like this woman did.

4/14—During the goal-setting group, clients discussed the goals they wanted to achieve in their lives. Most clients said they wanted clean time, meaning time away from drugs. Others wanted to get back to living normally again, and others spoke about financial success. When listening to their stories, I realized that they needed to learn how to write down their goals in short- and long-term formats. I got a sense that these goals they set for themselves were goals they wanted to achieve immediately and did not understand the steps involved or the time they needed to invest in themselves to achieve these goals. People with addictions sometimes want instant gratification and usually are often not willing to wait.

Many clients have difficulty seeing the bigger picture and understanding what is really important because drugs or alcohol have distorted their perception. They do not know how to plan for the future because, for most of them, there is no future. If they could use the conviction they have when they seek drugs to enhance their lives in a positive way, they may be able to achieve more goals. It helps to teach them that everything needs to be done in small steps. There are so many skills that people have never developed or lost because of drugs or alcohol that need to be rekindled or learned.

4/15—There are a couple of young people on the ward that I feel are not really serious about their recovery. They come from broken families, like most of the clients here. Older clients, who have been addicted for many years and have been in and out of detoxifications, have basically run out of excuses and understand that, to fully recover, they need to surrender to their addiction and ask for help. These younger people with addictions do not understand surrender and are full of excuses. Two young clients are friends on the outside and basically came here because they have no place to live and thought it might be fun to go to detoxification together. I have tried numerous times to help them make the most of their time here and not waste it by playing pool all day and not attending groups. I think they need to learn for themselves, and no matter what I or anyone else says to them, if they are resistant, intervention will not work. I hope for their sake that they learn sooner rather than later.

4/20—I met a client today that reminded me so much of a friend I once had. He was the type of person who was not comfortable being himself and needed drugs to be someone he thought he should be. It gave him courage he felt he did not have without drugs. He told me he has been in detoxification 15 times and never follows through with aftercare once he leaves. This is why he constantly comes back. He has snorted heroin for 20 years and is 33 years old. He has a job, a wife, and a 15-year-old son. He talked about having nice things such as a nice car, jewelry, and money. All his friends do heroin, and he feels this is all he knows. He does not want to go to rehabilitation because he works off the books and does not want to lose his job. He says he is too proud to ask his family for financial help. He feels very trapped with no other options. He is like a lot of clients I have met here, who say they want help but do not follow through when people suggest what to do. They stay in detoxification for five days, get their head cleared, and then say they can do it on their own. This very rarely works. If you are doing drugs for 20 years, five days of detoxification is just the beginning of a very long road you must go down in order to recover. Your whole attitude about yourself needs to change. This does not happen in five days. It does not even happen in five months. It takes years for you to think differently about yourself and the world around you. This is what rehabilitation and aftercare can do for people. It gives them a new perspective about themselves and their lives. It gives people a place to express themselves and share their experiences with others that have been through similar experiences. Self-awareness is a big part of recovery. In working with clients, I try to help them look deep inside themselves and accept what they see. Acceptance is a very hard thing to do but is crucial if people are serious about their recovery. It helps people work with their feelings instead of masking them behind drugs or alcohol. It helps people follow through with the help they need. As for this client, he may require long-term care. Otherwise I think that detoxification will just be a revolving door for him.

4/21—I ran a craft group today. After instructing the clients how to do the craft, all of them still required constant cueing throughout the task. Their memory is very limited, due to the effects of the drugs they have taken. They were all very impatient and wanted to finish the project as quickly as possible. They did not understand that this is something they can do to relax and be creative. I tried to help teach them this by allowing them to experience tranquility through focusing on the craft.

4/22—I did an assessment today with a female client who is about 55 years old. She has been drinking for about 30 years and started to abuse heroin for the last seven years. She suffers from depression and takes antidepressant medication for it. When she is noncompliant with her medication, she falls into a depression and starts to drink heavily.

When we were speaking, she told me that she was very depressed that one of her daughters has not spoken to her for the last year. She said her daughter was tired of her going in and out of the hospital for her substance abuse. The woman could not understand her daughter's anger toward her, because she thought she was only hurting herself, not her daughter.

Some family members may benefit from learning more about addiction in order to learn how they can deal with the problems that occur because of the addiction and to understand what their loved one is going through.

4/26—Today, I visited an outpatient program called Support House, where people can go after they leave rehabilitation to attend meetings and participate in different groups. I sat in on a self-awareness group attended by people who were at different stages of their recovery. Some people were new and some had 20 months of sobriety. One member spoke about his fear of moving from a drug-infested environment to a drug-free residence. Group members offered him support and encouraged him to do what was right for him.

I was happy to see some clients I had worked with in detoxification following through with their recovery at Support House. It is encouraging to think that maybe something I said helped them to take that step forward. It is important for people to have these types of places to go to once they leave rehabilitation, to discuss their issues with others. Some people do not have family members or friends that they can talk to or can help them.

4/27—Today I visited the Dual-Diagnosis Program here in General Hospital. The program is made up of mentally ill chemical abusers (MICA) clients. I met with an occupational therapist named Joanne and sat in on a couple of groups that she ran. Dual-diagnosis clients are very different from clients on the detoxification ward. Although they are mostly substance abusers, they also have psychosocial issues that need to be addressed. If MICA clients are not compliant with their medication, they tend to relapse.

The first group I observed was a task group. It was interesting to see the clients work together and choose which activity to engage in. It is sometimes easier for people to express their feelings through drawing than talking. Creative drawing and painting allows you to "see" how clients are feeling at that moment. Clients got a chance to engage in an activity that they could create and keep. The second group was a living skills group, focusing on how MICA clients can benefit from becoming aware of their emotions and being able to control them in different situations.

4/28—Today I ran my stress management group. Clients went around the table and spoke about what stresses them. Each client had a different stressor. One client spoke about how she was recently raped by two men, which in turn caused her to relapse. She now is very bitter and does not know whom to trust. Another client, who is about 21 years old, spoke about his parents and how they threw him out of his house because of his drug use. He feels stress about being homeless and wanting to gain acceptance from his parents again. A gentleman, who is 53 years old, was stressed about not being where he would like to be in his life and career. He has been drinking to suppress his feelings of failure.

As people are different, so are their problems and experiences. I have learned throughout my experience at General Hospital that substance abuse does not start out as the clients' main problem but may be a result of other problems that the clients have. Substance abuse only compounds the existing problems. Clients may benefit from learning ways to deal with the stresses they have in their lives other than abusing drugs and alcohol. These tools are taught again in rehabilitation once they leave the hospital. I handed out an exercise that would help clients become aware of when they were stressed and things they should do when feeling that way. Activities such as reading, taking a walk, or talking to somebody about problems can all help in reducing stress. Clients were aware of these exercises but did not use them. To them, it was easier to use drugs to relieve their stress. They all agreed to work on using healthy, effective stress-management techniques in order for their recovery to be successful.

4/29—I interviewed a client today who is 26 years old. He comes from a middle-class family that lives in New Jersey. Both his parents are professionals. His siblings are also successful in their careers. This client lives on the Lower East Side of New York City in a squat. He tells me that he is very comfortable there and feels accepted and loved. He does not feel this way when he lives with his parents in New Jersey. He is very confused about what to do but does want to get off heroin because he is getting very tired of this lifestyle. We sat and spoke for a while and tried to figure out what was so bad about his life at home. He said his parents did not make time for him when he was young, so he ran away. He feels that he is needed in the squat where he lives, because people come to him when they need things like drugs or money. He likes that feeling of power. I tried to explain to him that, if he wants to get off of drugs, he cannot go back there and should get into a rehabilitation program followed by a residence in a halfway house. He said that the idea of not being able to go back to the squat hurt, because he has grown to love some of the people there. He also said that, if he does go back, he would continue doing the same thing.

Environment plays a big role in a person's recovery. People in recovery need to be around people who are positive and not on drugs. People in the early stages of recovery are very vulnerable and can relapse very easily. They need a support network they can go to that can help them during times of stress and depression. These groups can be found in aftercare programs and groups like Alcoholics Anonymous (AA) and Narcotics Anonymous (NA). A sponsor or someone to talk to can be invaluable in a person's recovery.

4/30—Today is the halfway point in my fieldwork II experience. I find it important to reflect on my feelings regarding my experience at General Hospital so far.

This experience has changed my perception about people forever. Coming from a loving and caring family, I feel I have been sheltered in my experiences with meeting different people. The clients I have met here are nothing like the people I have known in my life. I come from a middle-class family in an all-white neighborhood in Queens, New York. My life, compared to the lives I have learned about from talking to clients, in my opinion, is an easy one. All the problems I think I have run into in my life are nothing compared to the problems I have heard about in detoxification. I am humbled by the stories they have told me in the last six weeks I have been here.

I have often passed people lying in the street dirty and homeless and have said to myself, *Why doesn't that person get his act together or get a job?* Now, I have had the opportunity to meet these same people in the hospital and find out what they have been through in their lives. Some of their lives have been filled with abuse, neglect, misguidance, or no guidance at all. They come from an environment that is riddled with drugs and illiteracy. There are so many things this population has never learned yet is able to survive in the street with no one guiding them. People with substance abuse are survivors and able to endure many things others could not. Their addiction stirs a drive in them that most people never experience. The problem is that the drive leads to self-destruction. They have lived two lives in one lifetime. They have lived "normal" lives, and they have lived an addicted life. They have experienced things people would have nightmares about, yet they live those nightmares every day.

5/4—A big problem, I think, that clients have with recovery is that they do not know how to follow through with the goals they set for themselves in detoxification or rehabilitation. Clients more often than not tend to forget what they went through to get 30, 60, or 90 days of clean time. When some clients start to feel good about their sobriety, they tend to slack on their responsibility of going to aftercare or attending meetings. They forget that the support of others helped them through the tough times in the beginning of their recovery. People benefit from remembering that they need help from others in order to stay sober. This is not a disease that can be treated by oneself. I suggest to clients that, when they think they may be on the verge of a relapse, to try to remember the effect that drugs or alcohol had on their lives before. Hopefully, this will deter them from relapsing.

5/5—Attitude is a big part of recovery. The attitude clients have about themselves and others dictate how well they will do in their recovery. Some people have a problem with authority figures. This can hinder a person's recovery, because the people with the knowledge to help recoveries are in positions of authority. If clients do not respect or trust people in positions of authority, then they start to develop what is called *selective hearing*. Selective hearing develops when people are being told something they do not want to hear. They do not hear all the things they should hear because they are listening for something that will give them an excuse to leave or argue. Clients may benefit from learning who they should take advice from and who not to. Most of their lives, they have listened to the wrong people and the wrong advice. Now that someone is giving them good advice, they do not know how to take it. I try to work with clients to develop their trust and point out the need for an open mind so that their recovery can become successful.

5/10—One thing I have noticed while working in detoxification is the clients' lack of knowledge about the benefits available to them. I was speaking to a client today while I was doing an assessment with him, and I asked him if he was depressed. He said, "Yes." I asked him what he did when he was depressed. He said that he drank. I remembered that I asked a few clients the same question and they replied that they either drank or took illegal drugs to combat their depression. I then asked them if they ever saw a doctor or psychiatrist regarding their depression. Eight out of 10 clients said that they never consulted a doctor about their depression. These numbers tell me two things. Either they do not know to consult a doctor about their depression or they are too embarrassed to do so. I think it is a combination of the two. One client told me that, before he came to detoxification, he was at another hospital and a doctor gave him some antidepressant pills and referred him to our hospital. The client told me he felt great and did not have the urge to drink on the way to the detoxification. I told him to ask the doctor in our detoxification about getting a prescription for antidepressants. He said he would. He was not going to do so if I did not suggest it. Clients may benefit from becoming more aware of what they can do or take in place of illegal substances to control their psychosocial issues.

5/11—I finally met my first client that had returned to the detoxification unit. He was here the first time during my second week of internship. We spoke, and he had told me that, when he had left the hospital the first time, he had to go to a holding station before he could be admitted into a rehabilitation center. A holding station is a place clients go to live while they are waiting for a bed in a rehabilitation center. Here, clients are given a bed and three meals a day. They participate in groups and meetings. This particular client ran into a person he knew and decided to get high with him. He never reached the rehabilitation center. Speaking to him now, he said that he is tired of getting high and really wanted help. We worked together for two days, and then the weekend came. I found out today that he had signed himself out Friday afternoon without completing his detoxification. I am learning that whatever clients say means nothing without actions to back them up. Clients are often humble and tired when they come to detoxification, but when some of them get a little rest, they forget the pain and go right back to the street.

5/12—During an ADL [activities for daily living] group today I learned how people really do not take care of themselves like they should when they are using drugs or alcohol. Clients checked off on a list that was given to them all the ADLs they should perform in their everyday life. You really get a good understanding of how debilitating addiction can be based on how people filled out the questionnaire. People hardly brush their teeth or do not take showers as much as they should and certainly do not get up on time. Addiction takes away the will to do any of these things, and people start to neglect their everyday duties. By not doing these things, people develop low self-esteem and self-worth.

Joan, who is also a dental assistant, talked to the clients about proper oral care. Many of the clients knew about how to take care of their teeth but did not do so when they were getting high. In fact, many of the clients I have met in detoxification have bad teeth or no teeth at all. Joan really gave them good pointers on how to take care of the teeth they had, and the group came away with some useful information as well as a new toothbrush that Joan had supplied.

5/13—I have run into quite a few MICA clients on the detoxification ward since I have been here. They are quite difficult to work with and get through to. One reason is that they are not getting or taking the proper medication. Doctors and counselors have stated that MICA clients usually do better on a psychiatric ward, where they can be monitored more carefully and efficiently. If they get the proper medication first and become stabilized, it is usually easier to help them with their substance abuse.

5/14—I worked with a particular client this week. I think I really touched and helped at the same time. He has been an alcoholic for 25 years and was abused as a child. He started drinking when he was 12 years old. He comes from a family of 12. His father used to beat his mother and she used to send him out for liquor. She would let him drink as well. He feels this is all he knows and is afraid of changes he will have to go through if he wants to recover from his disease. By getting to know him, I came to realize how the years of drinking have stunted his ability to think and rationalize in a normal way. He was somewhat hostile at first, with a low frustration tolerance. He did enjoy playing pool while he was here but became impatient with that. Patience and stress management were two of the things we worked on while he was here. Pool was a great tool to help teach this, and he did become good after playing with various clients on the ward. When he left today, he thanked me for my kindness and friendship and promised that he would use the tools he learned from me and apply them to his rehabilitation.

5/21—One day this week I was sitting with a client and he was telling me how he had it all one day and lost it all the next. He owned an auto body repair shop and a car towing company, which did very well until he started using cocaine and drinking. As his use of cocaine became more frequent, his business suffered. He would not show up for work, and started to take money out of the business he should not have. He even started to borrow money from loan sharks to buy drugs.

Within a very short amount of time he had to sell his business and tow trucks to pay off the loan sharks and eventually lost his house due to a lack of money. His wife left him, and he wound up living in a men's shelter with only the clothes on his back. He told me he fell into a deep depression and drank even more. One day, he realized he could not go any lower and decided to get some help. That is when he decided to go to a detoxification center for help.

He never thought this could happen to him. But, then, again, no one does. I have never heard of a story where, by using drugs or drinking, people's lives turned out better than before they started. This client told me he got caught up in the fast life of drugs, alcohol, and women. He thought he could handle it but in the end it handled him.

5/28—There are an infinite number of reasons why people use drugs and alcohol. People often start using drugs when they are of school age. They start for different reasons. Some children feel the need of acceptance from their peers. They or someone that is older often pressures them. Others do it out of curiosity. They may see a parent or older sibling drinking or smoking marijuana and want to try it.

As people get older and continue to use, they often find it hard to stop. Counselors say that the day you start using drugs is the day you stop growing emotionally. If this is true, then it is very hard to stop because you are a child trying to deal with adult problems when they arise. What also happens as you continue to use certain drugs, such as heroin and alcohol, is that you develop a physical dependency on those substances. If you do not give your body those substances, you start to get sick. When people withdraw from heroin they get what is called *dope sick*. They develop flulike symptoms, only more severe. These symptoms will quickly go away once that person starts to use again. People that become alcoholics also develop a physical dependency. They may suffer hallucinations and also become ill once they stop drinking. For these reasons, when people decide to stop using, it is helpful to be under a doctor's care.

Some people start to drink or use drugs when they get older. Some reasons why they start can be the loss of job, a divorce, or the loss of a loved one. These stresses of life are often too much to bear for some people. The problem is that the drugs and alcohol only suppress the feelings people should be dealing with so that they can go on with their lives. It can be helpful for them to learn other ways to deal with problems and emotions. By drinking and using drugs, they develop their own world in their minds and do not let any one in. I hope they can stay on the road to recovery.

CLIENT-CENTERED REASONING QUESTIONS FOR CHAPTER 11

1. Do you think alcohol is a drug? Why or why not? Use quotes from the log and narratives to support your answer.
2. Substance abuse is not always as obvious as it is in the preceding narratives. Often in the earlier stages of addiction, people deny or underestimate their use. As a practitioner, it is helpful to identify undiagnosed substance abuse that may be affecting intervention. How do you know if people are abusing

substances if they deny it? What are the physical, psychological, cognitive, verbal, and functional signs of substance abuse? Are they different for each type of drug? How?

3. What precautions would you take for this population and why?

4. What are some forms of intervention that would help this population? Describe how each form of intervention would be helpful. Use the narratives as case studies to write goals for each person.

5. What barriers to intervention do you think you may encounter working with this population? Why?

6. How would you respond if a client who abuses substances asked you if you are in recovery and if you have ever used drugs or alcohol?

7. How would you respond to a client who said, "You cannot help me because you have never used drugs or alcohol; you have no idea what it is like?"

8. Do you think you can help a person who abuses drugs or alcohol if you have never tried them or if you have never been addicted? How?

9. Have you ever been addicted to anything? How did you know? What did you do about it?

CLIENT-CENTERED REASONING
ACTIVITIES FOR CHAPTER 11

1. Pick one client from the narratives or log above and complete the following activities, which will then comprise a case study. Present your case to the class.

   - Write an occupational profile.
   - Write a questionnaire.
   - List additional assessments you would use with this client.
   - Write an occupational performance analysis.
   - Write an intervention plan, picking the setting of your choice that you think would be the best for the client, and state why.
   - Write a discharge note.
   - Make referrals to other services.
   - Write a group protocol for a group that would meet the client's most important goal.
   - Identify the types of clinical reasoning you have applied in writing this person's assessment, occupational performance analysis, intervention plan, discharge plan, referrals, and group protocol.
   - What frame of reference or theory have you applied in creating this person's assessment, occupational performance analysis, intervention plan, discharge plan, referrals, and group protocol? Provide support for why this theory is ap-

propriate for this person's needs. What other frame of reference might be appropriate and why?

2. Finish the narrative for each person.
3. Write your own client-centered reasoning questions and activities for each narrative and log.
4. Trace Philip's maturation in his log.

12

Violence, Aggression, and Hypersexuality

As practitioners, we like to think that our clients will not be violent, aggressive, or sexual toward us, yet almost every practitioner can relate at least one incidence of these. You may never experience it during your career, but it is important to learn about aggression: how to manage aggressive clients, the signs of escalation, how to avoid aggression, how to predict it, and how to speak up when feeling threatened, even when you are the only one experiencing the threat. Violence is not always predictable or avoidable, but the more you know about it, the safer you will feel and the better equipped you will be to handle a dangerous situation should one arise.

This chapter begins inside the mind of a violent person and then moves through the minds of interns as they experience aggression first-hand.

NO REMORSE

Anonymous

> I feel good. I feel in control. Growing up, I was lucky. Growing up, there were a lot of accidents, lots of people getting killed, and people hurting each other. But the Lord watched over me. All I can do is turn to God. I carry so many men on my shoulders, dead or alive. They wanted me to do so much. A lot of the time, they did not want me to. The first time, I was in a drive-by. I was 9 years old, but no one got hurt. They just kept driving, no one retaliated, just kept on doing what they were doing. I found a 44-mm gun. I did not know what it was. Mr. T., who was like a father to me, took it from me.
>
> I do not know what to do with my mental illness. When I did not have any control, I was doing a lot of things. I did not have any remorse for people. I was very cold-blooded. They had to call the police to bring me to a psychiatric hospital. I was in a state hospital for the criminally insane. There were at least 10 fights a day. Craziest criminals. Craziest things. Now I am getting in

control of myself. Before, I was being persuaded, lured, enticed, and aggravated by the devil or evil forces around me. I used to rob banks, stuff like that. It no longer haunts me anymore. I do not know if it is the effect of the medications.

I have been dealing with this for five years now. I was getting my bachelor's degree when I started hearing voices. Voices are giving me secret messages. I cannot control them. I heard my brain crack one day while reading the dictionary in jail. I think I broke my brain. Anyway, I beat up the dean because he called me a monkey. He was hindering my ability to grow. I went to my car, let the top down, lit a cigar, and watched the ambulance go by. I went home, told my brother as little information as possible, packed my things, and left. For five days and five nights, I was on the news. They used my driver's license picture. The CIA questioned my mom. They thought it was a part of a big organization. Was it a planned hit? I was on the run for a few months. I stayed on the streets living out of my car.

I got into a fistfight with the police. It turned into a mutilation. I went back home, and my sister locked me out of the house. I went to my car and got my machete. I was waving it around when the cops came. I told the cop, "You do not need to mace me." He used mace on me. Then, he tackled me on my back and somehow he fell with one handcuff still on me. So, I smashed his head on the cement every time he tried to get up. He did not get up. I knocked him out, I guess. I just sat there and looked at him until his partner came around the corner. Arrested. I was angry that day. I do not know. He would not let me talk. I can tell he was scared of me. One thing led to another. Opportunity came and I took it.

I would like to have a professional education and own a small business. I have the knack to sell things. I would like to start my own grocery delivery chain, a mobile store where people can buy vegetables, not an ice cream truck, because in the neighborhood that I was from, we have an understanding. I want to help my neighborhood. I also want to train to be a history teacher. I am hoping public schools will have African American studies or a choice between African American history, American history, and Asian American history, so people will not want to hurt each other or murder each other. If someone puts a rumor out on you, due to ignorance, then people will want to hurt you.

We have to realize that, in a multicultural society, we are all equal but not all the same. It is important that people know that. We need to break down the barriers because racism can hold you back. Prejudice equals prejudgment. Stereotypes are never good. If you do not work together, you will never make it. Name callers and name labeling are destructive. One thing I do not like is when someone is prejudiced and says, "Hey, I have a friend who is black." He is African American. Color is only skin deep. African Americans can be albinos, too.

Client-Centered Reasoning Question

How would you work with a person with a history of violence such as this? Read the following interns' narratives to gain insight into this question, and then respond to the questions and activities that relate to all the narratives at the end of this chapter.

OVERVIEW

LILIANA MOSQUERA

Lately, we have had many clients that have the tendency to be explosive and violent. They are coming in with forensic histories, some with assault and battery. Having so many clients with histories of violence makes everyone on the unit nervous. There are no daytime male nurses on the unit to help if something were to occur. But, on a unit such as ours, I think it is essential to have male nurses. Many of the clients are male and have a large stature. Therefore, it would be hard to try and control a situation that might escalate. I do not think any of us would physically get in the middle of a fight, but since we are on the unit most of the day and have so much contact with these clients, we need to feel safe. It can be slightly frightening knowing someone has a past history of violence. Sometimes, we find ourselves looking back when we leave a room or walk down the hallway.

On the other hand, there is a level of comfort on the unit that we have established with the clients. It is hard to express and identify, but since we are there so often and have a lot of interaction with them, we are able to pick up signs of potential aggressive behavior before it happens. Also, I think that the clients do not see us the way they see the other staff members. I think this has to do with the fact that we interact with them on a daily basis, and at some level, they can identify themselves as individuals with us. Since violence has been a topic over the past couple of days as it was once before, we brought up the idea of having an in-service with security again. I am not sure if other staff members took the in-service seriously or what their reaction to it was, because I felt it was spoken about briefly and then quickly brushed off. However, we are not the only ones that are concerned with the safety issues on our unit. When thinking about potential violence, it seems that we deal with it every day but sometimes do not realize it. It is as if we have innate reactions that help us to make decisions when incidents come up and when we find ourselves in the situation. I think having the experience of being on the unit and having knowledge of different types of clients and symptoms can be helpful in identifying potential violence. Even so, working on a psychiatric unit or in the area of mental health can be dangerous and constantly keeps one on his or her guard.

HE WAS NOT HIMSELF

ANONYMOUS

Today was a little disappointing for me. Two of my favorite clients were not doing well today. Chan was not himself. Normally, he is disorganized but always in a happy but preoccupied kind of way. Today, however, he was angry and hostile, mumbling and cursing under his breath and aloud. It was upsetting to hear him like that, and when I tried to talk to him, he dismissed me completely and continued on with his tirades. I was sad because it reminded me of a bad day he had last week. He walked through the halls looking as if he were going to fall on his face. He appeared so sedated, and he seemed to be fighting his exhaustion with everything he had. Finally, one of the social workers took him gently and led him to his room. She spoke with him softly, telling him that she thought he needed to rest and that it was all right to take a nap. He finally did. Today reminded me of that day.

FEAR

FRANCIA BRITO

During a staff meeting we were told that Mr. Cotto hit a staff member and was put into four point restraints, which he then chewed himself out of. This incident really terrified me. Even speaking about the upcoming in-service to teach us how to restrain a client scared me. It stirred up all of the feelings I had about an inpatient unit. It stirred up the feelings about clients lashing out. It is scary, because I was thinking about myself or possibly others getting injured. What if they are not able to calm down such an incident? What if it gets so out of control that the staff could not handle it safely? What if the out-of-control client hurts others, then himself? These are the things that terrify me.

During team rounds, we visited Mr. Cotto. As we entered his room, my anxiety level rose. My heart started palpitating. I thought that my anxiety must be obvious to others. My feelings tend to show up in my facial expressions. I was standing right in front of him. The attending doctor and psychology intern proceeded to speak to him. He arose from his bed, began getting very agitated, and went on a tangent about racial issues. As he got more and more upset, a student standing right next to me was smiling. I think she was nervous. Her smile made me even more anxious because I was afraid that he would notice it and get angry.

ESCAPED AND DANGEROUS

ANONYMOUS

During team meeting, there was uproar on the unit. A client that had been brought in a couple days before was very agitated because he had a court date today that he could not miss. This client was brought into the hospital because he was found between subway cars, attempting to hang himself with his belt. A few days after he was brought in, he punched a nurse in the face and was put in restraints and seclusion. During the team meeting, the client proceeded to escape from restraints. When he got out, he somehow broke the top off a table and used the legs to try to break out of the exit door. The nursing staff, with the help of security (who arrived about 7–10 minutes after the fact) got the client back into his room and back into restraints. Not 10 minutes later, he was out again! This was really scary, not only for the other staff and me but also for the clients that were roaming the halls during the incident. We tried to get all the clients away from the scene. What if we were not quick enough? What would I do if the client came toward me? Yes, I would run, but what about the clients? They could not react as I or the rest of the staff could. What is even more unsettling is that most of the clients did not even know that this was going on. If the client approached others who were not attentive, someone else might get hurt.

I feel a little better about the safety issue with violent clients. Violence was discussed in the staff meeting, and restraining techniques will be taught to all. Even if I never have to help restrain someone, I will feel safer on the unit knowing that all of the staff members know how to manage a violent client. It will make the unit safer for the staff as well as the clients.

SIGNS OF ESCALATION

FRANCIA BRITO

One of my biggest fears, that a client will lash out at someone, almost came true today during team meeting. A Spanish-speaking client's (Jose's) anger escalated while speaking to one of the male nurses. Jose was trying to communicate to the nurse that a nurse had given him the wrong medication. The nurse tried to explain to Jose that he [the nurse] did not understand Jose. Jose became angry. As I sat in the team meeting room, I saw his anger escalate, demonstrated by the tone in his voice, his choice of words, constricted pupils, and clenched fists. I turned to one of the psychology interns and stated that I thought that Jose was getting very upset. As a nurse entered the room, I asked him if he wanted me to tell him what Jose just said. I began to translate into English what had just happened. Jose entered the room and screamed at the nurse. Jose told the nurse that he [the client] did not know why he [the nurse] could not understand what he [the client] was saying about medications now because he [the nurse] was able to before. I was able to tell the nurse why Jose had been upset. At this point, the nurse turned to Jose and stated that he understood. As the nurse was sitting down, Jose then approached him and put his fists up to the nurse's face. Jose asked him in English, "What the hell do you understand?" The nurse stood up. We all stood up behind him. Jose yelled and made gestures as if he were going to punch the nurse in the face. Jose yelled at the nurse and said that he was going to hit him in the face and that he was not crazy. The nurse calmly left the room to call security, as the attending doctor calmed Jose. This was such a close call. Jose was right in the nurse's face, ready to hit him, but did not do it. What stopped Jose from hitting the nurse? Was it the fact that all of us in the room were standing around, just in case something did happen? Or, was it that, in his mind, he really did not want to hit the nurse, all he wanted to do was get his point across?

One of the reasons why I believe that it escalated as it did was due to a language barrier problem. Jose was trying to express some feelings he had toward the medications, but the nurse stated that he did not understand Jose. Jose also expressed that the nurse was able to understand him before, why not now? This may have been frustrating to Jose and also to the nurse. One of the psychology interns expressed that if you do not speak the same language, many cues can be missed. For example, I was able to pick up verbal cues in his choice of words that led me to believe that his anger was escalating. So, for two to three minutes, my fears of violence flashed before my eyes. I really thought that someone was going to get hurt. No one did. And the situation was kept in control.

HYPERSEXUALITY

FRANCIA BRITO

There seems to be a lot of hypersexual behavior among many of the clients. Many of the clients are kissing and touching one another inappropriately. Some are even dressed inappropriately, expressing sexual desires. A client even touched my arm in a sexual manner, asking me what I felt as he touched my arm. As this occurred, he and I discussed inappropriate behavior, and why touching others may have consequences. He was receptive toward what I explained to him, and he acknowledged and agreed that his behavior was inappropriate. But why are so many of the clients on the unit acting this way?

POTENTIALLY VIOLENT

SHEENA SETHI

My second day on the inpatient psychiatric ward, I was introduced to a middle-aged African American man by the name of Bob. On approach, Bob was pleasant, animated, playful, and talking to himself extremely loudly. Bob was the first client that I had a conversation with. While observing a leisure skills group led by the previous intern, Bob approached me and asked if he smelled; I then asked him if he had taken a shower earlier. He said no, then got out of his seat and quickly walked to the door, my initial reaction being, *great my first interaction with a client and I already messed up.* I felt my face drop, my head spun with thoughts while my body temperature rose and my heart raced. After the group, I spoke of my thoughts to the intern. She consoled me and told me not to worry about it.

This interaction made me obligated and motivated to learn more about this client, since I was already on bad terms with him. I went to the nurses' station in search of Bob's chart, which I signed out. I sat in one of the group therapy rooms and analyzed and compiled detailed information regarding Bob.

Surprisingly, his evaluation was done using information from the chart secondary to Bob's refusal to give the information himself. Apparently, Bob stated to the intern, "Get out of my room or I will beat you up," at the time of his admittance, approximately three weeks before I arrived. This was shocking enough for me; I could not understand how such a pleasant, cooperative man could have refused his interview. I felt that this pleasant psychotic person could not hurt a fly. I was intrigued. I continued reading in the chart:

> Pt. is a 42 y.o. Afro-American male, unemployed with a h/o noncompliance with meds. and a h/o paranoid delusions. Pt. has had multiple psychiatric hospitalizations and a h/o ETOH, crack and marijuana. Pt. spent most of his life in an orphan home and was apparently beaten by foster mom. Pt. has h/o suicide attempts and hears voices telling him to harm himself. Pt. was BIB security from Samuel's Clinic (HIV facility) due to an infected cut on his right 5th finger. A nurse made an attempt to assess the cut, pt. refused consultation and became hostile, threatening, cursing, and yelling. Pt. is internally preoccupied and is seen talking loudly to himself. Pt. onset of HIV was in 1991. Pt. is uncooperative, restless, increased psychomotor activity, loudly threatening, poor eye contact, and tangential. Pt. is disheveled, poor hygiene, and wearing a hospital gown. Pt. has been diagnosed with an acute exacerbation of schizophrenia.

I felt alarmed after conducting this chart review. I remember turning to the intern and stating, "Bob has been diagnosed with HIV." Before coming to this ward I had never come in contact with someone with this horrifying disease. The intern then discussed the reality of this disease on the ward. Approximately 90% of the patients on the ward were indeed HIV positive. I took a sigh and realized that I had to be extra careful to use universal precautions. I cannot explain in words the harsh and insecure feelings that I had, knowing that I was working with HIV-positive clients. After being able to push these feelings aside, I thought that this could not be the same Bob I just met. I now felt that Bob leaving the group would result in hatred toward me, and after reviewing his chart, there was no way I wanted to be on his bad side.

I saw someone watching through the window of the activity room. Sure enough, it was Bob. He waved and told me to open the door. I thought my heart was going to jump out of my body as I slowly approached the door. When I opened the door Bob's hand was pulling up the bottom portion of robe displaying his legs. I was confused because I did not know what to say or do. Bob then said, "Well, are you going to tell me they are pretty?" Confused, I replied, "What do you mean?" In a jolly manner, he stated, "Ugh, I cleaned them." Laughing at Bob I said, "So you took a shower." I then smiled and said, "You look very clean and pretty now." Bob said, "Thank you," and returned to his walking and talking routine.

This was my first experience with a manic person, and I have learned not to underestimate the severity of a person's symptoms. So what if he has HIV or is hostile? Sometimes clients are not able to control themselves. Their violence is part of their illness. THANK GOD for psychiatric medicine, because I cannot imagine these clients without them.

BUT SHE DOES NOT LOOK DANGEROUS

SHEENA SETHI

In team rounds, the resident gave a brief review of a new client. Jenny is a 64-year-old single white woman who was brought in by the police in handcuffs. She carried a diagnosis of paranoid schizophrenia for a long time and for the past four months she has not taken her medication. She has lived in her residence for the past year and a half, recently exhibiting hostile, belligerent, and agitated behavior—and she beat up her case manager.

I decided to evaluate her right after rounds. I knocked on her door and got no answer, so I walked in. I called her name once, and she turned around; I then asked her if she minded if I talked to her a little while. She was very inquisitive, wanting to know who I was and why I wanted to talk to her. I explained that I was an intern who wanted to find out a little about her so I could assess her facilitators and any barriers that she needed help with. I wanted to help her maximize her level of occupational performance and maintain her health. She asked me how I could help her specifically, and I told her that, after the interview, we could chat about what goals she has and find out what she needs help with. I could utilize purposeful activities to help her with daily living skills, develop leisure activities, and enhance her functional performance. She thought it was interesting and then agreed to let me evaluate her.

To my surprise, Jenny was pleasant and highly educated. She graduated with a literature degree from Paris and then furthered her education at New York University. She explained that she is fully able to maintain her activities of daily living, including showering, dressing, grooming, sewing, cooking, cleaning, laundry, and money management. She expressed the need to be discharged because her absence at work will prevent her from paying her bills. She claimed to work as a record keeper and a translator for a well-known law firm. She translates Spanish and French. She claimed that it is so hard nowadays to maintain money and pay bills: "The world now is too expensive," she said. She claims that she does not have insurance and will not be able to pay her hospital bill.

I was confused after the interview. Jenny seemed normal to me and reminded me of my grandmother. She was so sweet and pleasant; she is 64 and looked not a day over 40. She maintained her skin so beautifully, and there was no sign of agitation or frustration. On her occupational performance analysis, Jenny received a within normal limits score in the categories of: personal hygiene, grooming and dressing, management of personal space, mobilization, concentration, organization, following directions, neatness and attention to details, and rate of performance. For the categories of problem solving and frustration tolerance, I really did not know how to assess these areas. Although she had a recent history of violent behavior and currently was in special care, she seemed to be calm and relaxed. On approach, she was pleasant and seemed to maintain her frustration tolerance; however, her chart says that she was agitated, belligerent, and hostile. I finally decided to mark her with a number 2, which states that she has moderate difficulty with problem solving (beating up her case manager and not taking her medication for four months) and frustration tolerance. This was a hard case to assess, so I decided to wait a couple of days to see if she changed.

The very next day, I went to her room to see how she was doing and asked her to attend groups, thinking that she would be compliant. To my surprise, she told me that she was tired and did not feel like it. I then advised that she come to group because, not only will she wake up, but also enjoy it. She began to yell, "I told you people to leave me alone, and it is not your job to argue with me." I said, "Jenny, it seems like you are upset with me; can I do anything to help you?" She claimed that she hates the hospital and cannot afford it. I told her not to worry, everything would be all right and advised her to talk to her social worker. She agreed; however, she still refused to come to group.

Later that day, she approached me in the hall and stated, "I think you should participate in grooming group, it will really help you." It just so happens that we just finished grooming group and that was the group I wanted Jenny to attend. I thought that she might have confused her words, so I asked her if she needed grooming supplies. She stated again, "I think you should participate in grooming group." I asked, "Why do you feel that way?" She told me that long hair is unacceptable in society and that I should chop it off. I told her that my religion is Sikh, and it was against my religion to cut my hair. She paused a minute and then said, "I knew you were Indian," but then she went on and in a hostile manner stated, "Well, it would be easier for you to strangle yourself with your long hair, then they will never let you out of here." I do not know why, but I asked, "Would you be upset if I harmed myself, because it seems like you are looking out for me?" She then screamed, "*No*" with all her might and forcefully walked away not awaiting a reply from me.

At this point not only was I perplexed but hurt. I really liked Jenny, and I felt that she had betrayed me. All this time I thought she was a pleasant psychotic person but I was wrong.

AFTER THE ACT: DEALING WITH REACTIONS TO VIOLENCE

ANONYMOUS

Today was the first day that I have felt any aggression from a client directed at me. I was leading our leisure skills group when someone began knocking on the door and just kept knocking. I turned around to see that it was Edward, a 20-year-old guy with a really nasty attitude toward all the staff. Now he was directing it at me. I try very hard to appear to clients as if nothing they say or do bothers me, but he does bother me, so I played my poker face as usual. When I opened the door, he asked in a very challenging manner if he could come in. I told him that our group was almost over and that next time, he should come on time and knock only once. I closed the door, but he began to knock again. I kept my back to him, ignoring him until he finally went away. This incident made me nervous because he is one of our more dangerous clients, and now I have to be even more careful than usual. Surprisingly, I have felt very comfortable on the unit up until now. It is quite unnerving knowing that I have someone with such a dangerous reputation acting aggressively toward me.

Later that day, he once again was inappropriate with me, mouthing off to me and not following safety instructions during a movement group. Also, I observed him watching me through office windows with his menacing stare.

When I went home last night, I did not tell my husband about any of it. He is not happy about the site I am at for many reasons: the location, the type of unit, and the homicidal and suicidal tendencies of the clients. The last thing I need to do is tell him about a very aggressive client acting provocatively toward me. I am angered that I feel like this. If I tell my husband the story, my own frustration and fear may come through and that will upset him more. The doctor, who is Edward's team leader, and the social worker on that team said that I should really watch it. I do not like having to watch it any more than usual, and I resent being made to feel unsafe. Now, I am just waiting for him to be discharged, but that is not a realistic option. He is a danger to others, which is why I have to watch out for myself, so he is not being discharged.

I think I need to take some time to allow myself to deal with this feeling so that I am better prepared to deal with the future Edwards.

The next day was the first day that I actually witnessed violence on the unit. The other interns, Lisa and Sheila, were sitting with me in a conference room doing paperwork and talking. The conference room door has a window, and we could see the staff office door from there. Out of the corner of my eye, I see Dr. Brine at the office door. All of the doors on this unit are locked and you must use a key to get inside, so it takes a few seconds to get yourself into a room. All of a sudden, I hear a male scream and then someone is on Dr. Brine attempting to punch him. This client's fist came down and grazed the side of Dr. Brine's face, and then the client lunged for the housekeeping cart that was a couple of feet away and grabbed a broom. Just then, two maintenance workers grabbed him and the broom. They wrestled the broom away from him, got him on the floor, and pinned him until security arrived.

It all happened so fast. By the time I got out of my chair and ran for the door, it was all over. The maintenance men waved for me to stay in the room. I just stood there. I found myself saying over and over, "I just cannot believe what we just saw." Lisa said that she thought she was going to cry, and I had a bout of nervous laughter with Sheila. The three of us said, "Can you believe what just happened?" at least 100 times. It did not feel real.

I reluctantly told my husband about what happened. When I leave here at night, I find myself wanting to talk about everything with anyone who will listen. It is just such a wild place, in good ways and bad. My husband was less than amused or entertained by the story. He was kind of angry, again telling me that if anything happens to me while I am here, my school should be held responsible for sending me to such a place. I really cannot blame him for his thoughts and perceptions on the hospital and the unit. He is a regular person, who has never dealt with or been exposed to any type of psychosocial issues. This is the type of attitude most of society has concerning psychiatric hospitals and psychiatric clients. He thinks that staff is actually crazy if they choose to work in mental health, and he is not the first person I have heard say that. In fact, up until my internship, I have to admit that I shared a similar opinion.

I kept saying to him that I wish I could bring him in with me for one day. I just wanted him to see what I do and see for himself the human side of psychosocial distress. He always replied, "I do not want to know."

Later that same day, Larry apparently had caused some situation that resulted in his being put into restraints. He is a very small man and he managed to slip himself out of the straps and proceeded to refuse requests for him to stay in his room. Security was called, and three very large men assisted in the procedure.

I was down the hall in the solarium, unaware that any of this was going on. We were setting up for a group, and I walked out to begin to gather clients for the group. As I walked down the hall, I saw a crowd of people standing around the phones; there was a person sitting on a chair, but I could not see who it was. My supervisor, Pam, came down the hall to observe our group. She saw the person in the chair and described his physical characteristics to me; then I knew it was Larry. Pam hung around the crowd because she had noticed that the security men were armed. Guns are not allowed on the unit due to safety issues. A client could pull a gun out of the guard's holster and shoot someone. I really felt that I should leave and give this kid some privacy during this ordeal, but morbid curiosity and the thought that, as a staff member, I may be required to assist kept me planted close by. And then it happened: The crowd of staff converged on him and he began to kick and punch. Staff members had his legs and arms, and he was flailing his body around in a manner I had never seen before. The crowd moved as a unit down the hall with this kid spread-eagle in the middle of them. They placed him on a bed at the end of the hall and held him still while nursing staff put on the straps. The attending doctor gently said, "We are not going to hurt you Larry." And that is when what I saw hit me. I stood there really not knowing what to do with myself, feeling that I wanted to cry. It is so sad to see this good-looking young kid so messed up in the brain. It made me think of the time I was a teenager. I was every parent's nightmare; I toted around the same bad attitude that this kid totes around. But there is something different about what is happening in his brain. I grew out of it, but he ended up in restraints in a psychiatric hospital. It is a scary thought. Mental health problems are sometimes subtle, sneaky disablers that get you when you least expect them. I stood there, feeling frozen and feeling really bad for this kid who really does not understand or maybe is not able to control these acts of rule breaking and defiance. I felt embarrassed for him, too. He is now strapped to a bed in the hallway, unable to move and probably feeling some fear, surrounded by strangers who, he thinks, do not care about him even though they really do, all alone. A nursing attendant will sit next to his bed to monitor him, and she will probably read a book as most of them do. His next stop will be the seclusion room for a cool-off period, but not until the sedative kicks in so that it is safe to move him; he will remain there until it looks like he can handle himself in an appropriate manner.

This whole experience really hit me hard. It was the most emotional moment I have had since I have been here. I really hope I do not ever have to see one of the clients that I know go through that, it was very traumatic for me, and I can only imagine how traumatic it is for them.

WORKING WITH PSYCHOTICALLY INDUCED HYPERSEXUAL AGGRESSION

SHEENA SETHI

It is 9:30 on Friday morning, the standard meeting time for team rounds. It is my seventh week out of a 12-week internship. The attending doctor came into the meeting distressed, commenting, "This case is from hell," and asked the resident to report information about the new client. Jim is a 19-year-old Hispanic man with no previous psychiatric history. His family brought him in secondary to bizarre behavior. Jim presently appears disorganized, delusional, paranoid; and he experiences hallucinations (auditory and visual). Jim is mildly retarded and is currently in the 11th grade. His parents do not understand what has happened to him. Jim came home after hanging out with his friends prior to admission. He was panicky and gazing out of the window. His parents seem to believe that Jim's behavior was due to drug use. Jim denied any alcohol or substance abuse. Ever since he arrived on the ward, Jim has been in four-point restraints, secondary to his hypersexual and delusional behavior.

After hearing this report and the comments made by the staff, I felt that I needed more information about Jim to understand better what was going on. I went to Jim's room to observe him. I found him lying down in restraints, shaking his head. I went in closer to his bed and introduced myself. After a few seconds he yelled, "Valerie why are you doing this to me? I miss you. Come and give me a kiss." I could clearly see now that he was delusional and possibly hallucinating. I tried to orient him and explain that I was his intern and not Valerie. He was waxing and waning in concentration, and I knew that this was not the time to talk to him due to his psychotic state. This was the first time that I have seen an initial onset of a psychosocial problem. I wanted to know more about this case, and I already wanted to see Jim's final baseline on discharge.

It was now visiting hour, and Jim's family had come in to visit. There was a mother, sister, brother-in-law, and father. The nursing staff did not want to shock the family with the view of Jim in restraints, so the family members were told that they needed to speak to a doctor first. A nurse then called me over and asked me to set them up in an activity room. Looking at the mother's condition at this time made me feel terrible. Apparently, one of the nurses had told the mother that Jim was psychotic at the present time, and they currently could not see him. The mother started to cry hysterically; I honestly thought that she was going to hyperventilate. I went to the attending physician and asked him if I could sit in on the family meeting that he was about to have. He was a little hesitant because he said he does not know much about this particular client and has not in fact seen him yet. He stated that he only had five minutes to talk to the family, but I was welcome to observe. I jumped at the chance and attended the meeting. Jim's family was clearly a loving and supportive family. There was no previous psychiatric history within the family. They mentioned that this problem he is facing must be due to drug use or the liquid diet beverage he was using. Apparently, Jim was taking this diet beverage and lost 50 pounds within a month. Its manufacturer, due to a mistake in the product, recently recalled this beverage. Jim's eyes appeared red during this month, as if he had taken drugs. Recently, Jim has been hiding the fact that he needs candy, chocolate syrup, pancake syrup, and plain sugar from his family. Jim went out with his friends. When he returned, he was panicky, yelling, and paranoid about someone named Valerie. What surprised the family the most was that he began speaking Spanish. Jim never spoke Spanish with his family or friends, and they were amazed that he was speaking only Spanish instead of English.

The doctor was confused at the time about what was going on, because this was all new to him also; the doctor empathized and expressed concern for Jim. He then left the room to go assess Jim's condition at the present time. While the doctor was gone, the family vented their feelings to me, and I assured them that the staff on the ward was excellent and that they would help Jim.

Later in the day, Jim was let out of restraints. I was in one of the activity rooms actually writing up Jim's evaluation with the information that I compiled from the family, staff, and my own observations. All of a sudden, I heard loud screaming, but I could not make out who was screaming. I opened the door and peeked out into the hallways and saw Jim walking around screaming with a nurse's aide following him. Jim seemed to be disorganized, confused, and hypersexual. He was sexually touching the nurse's aide and calling her Valerie. I then saw other staff members trying to calm him down, while waiting for security to come to the floor. Jim made eye contact with me, and my heart suddenly started pounding, as I knew he was headed in my direction. My first impulse was to shut the door. Jim approached the door and looked through the window, saying, "Blow me and kiss me." My heart was racing. Jim went on, "If you do not talk to me, I will kill somebody and then hide in the church." I had to speak now, so I asked Jim who he was looking for. Jim then stated, "Val, I am going crazy, why are you not talking back?" Jim was now tonguing the window and banging on the door. I did not know what to do. I knew staff was aware of what was happening, but I was in the room all by myself. I explained to Jim once more that I was not Valerie but a staff member. Jim continued to be sexually provocative and lick the door. Suddenly, the other door to the activity room opened; it was another intern. I was so relieved and felt more secure. Jim did not stop and now believed that the other intern was Crystal. This drama went on for about 25 minutes, then I heard a long moment of silence. I looked down the hallway, noticed it being empty, grabbed my clipboard, and rapidly walked off the floor. I was so relieved once I shut and locked the main door. At this time, my mind was boggled and this scene stayed with me for the entire weekend. I now knew what the doctor meant by "this is a case from hell."

I definitely felt scared when I left; however, regardless of what happened, I came in on Monday with an open mind. Before the team rounds, I briskly walked by Jim's room and found that he was out of restraints but under constant observation. I approached Jim and said, "Hello." He said, "Hi, didn't you go to school with me?" I then stated again that I was an intern, and the first day we met was on Friday. He looked confused but held himself together. I was shocked. I was now anticipating the team rounds so I could hear the weekend report on Jim. The nursing report stated that Jim was responding to his medication. He was not at this time sexually provocative to any female staff members. He was still delusional about Valerie. He thought that the nurse's aide who was assigned for constant observation was indeed Valerie. I was happy that he was already slightly better and responding well to medication. He was clearly unable to attend groups and even work one-on-one with the therapist at the present time.

A week has gone by, and Jim is much better than when he came in. He wandered into our movement group and stayed with his nurse. I was glad that the nurse participated in the group along with Jim. He joined and surprisingly did well. This group consisted of about eight clients and three staff members. We were doing an open exercise and dance movement group. We threw around a small cushioned ball to participants in the group. The person receiving the ball had to do a movement to the music that was being played. Jim was able to concentrate for 30 minutes, organize his behavior, appropriately interact socially, and attend to the details of movement and catching the ball. After the group, Jim was even able to express his feelings regarding the group. He mentioned that it had been a long time since he had some fun exercising. That statement alone made me excited.

I thought that the team would be as delighted about Jim's progress as I was. Unfortunately the attending physician was not. The physician thought that Jim did not belong in groups, regardless of his trial run, even with his nurse beside him. I did not want to break the news to Jim, so I asked his doctor if he would do so. The next day, Jim wanted to participate in a self-awareness group. I was upset that I had to decline him. Jim now looked very sad. He was able to maintain his frustration and followed directions. I was so proud of him. Later on, I spoke with him and discussed some goals that he had for the future. He told me that he wanted to graduate college and hold a job. I then decided to give him a job on the ward without him attending the community task group. Jim's job was to clean the tables after snacks. I felt that I had to keep this client motivated. I knew that this was his first break, and I tried to be sensitive to the way he was feeling. He expressed to me that he was upset that he was different from everyone else. We then discussed that everyone was different and no two people in this world are the same. He expressed that he was always picked on due to his mild mental retardation and that he went to a special school. I empathized with him and told him that he did not seem retarded. I assured him that he has many good qualities— good family support, motivation to pursue school and maintain a job. I assured him that, if he stays motivated, he would definitely do well. I discussed with him about how I thought he had done wonderfully in the group that he did attend and he has the potential to pursue his goals.

Jim kept up with his job of cleaning the tables. After our grooming group, which he was not able to attend, he came in and wiped down the tables with absolutely no reminders. I brought up in team again that I think he should be able to participate in groups. The doctor decided to take him off constant observation to see how he does first. Jim did fine and was slowly introduced to the groups on the unit.

On his third week here, he was planning for his discharge. Jim's family was slowly learning about Jim's schizophrenia. The social worker had a family meeting scheduled yesterday, and of course, I asked to attend. Before the social worker arrived, I got a chance to talk to the family and reassure them that Jim was doing much better than when he came in. In the meeting, the social worker discussed issues regarding the illness, medications, follow-up, and support groups. The family responded well and was able to absorb all of the information. The social worker made an extra effort to include me in the discussions and even gave me time to give a more functional perspective of his facilitators and barriers. The discharge date was the next day. I was scared. The team had decided to let Jim go, but I feel bad because he is still confused at times and currently showing psychotic symptoms. I hope that his day treatment center can continue to help him.

RESOLUTION

FRANCIA BRITO

My first feeling as I came to this inpatient psychiatric unit was fear. I was afraid of psychiatric clients because I had many misconceptions about them. I believed that there would be a lot of people running around, screaming, hitting, and assaulting one another and staff members. I also believed that the clients would be too psychotic to even understand or attend to any treatment provided them. I was afraid that the unit would get out of control, and no one would be able to handle it. Well, I was wrong. As time went by, I began to realize how wrong my misconceptions were. I also came to realize how many obstacles these people have needed to face in life, especially with the stigma of having a mental illness. I also came to realize how much the clients were aware of their surroundings and what was happening to their lives. Do not get me wrong, there was a time when many of the clients were so low functioning that they were not really related during groups; but during individual sessions, they were able to raise important issues in their own unique ways. As I progressed, I got to know each one of them well, and now I understand that they are people, too. They would often say in groups, "We have feelings, too, you know. All we want is some respect."

I have been able to identify culturally and socioeconomically with many of the clients, which aided in building a relationship and rapport. Occasionally, there was violence on the unit, but it was dealt with in a professional, effective manner. I learned to see beyond the anger, aggression, violence, and agitation that many of these clients possessed. As I looked beyond the violence, I saw clients who were scared, upset to be ill, vulnerable, and frustrated about their illness. Because I was able to look beyond this and view them as people who are hurt, scared, vulnerable, and confused, I was able to understand them better as people. I came to realize how sweet and caring these people really were. I believe my anxiety and fear decreased because of this realization. Someone on the unit once told me that I had a high threshold for danger and that he would be scared. It is not that I am no longer scared, it is just that I can look beyond what is going on, on the outside, and try to understand some of their problems. Understanding them as whole people has helped to decrease my fears, misconceptions, and anxiety. Before I started this internship, I had made up my mind that I was not going into the mental health field. But, because of the insight, knowledge and experience I attained working with the clients here, I am now considering a career in mental health.

CLIENT-CENTERED REASONING QUESTIONS FOR CHAPTER 12

1. This chapter tells of 12 acts of aggression, potential situations for violence, or sexual promiscuity: two in the first narrative by the anonymous author followed by Chan, Mr. Cotto, a client, Jose, another client, Bob, Jenny, Edward, Larry, and Jim. For each story, answer the following questions:

    *   What was the act of aggression or potential for aggression?
    *   What were the signs of escalating irritation?
    *   Was there a history of violence? If so, under what circumstance(s)?
    *   How did people respond to the aggressor before, during, and after the act?
    *   What would you have done differently, and what is your clinical reasoning for each action?
    *   What are your feelings, thoughts, and reactions to the act of aggression?

2. Use one of the narrative quotes below as a topic sentence. Develop the theme of the topic sentence as far as possible, resulting in a new narrative that addresses the etiology of violence. Express your writing in the same character as the quote portrays: "sometimes clients are not able to control themselves. Their violence is part of their illness" (Sheena Sethi, "Potentially Violent"); "I do not know what to do with my mental illness. When I did not have any control, I was doing a lot of things. I did not have any remorse for people. I was very cold-blooded" (Anonymous, "No Remorse"); "But, there is something different about what is happening in his [the aggressor's] brain" (Anonymous, "After the Act: Dealing with Reactions to

Violence"); "I heard my brain crack one day while reading the dictionary in jail" (Anonymous, "No Remorse"); and "Now I am getting in control of myself. Before, I was being persuaded, lured, enticed, and aggravated by the devil or evil forces around me" (Anonymous, "No Remorse").

3. Respond to the following narrative quotations. In your response address the questions that follow each quotation.

   - "Why are so many of the clients on the unit acting this way [hypersexually]?" (Francia Brito, "Hypersexuality"). What are some of the reasons for hypersexuality in psychiatric clients?

   - "Jose was right in the nurse's face ready to hit him but did not do it. What stopped Jose from hitting the nurse?" (Francia Brito, "Signs of Escalation"). How is it that the majority of us can stop ourselves from hitting someone while some people cannot? Can this change throughout someone's life?

   - "It reminded me of a bad day he [the client] had last week" (Anonymous, "He Was Not Himself"). What is a bad day in mental health terms, and what may it be a result of?

   - "I am not sure if other staff members took the in-service [on violence] seriously or what their reaction to it was because I felt it was spoken about briefly and then quickly brushed off" (Liliana Mosquera, "Overview"). Is it possible that staff members feel more comfortable with violent situations than interns do? Is it possible to get used to a work environment where there is the potential for outbursts?

CLIENT-CENTERED REASONING ACTIVITIES

1. Work in groups to prepare and present the following seminars on clinical aggression management to your class. When material from the narratives is insufficient, research the topic area and use your own ideas. Choose one seminar per group. List and explain the types of clinical reasoning your group used in preparing the seminar. What frames of reference did your group use? Provide support for why this frame of reference is appropriate for your seminar. What other frames of reference might be appropriate and why?

   - Aggression prevention seminar: Methods to keep aggression from occurring. Goal: After this seminar, class members will be able to identify techniques that they can use on their internships to prevent different types of aggressive situations from occurring.

   - Aggression management seminar: Managing an aggressive situation as it is occurring. Goal: After this seminar, class members will be able to identify techniques that they can use on their internships to manage different acts of aggression.

- Hypersexuality seminar: How to work with a hypersexual person. Goal: After this seminar, class members will be able to identify techniques that they can use on their internships to manage hypersexual behavior in their clients.
- Reporting threats of violence: How to speak up when you feel threatened. Goal: After this seminar, class members will be able to identify why it is important to tell other practitioners if they feel threatened by a person they are working with and why; and how to be assertive enough to speak up even if they are the only ones experiencing the person as threatening.

2. Write a group protocol for anger management. Include three in-depth intervention sessions for the first three groups. What frame of reference did you use? Provide support for why this frame of reference is appropriate for this group protocol. What other frame of reference might be appropriate and why? What types of clinical reasoning did you use in creating this group protocol?

3. Write a protocol for anger management intervention to be administered during individual sessions. Include three in-depth intervention sessions for the first three meetings. What frame of reference did you use? Provide support for why this frame of reference is appropriate for this group protocol. What other frame of reference might be appropriate and why? What types of clinical reasoning did you use in creating this group protocol?

4. When would you use one-on-one sessions with someone working on anger management instead of a group? When would it be more appropriate to utilize a group setting?

5. Choose one intern's narrative and identify that intern's types of clinical reasoning.

13

Analysis of Logs I: Growth Throughout the Internship

Learning client-centered reasoning on an internship is a dynamic process. Most interns progress through various stages and various themes that occur despite different settings and the differences among interns. Learning takes place each second. Each experience shapes the growth process and the decisions made, which in turn affect how the next experience will go. Much of this process occurs without the conscious awareness of the intern. Many interns expressed surprise at the end of their internship that they learned so much. They were unaware that they had acquired such an extensive skill and knowledge base until they oriented new interns. They were, however, able to recall specific things that shaped each of their experiences when asked.

The more awareness of this growth process interns can have before they begin their own internship, the better they may be at identifying their own growth process as it happens in their internship. This ability to recognize their own process of growth as it happens will give them ongoing insight and reflection into what they are feeling, thinking, and doing; the reasoning behind their intervention decisions; and how to overcome barriers to their own growth when they get stuck. This self-awareness may help them communicate their needs to their supervisors in a more expedient and thorough manner, enabling them to get the most out of their internship.

This chapter is dedicated to helping students identify the growth process of other interns in order to become more aware of their own. To achieve this objective, two logs are presented. In the first, various stages and themes of growth are identified in bubble inserts. The second log has no such inserts so that the reader can identify the stages and themes in the same fashion as in the first log.

MARSHA EISERMAN

Client-Centered Reasoning Activities

1. As you read Marsha Eiserman's log take notice of the editor's information bubbled above her words. These are stages that

interns usually progress through during their internship. They are listed in the first chapter of this book, which you should review at this time.

2. Most of the issues presented in the previous chapters re-emerge throughout the logs. See if you can identify them in the log to follow. How do the authors deal with each? How would you deal with each and why?

3. Identify types of clinical reasoning. Asterisks mark examples to label. Some asterisks have been omitted in order for you to find additional examples.

Log 1. 6/1

1. Preconceived ideas about clients

Dealing with people who have psychosocial issues is not a new experience for me. For six years, I lived near a residential home for emotionally challenged adults. A few of my friends or their children have mental health issues. Additionally, two extremely close friends of mine come from troubled homes, where at least one parent has psychosocial issues.

As a prospective neighbor of a home for emotionally challenged adults, I was forewarned of its moving on the block. At that point, I made a decision to treat its residents like any other neighbors on the block, greeting and asking questions concerning their welfare as they walked past me. My children, ages 1 through 6, would also be taught to treat them like anyone else. I wanted my children to feel comfortable with this population. As time went on, some general rules were set and explained to my children, such as not giving them money at any time, since begging can be a barrier to their wellness. Over time, my children and I developed strong casual relationships with many residents. (My husband was not involved, since it is I who spent a good portion of each day watching the children as they played in the front yard of the house.)

2. Fear

The slight apprehension I had prior to starting my internship was connected to procedural details—arriving at the clinic on time and getting the documentation done in a timely manner. I was not too concerned about building a trusting therapeutic relationship. That was a major focus when I did my prior internship, but now I feel confident in my abilities to do so. That was until I met Leah.

3. Shock

Leah noticed me when she entered the hallway from the solarium. She approached me and asked me in Yiddish if I am a religious Jew. My initial reaction to this encounter was a strong feeling of sympathy. Not that I do not feel the pain of other clients, but she is one of my own. Although I do not know her personally, the Jewish people automatically feel connected to one another, viewing each person as a crucial member of the fold. From early childhood, an Orthodox Jew is taught to feel as if the entire Jew-

7. Sympathy

6. Overidentification

7. Sympathy

ish nation is one body with each of its members acting as a crucial portion of this body. Therefore, if one member is in pain, other members who come in contact will feel part of the pain on their own level.

In addition to the strong feeling of sympathy, many other thoughts flood my mind. My main concern is the way I should handle her in the future. Knowing that the religious Jewish community is very close knit and considers mental illness to be a stigma, I am not sure how to approach Leah the next time I see her. (It should be noted that a serious mental health problem carries a stigma in all ethnic, cultural, racial, social, and economic classes. It is not specific to the Jewish community.) Does my presence on the ward make her feel uncomfortable? Does she realize there are laws pertaining to confidentiality? I made three decisions: (1) Leah would need to initiate the encounters with either a verbal or facial expression (*); (2) I would mention that I am bound by laws of confidentiality not to disclose her case to anyone (*); (3) I would notify the staff at the next meeting of possible consequences of my presence on the ward (*).

There are some funny moments also. A client, Rob, considers it his duty to welcome the new interns to the ward. Among his many comments is an invitation to join him for dinner after he leaves the ward. The primary theme of his monologue concerns the dullness of working as a professional, attending meetings, and doing whatever. After about 10 minutes of his speech, I am ready to move on. I mention to the other interns that were waiting with me that I am going to walk to the other meeting room to check on its status. Since no one else cares to follow, I walk on my own. I realize I am losing my patience and need a break.

I have no qualms about departing, since I know my limits. Even when speaking with friends, I am able to listen for long periods of time; however, once people start repeating themselves frequently or add a tremendous amount of unnecessary details, my interest wanes. Usually, I would try to refocus the person; however, here I am, new on the ward, not knowing anything about the client, and feeling that it is appropriate to set limits.

16. Understanding symptomatology as it relates to diagnosis and functioning

Rob is also moving his feet constantly while talking. It is not very irritating but very puzzling. Which diagnosis would present with this symptom? I convey this question at night when speaking with a fellow classmate. I discover that the "moving feet syndrome" is caused by medication, not an illness. I am too busy trying to figure out clients' diagnoses based on presenting symptoms that I completely forget about the possible side effects of medication.

The last hour of the day is spent observing an evaluation and documenting it. Any information given during the interview does not scare or shock me. The client is cooperative throughout the interview.

Log 2. 6/2

The community meeting is very interesting. Compared to my previous internship, this meeting dwells more on the clients' voicing complaints and worries than on anything else. At the previous site, the meetings lasted for exactly half an hour. The first 10 minutes were devoted to making announcements, by both staff and clients, regarding different events going on in the transitional day treatment program (TDTP). The next 10 minutes were set aside for voicing complaints and concerns. The last 10 minutes were for clients to mention positive accomplishments during the week. Another important difference is that, at the other site, the clients felt complaints were being addressed. During this meeting, even I feel that complaints are not getting answers. It seems to me to be a futile meeting. If the clients want more activities, why is no one offering to look into it? If the clients are complaining about poor communication between the doctors and clients, why are the doctors not stating they would be clearer or pointing out to the clients that often they do inform the clients of different procedures, but that the medicine or illness may be affecting the clients' ability to remember?

> 11. Anger when limitations are not solvable

During the staff meeting, the happenings at the community meeting become clearer (*). The staff, particularly the nurses and doctors, addresses most of the clients' issues. Additionally, it seems the long list of complaints is a reaction to just going through a long holiday weekend. Hence, some doctors were not on floor for the previous four or five days, leaving the clients with feelings of abandonment and poor communication with the doctors. As a rule, fewer activities are scheduled during a weekend, thus adding boredom to the hospital stay.

I have a few minutes free in the afternoon; therefore, I am spending time trying to meet more of the clients that are in the solarium. I speak with Felicia, who is focusing on getting her children back into her custody. She feels that her answer to all her problems is completing her major in college. Maybe a half-year ago, I would have felt saddened by the fact that her children are with her husband, but seeing her in the present condition makes me wonder if the children are not safer with him (*). If she were to tell me that the answer lies in her ability to learn to manage her barriers, I would feel differently. Now, I am beginning to understand one main difference between clients in a locked ward and clients in a TDTP. A larger portion of the clients in a TDTP accept their illnesses, whereas those in an inpatient unit seem to be in denial.

> 16. Understanding symptomatology and pathology as they relate to diagnosis and functioning

Jean, during a group session, mentions that she wants to leave the hospital so that she can go back to her business. To find out whether it is a real business (it is possible for people with psychosocial issues to run a business) or a symptom of an illness, I decide to approach Jean rather than read her chart (*). Within five minutes of speaking with her, it is quite obvious she is in either a hypomanic or manic state (*). This conclusion is based on the fact that the business begins after she is hospitalized, the orders are from staff members, and her goal is to have a wreath hanging on every front door in America. It is a boost to my confidence that I am able to interpret data correctly.

When documenting observations as a hospice volunteer, I had to use the terms *it seems* or *it appears*. Although I am now closer to being called a professional, I still do not feel comfortable deleting the terms *seems* and *appears*. An occupational therapist intern's level of knowledge is quite limited when compared to a social worker, psychologist, or psychiatrist. Fellow classmates during seminars frequently express this feeling of inadequacy also. The encounter with Jean confirmed that, as an occupational therapist intern, I know much more than I realize.

4. Inadequacy

Leah is still a concern of mine. At the staff meeting, a social worker mentions that my presence may have a positive effect on alleviating her stigma of the illness. I thank the staff member for her suggestion, for I clearly am not thinking in those terms. My resolve not to speak to Leah until spoken to is changed to treating her like everyone else on the ward (*). I will greet her if she does not initiate; however, it will be her choice to respond. Alas, Leah does not take notice of my presence even when greeted. She is very upset today, avoiding eye contact with the staff, possibly because her clothes are not yet returned to her since she is not complying with the ward's rules and regulations.

12. Focus

I meet with Dr. B. today to discuss the stigma related to psychosocial issues (*). I have two basic questions: How does one know when a denial or nonacceptance of an illness is considered within normal limits or a clinical symptom? If Leah has been in denial for 30 years, how can my presence make a difference? Also, what is the likeliness of insight changing in any person who has been in denial for such a long time? The details of the discussion are not important to this log; however, what is important is that Dr. B. is available for staff to discuss issues related to the work on the ward.

12. Focus

The last group of the day is a movement group. I find myself comparing this group to the movement group I ran on my prior internship. On the one hand, I am surprised that the demands made in the inpatient unit are more physically strenuous. On the other hand, a smaller percentage of the client population attends this group than my group at the TDTP. I am not sure if the poor turnout is as a result of the more strenuous demands being made or that an inpatient population is on a lower functioning level, meaning there would be no difference in turnout even if the exercise were less demanding.

Log 3. 6/3

Today Leah appears to still be very upset and angry at the world. It, therefore, is not surprising that she does not initiate conversation or respond to my greetings. (At some point during the day, I find her in bed, crying.) Although fellow interns recommend not reading charts, I feel it would be beneficial to review Leah's chart to gain more insight about her as a person.

8. Empathy

By the end of the day, I finally realized my presence on the ward is most probably not an issue for Leah but for me (*). On the first day, I try looking at the situation from her standpoint, applying general views that exist among the Orthodox Jewish community, specifically in the Chassidic sect. I am employing hypothetical reasoning; however, I am ignoring some blatant cues displayed by Leah. This realization, in combination with chart review, causes me to look at the situation from a different standpoint.

Initially, I assumed my presence would make her feel uncomfortable, based on the notion that she and her family would still be trying to keep her psychosocial issues as hidden as possible. I failed to acknowledge the fact that Leah did not withdraw or appear anxious on hearing that I was religious. In fact, she continued the conversation without a noticeable change in tone of voice, mood, or affect. In addition, she insisted on conversing in Yiddish, even though I responded in English. Last Tuesday, Leah stood in the hallway when making a loud blessing over a snack (a Jewish law). Today, when asked to sign a sign-in sheet at the end of a group session, she wrote her name in Hebrew.

The actions that occurred on the first day of the internship are safely stored in my memory but not utilized in the thinking process. As I witnessed her Hebrew signature, I began to explore other possibilities. Maybe she was doing this to make a common bond. We both are religious, make blessings, and speak and understand Hebrew and Yiddish. Possibly, she was trying to make the hospital feel more comfortable and hospitable; she might feel she is not totally alone since there is a natural bond between fellow Jewish people. It is conceivable she was using this as another way to deceive herself and deny her issues or to test and manipulate me. Only time will tell.

Although I observed more group sessions today, the only other major event that came to mind is the nightmare of all health care providers—documentation. Within the third and fourth day of the internship, I am responsible for writing progress notes on seven clients, many of whom I have not met yet. From the moment it is announced in orientation on the first day of the internship, I am a little concerned, since I know it takes me a while to put names to faces.

Using suggestions made by fellow interns (*), I am almost able to glide through documentation. One recommendation is to visit my clients in their own rooms for 5 to 15 minutes. In that amount of time, I am able to make many observations about orderliness of personal space, personal cleanliness, responsiveness to staff, facial expressions, frame of mind, and so forth. The most important accomplishment is that I am finally putting together names, faces, and personalities.

Michael, one client I visited, and I had already met two days ago, during the initial evaluation session. He was still in a special care room due to suicidal ideation. No improvement in mood and affect was noticed. He was spending most of the day in bed and still feeling as if his organs do not exist and that he is dying. He asked me to explain the role of my occupation. One question led to another, and by the end of the visit, he said he wanted to get out of bed and visit the television room. I was happy that he was taking this step by himself. I did not realize that his motivation to engage in a purposeful activity might be due to my intervention just now. My supervisor helped me see this and suggested that I visit him more often and note his progress (*).

There are a few reasons for the lack of visits to Michael after the interview. Since most of the clients on the ward were strangers to me, I am trying to meet those I do not know. I meet many clients as they pass by me in the hallway or at group sessions, two locations that are off limits to a client in special care. Additionally, I am avoiding the special care section. Recently, there had been two incidents of violence in that section; and frankly, I do not want to be there in case it should occur again. When I actually went to visit Michael to write a progress note, these factors did not enter my mind. My ability to enter the special care area might be due to the fact I am concentrating on fulfilling my responsibilities. Now that I actually entered that section again, I realized that, as long as I am going to the room of a nonviolent client, I am not so worried. Maybe this is somewhat foolish, for who says the violent client will stay in his room (*)?

2. Fear

Log 4. 6/4

Leah was in better spirits this day. She still did not have her clothes returned to her, she still was noncompliant with her medication, but she initiated a conversation with me. Again, she spoke only in Yiddish. I was surprised at how well I understood her. Years ago, I developed a mental block against Yiddish and, for that matter, any foreign language. When people in my neighborhood approach me for information, I always ask them to speak in English. I am not sure why I was able to understand her. It may be because she spoke more slowly than the average person. Possibly, I guessed the meaning of some words based on context, since the conversations revolve around hospital issues. Our conversation was shortened by a visit from one of her relatives. It left me in a quandary as to whether I should go over to her to wish her a Good Sabbath before leaving for the day. I decided against it for I felt it was not appropriate in this situation (*). In her present state of mind, she might take it as preferential treatment or misconstrue it for something else, since her use of religion is a symptom of the illness.

I would like to note here that it seems to me that it is very common for people with psychosocial issues to use religion in the wrong ways. Some see themselves as a savior; others think God is talking to them. On some level I understand why this happens. Religion, by definition, has a spiritual component while the nature of some psychosocial issues obstructs abstract thinking and maybe even concrete thinking (*).

At team rounds, I learned that Sharon, a client I am supposed to evaluate today, may be depressed. All I know is that, when I approached Sharon yesterday, she refused to talk. Later that day, I was given a message from nursing not to approach Sharon for the rest of the day, per the client's request.

16. Understanding barriers as they relate to diagnosis and functioning

I am learning new things every day. At today's meeting, I was told that her crying bouts and refusal to speak with me yesterday are symptoms of depression. I had thought the crying was a side effect of medication and her refusal to speak a form of anger against hospitalization.

Later in the day, Sharon was "forced" to attend an arts and crafts and skills development session. A nurse got her to agree to attend the group, but Sharon left the room within minutes of the nurse's departure. I immediately informed the nurse, since he officially told the client to work with me. The nurse brought her back to the room. This time she spent the first five minutes staring at the paper in front of her, refusing to have anything to do with it. Eventually, she picked up a crayon and started coloring in the picture. She worked very slowly, doing only a minute section of the picture, and leaving about halfway through the session. While some behavior might be caused by depression, I still feel a certain portion of it was caused by anger and the need to gain some control of the situation (*).

Jose is a mystery to me. This person has a reputation of being a loner who walks the halls and responds to auditory hallucinations, or so say fellow interns working with me. To me Jose is a person who interacts. Since my first few days here, he always smiles and says hello to me when I greet him. Even as he passes a doorway to a room I am working in, he smiles at me when our eyes meet. One day, he even initiated contact and asked me if I am a happy person. When I ask what makes him think I am happy, he replied because I always smile at him when I say hello.

I wanted to protest today when the doctor and nurse were updating staff regarding Jose. They said he is as introverted as one can be, speaking only to his voices. I withhold my opinion because I realized he is only like that with me (*). As if to prove the point, Jose also stopped responding to me today.

What I gain from writing today's log is that I am left with many questions that need answering. (1) In the future, should I say "Good Shabbos" to Leah (*)? (2) In a similar vein, should I mention to one client that she and I share the same first name? Where do we set limits and boundaries? How much do we share of ourselves with these clients? At a TDTP, it is safe to share very superficial and obvious information, such as pointing out that a staff member and client share a common first name. Is it safe to do likewise in an inpatient setting (*)? (3) Is part of Sharon's behavior an expression of anger and need to control (*)? (4) What enables a client with Jose's history to open up to me (*)?

Log 5. 6/7

Today is going especially well. I left the building feeling accomplished and confident in my abilities as a professional in a mental health setting. I found it easy to converse with most clients, meet deadlines for documentation, and glide through my first interview. Also, I finally felt comfortable with the Leah issue.

I spoke with Dr. B. regarding the Good Shabbos question. Is it appropriate for me to seek out Leah Friday afternoons to wish her a Good Shabbos? May I allow her to continue speaking to me in Yiddish? Would it fuel her illness? Dr. B. responded that speaking in Yiddish or saying Good Shabbos would not affect her illness. It depends on my comfort level. He did mention, however, that he is interested in knowing why she insists on using Yiddish.

The next time I meet with Leah I asked her why she uses Yiddish when speaking with me. She replied that, in her neighborhood, all the religious people converse only in Yiddish. Based on this answer, I decided to allow her to speak to me in Yiddish and to wish her a Good Shabbos, since these are considered proper social etiquette in the religious community where she resides.

Another area that is troublesome to me is how to ascertain if a client is attending to his or her personal hygiene needs. Usually, I can tell by looking at the hair. This is not a solution when observing African-American clients, since their hair does not become greasy when dirty. Additionally, the interns, who were responsible for training me, tell me they use body odor as the determinant factor. I try to explain to them that body odor is not a possibility for me since I have a loss of smell due to allergies. Their only answer is that I need to learn how to smell body odor.

Fortunately, the entire staff works as a team. I, therefore, approach nursing for an answer. A male nurse explains to me that nurses use three signs to decide a patient's hygiene level—the eyes, nose, and teeth. I appreciate this advice for now I acquire tools that I can use (*).

As mentioned in previous logs, the availability of the different disciplines plays a significant role in my adjustment to this site. It means that I have many sources to glean information from. Schedule permitting, I would like to observe the dance therapist to learn additional skills.

Log 6. 6/14–6/15

4. Inadequacy

While the rest of my colleagues already feel comfortable working in the ward, I am still adjusting to the unit. I lost any confidence I had during my first week at the site. I constantly question my abilities, wondering if I am handling situations properly.

Documentation is also taking longer, since I no longer trust my ability to correctly describe clients' behavior.

Sharon was on the ward for approximately ten days. Excluding the initial psychiatrist evaluation, the client refused to speak with staff members or fellow clients. Initially, she pretended to be sleeping whenever I entered her room. Now she remains awake, but changes her sitting position so that her back is turned toward me. At least, she waits until approximately my fifth sentence before turning away from me. Since I am already feeling insecure, I investigated her behavior with other staff members.

4. Inadequacy

15. Discouragement around lack of progress, regression, or recidivism

Michael showed very little improvement since the initial evaluation. He is still having delusions but on a smaller scale. He rarely attends or participates in groups. Initially, I felt he was absorbing some of our individual discussions, since at the end of each visit, Michael got out of bed and walked into the hallway. I am beginning to feel frustrated with this client due to the fact he has not improved beyond this point. I constantly find him in bed no matter what time of day I enter the ward.

The one place I felt I was correct is in my description of Brian. Many staff members consider Brian to be delusional. Based on his verbal and nonverbal communication during my evaluation, I suspected he is putting on a show in order to get free room and board (*). He was a little too well focused and organized during the interview, choosing an image for his delusion and supplying answers to fit the image. Brian's physical appearance is also very good. He is well groomed and stands tall and erect when walking. He displays appropriate social interaction with other clients. Additionally, he had good eye contact during the entire interview, unless he discussed the delusion. This idea was confirmed today during staff meeting. Brian's primary psychiatrist felt the same way.

Log 7. 6/16–6/17

I am beginning to feel attached to these clients. Carolyn was extremely psychotic and restless when she first arrived on the unit. Although I am not her primary therapist, we have a very good relationship. Recently, she was cornered and physically handled by a male client who wants sexual contact. In response to Carolyn's expressed concerns, I explained that she did not do anything to cause this (*). She just happened to walk past him at a time he was looking for any female that was easy to corner. I also advised her to speak further with her primary social worker or psychiatrist. This small amount of giving to Carolyn further deepened my attachment to her.

5. Underestimating pathology

Brian was supposed to be discharged. However, right before his release, the doctor met with him again and found him in a hypomanic state. So much for my understanding his illness! This is the client I thought was faking an illness in order to get free room and board. I do not understand why he is considered hypomanic.

I feel it is a natural reaction to be excited, since he is about to be discharged. Once he was told he is going to remain for a few more days, he was saddened, another natural reaction in my mind. My only question is why is he speaking about his music business, a subject he had not referred to since the first two days on the floor. This did not fit into my understanding of the client.

16. Understanding symptomatology and pathology as they relate to diagnosis and functioning

My answer came the next day. I was fortunate to be able to accompany the team doctor, Dr. B., to court. During the taxi ride, Dr. B. allowed me to ask questions. I questioned Dr. B.'s decision regarding Brian's hypomania. After listing the symptoms associated with mania I am able to clearly see why he is hypomanic (*). I realize that I am using the wrong approach when trying to understand a client's status. I start from the assumption that mental illness is just an exaggeration of a normal response to stress instead of looking to see if the client's reactions fit the criteria for a particular illness (*).

As mentioned previously, Brian seemed depressed after hearing he was not going to be discharged. For the next few days, I found him spending most of the day in bed. Another client of mine was also not doing so well. Michael's depression did not seem to be improving, only worsening. The doctor is changing his medication, hoping to see some improvement.

6. Overidentification

As a clinician, I find it very difficult to work with these clients. I realize it is easier for me to deal with a client in a manic state versus a depressed state. Brian felt great in the manic state. I just know it is not a healthy or safe state, since the client lacks insight and judgment and, therefore, may hurt himself. The depressed state is much harder on me since Brian and Michael feel a tremendous amount of pain and sadness. As a clinician, I try to alleviate the pain by encouraging them to get out of bed and involved in an activity. It is hard to watch them struggle with their barriers and the pain associated with it.

Log 8. 6/18

Yesterday, one of my clients was in court. Sharon's case was presented in court because of noncompliance with medication. Although she delivered a very strong argument in her defense at court, the judge sentenced her to retention in the hospital and permission to administer medication against her will. As a result, Sharon decompensated before leaving the courthouse and had to be placed in a four-point restraint.

6. Overidentification

2. Fear

I have mixed feelings regarding Sharon. The main source of her sadness and anger is that her 4-year-old son is in foster care due to her hospitalization. I am a mother and feel her devastation at being separated from her child. Yet, I am also afraid of her. Initially, she was selectively mute. Whenever I met with her, she would turn her back toward me to signal the time for me to leave. The day before the scheduled court appearance, she became verbally abusive. Now that she is placed in special care with four-point restraint, I am afraid she

2. Fear

might physically hurt me. Although I asked the doctor to make sure it is all right for me to enter her room, I am still scared. I decided to wait until Monday to visit, since by then she will have more medication in her system (*).

I feel my fear may be classified as a phobia. Yes, there have been a few reports of violence on this ward since I have started; however, I think my fear is already irrational. I am still not ready to visit her until Monday; however, I am prepared to speak with the psychiatrist on my team to figure out guidelines for deciding when to be cautious and how to protect myself without running away from the situation.

Log 9. 6/21–6/22

I am acclimated to the clinic by now. I have led all my groups at least once. Documentation is taking less time to complete. I am already feeling very comfortable with this population.

5. Underestimating pathology

Some clients' conditions were very puzzling. Michael is not improving. His medication was changed twice since admission to the hospital; nothing seems to help. Brian is too comfortable in the hospital. From the start it seemed as if he was coming for a free ride. Within a few days after admission into the hospital, it became quite apparent that Brian has psychosis in combination with other disorders, a legitimate reason for hospitalization. What disturbs the staff is the fact he is too comfortable in the hospital and is not actively seeking discharge.

In my opinion, Michael is resisting intervention, since he is very anxious about going home to a wife and children (*). He stated he is afraid to take on the roles and responsibilities of a husband and father. Brian, on the other hand, is homeless; and the hospital is providing a safe haven with free room and board (*).

4. Inadequacy

Today was the first time I visited Sharon since her appearance at court. I felt very awkward during the conversation. All she speaks about is her desire to be discharged, how she does not belong in the hospital but in an outpatient clinic, and whether I am able to help her get released. I know I am supposed to tell her that, to get discharged, a client must abide by the rules and regulations of the unit, including such items as taking medication, showering and dressing daily, and attending and participating in groups. I am unable to convey this message, for I feel like the staff is in control. The staff developed the rules and regulations. Clients who play the "game" properly and comply with the rules get discharged. Clients who do not obey will not be discharged. All I could do was validate her feelings by stating it is hard for a mother to be separated from her child and that it is upsetting to be in a hospital against one's will.

Log 10. 6/23–6/24

I am still trying to define my role as an occupational therapist in the mental health field. I understand the purpose of all the groups the occupational therapists lead. I see positive tangible results in individual clients who attended groups. However, when working with clients one on one, I rarely see significant results. This may be because most of my caseload has been either extremely psychotic and delusional or uncooperative.

Yet, every time I enter the ward, clients surround me. Some are asking for assistance in obtaining a specific item. Others just want someone to listen to them. Most of the clients who approach me in the hallway are not assigned to me. The clients I meet with daily on a one-on-one basis do not seek me out. They greet me or ask for assistance only when we happen to meet in the hallway. I will start noting if there is a correlation between a client's level of illness or improved mental health and a client's desire to seek me out when I enter the ward (*). Do the other interns experience the same thing? Is only a select group of clients initiating contact with the interns?

Another issue that arose today was a client's transference issue. Eric tells me he does not like calling me by my name, Marsha. He asks if I have another name. My response is no, I do not, therefore, he has to learn to cope with my name as is. Additionally, I ask him why my name makes him uncomfortable. His response is that, as a teenager he loved Marsha Brady, a member of the Brady family on television. I am not sure how to respond, so I continue to listen. In the end, it seems he just needs to voice his feelings, for once stated, he no longer has an issue with it. He also stops greeting me with "Marsha, Marsha, Marsha!" a common way for people to greet Marsha Brady on the television show.

Log 11. 6/25–6/28

> 11. Anger when rescue fantasies are not possible and limitations are not solvable

> 9. Rescue fantasies

> 15. Discouragement around lack of progress, regression, or recidivism

I usually meet with each client once a day. Friday, June 25, I was able to meet with only those who approached me. I spent most of the day doing documentation, since many interns are out. It leaves me with an empty feeling.

The main feeling I am experiencing at this time is frustration. From a caseload of seven clients, only two improve. Matty is extremely psychotic, preoccupied with internal stimuli, and doing only what God tells her to do. Sharon refuses to talk to anyone unless she needs something. Sharon and Tom lack insight and awareness. They feel there is no purpose to their hospitalizations and are extremely angry. Brian is satisfied and comfortable with his hospitalization; therefore, he is not motivated to do anything. He also lacks insight into his psychosocial issues. Michael wants the medication to eradicate all of his symptoms without any work on his part. Carmine improves, but it may be due to medication only. Tyronne is my only client who actively works on impulse control in addition to the benefits of medication.

Michael is the most frustrating of all my clients. Beginning with the initial evaluation, he speaks as if he has insight into his illness. He lists symptoms due to depression, but then ends the conversation by saying he is a difficult client. Of course, I answer

5. Underestimating pathology

if he is difficult, it is only because he chooses to be so. It just seems to me that Michael talks in circles, discussing every symptom and detail of his psychosocial issues without really trying to fight his symptoms.

I really do not understand how any health professional enters the field of mental health. It seems that many clients are improving due to the benefits of medication but not through active participation by the client. I would like to know the rate of burnout with mental health professionals, especially those caring for the more psychologically unstable clients. The message for me is to accept the idea that I cannot cure anyone or everyone. My role as an occupational therapist is to provide the clients with ample opportunity to learn new skills or techniques that will enable them to return to their roles prior to hospitalization. Occupational therapists should also be involved in helping clients gain awareness and insight into their illnesses.

Log 12. 6/29–6/30

13. Intervention

One job I find myself doing as an occupational therapist in the mental health field is listening to the clients verbalize their feelings and thoughts, validating their feelings, pointing out inappropriate behavior or irrational thoughts, and interpreting their verbal and nonverbal communication. Indirectly, I am helping them gain insight into their illnesses. These tasks apply only to clients who are not psychotic or in denial.

My guess is that the extremely psychotic clients will not improve, no matter how much effort is put into their intervention (*), especially considering these clients are on a waiting list for a state psychiatric hospital. The extremely psychotic population never attends groups either.

Regarding the client population that is in denial, it seems that time is the most important factor. As medications build up in their systems, their symptoms decrease, the clients gain more insight into their respective illnesses, and they are more compliant with the unit's rules.

A small issue that arose during the staff meeting is that a doctor referred to the occupational therapist interns as PT/OT. This is the second time a staff member called us by this title. It also is the last day for the attending doctors at this site, since they are leaving to new jobs. I cannot resist correcting their misconception (*). I, therefore, mention in a polite way that the interns are all occupational therapists and that there is a difference between physical and occupational therapists. I feel comfortable making this statement, especially since I have established a rapport with the staff member who makes the mistake. Two points for us. If occupational therapists are not going to clear up misconceptions, who will? It just has to be said at the right moment in an appropriate manner.

This point leads to one difference between my colleagues and myself. Since the start of this internship, the other interns have disagreed with how I present myself to other professionals. Their opinion is that every movement we make is held against us, including our body language at a staff meeting. Therefore, the other interns will not chance speaking at a staff meeting. I, on the other hand, feel very comfortable among professionals and do not feel anything is wrong with speaking at a meeting, providing the statement is apropos and stated properly.

I spoke with fellow classmates to do a reality check regarding the situation. The conclusion we made is that age and maturity play major roles. For one, most of my close friends and associates outside college are professionals, including doctors, lawyers, and social workers. Second, as a parent and consumer, I build a strong rapport with each doctor that treats any member of my family. As such, I have learned how to speak and relate with professionals.

Log 13. 7/1–7/2

Today is the big day. There is a big changeover in staff. Many psychiatry and psychology interns completed their second year residency and, therefore, are going to new placements. In addition, the two attending doctors, who led the teams, are leaving this site for new positions.

18. Consolidation

While the change in staff is difficult for clients, it is also an adjustment for the remaining staff members. Since the teams are in the initial stage of development, all team members are acting more polite and accommodating than usual. The attending doctors lead team meetings following the format set by their predecessors. All this should change once the new interns and attending doctors are able to define their roles, needs, and goals better.

14. Hope

I feel better as a professional. To handle the frustration I feel, I pull back a little, telling myself that I cannot change people and just try to do the best I can. Some of my clients are finally beginning to show improvement in small increments. I feel comfortable expressing ideas to clients, even when I know it might cause the client to add my name to the black list of staff members.

13. Intervention

Michael was never able to develop and maintain a daily schedule, but he is finally willing to engage in a task instead of lying in bed all day. Ibrahim finally agreed to wear a hospital gown while his clothes get washed. (I should mention that nursing asked me to try to get him to agree to shower and wash his clothes. I am excited that I am able to work with nursing to help meet this goal.)

14. Hope

18. Consolidation

Sharon still refused to talk to me, but at least I am able to come up with a new way to approach her. (Due to lack of time, the new approach will not be carried out until my next day at clinic.) Brian agreed to dress in street clothes and attend groups, criteria for attaining the privilege of going on group walks. I will see if he follows through with his commitment. At least he is willing to listen and accept the rules this time. Matty was still psychotic, irritable, and disagreeable with everything, including denying that she has a large stain on her outfit. The doctors are waiting to transfer her to a state hospital, since she has a long history of noncompliance with medication and no improvement in her illness. Tom was still in a strong stage of denial, but I finally could state his problem clearly to him. This is an accomplishment for me, since I was leaving this undesirable job to the other staff members.

Log 14. 7/6–7/7

Every Wednesday morning, there is a staff meeting. This is the only time the entire staff meets. The ward, including staff and clients, is divided into two teams. A team meeting, whose purpose is to discuss treatment planning for individual clients, occurs on the other days. The focus of staff meetings is to discuss issues important to managing the ward.

During today's meeting, I presented a problem I encountered the previous day in a group therapy session. The discussion in yesterday's group centered on identifying the differences between passive, assertive, and aggressive communication styles and practicing assertive communication. A client mentioned her difficulty in expressing her needs to the nursing staff. After repeating the general guidelines I mentioned to the clients, I asked the nursing staff for their ideas (*).

4. Inadequacy

A few thoughts passed through my mind prior to posing the question. Will it lessen my credibility because I admit I do not have the answers to everything? Will it lessen the staff's respect for my profession?

The nurses addressed the issue in a serious manner, offering concrete suggestions. After mentioning a particular client's response to my guidelines, the nurses made an intervention plan for that client regarding assertive communication as it relates to interaction with the nurses. Not only did the nurses offer concrete suggestions, they stated how important it is to discuss this issue at

14. Hope

staff meetings. I walked away from the meeting feeling the question strengthened my credibility and role on this ward.

Log 15. 7/8–7/16

On Thursday, July 8, I received an emergency call during the team meeting, informing me of a death in my family. Since I knew I would be out for the following week, I focused on finishing as much documentation as possible. (When faced with an emergency, I hold myself together until the initial emergency is over.) Even though I told my colleagues I will be out until next Thursday, I did not warn the clients. My mind focuses only on the fact a family member has died, information I did not want to share with the clients. Now, looking back at the situation, I realize I could have told them I was going out of town for a week, without offering an explanation. However, during the emergency, I could not think fast enough.

Thursday, July 15, feels somewhat like the first week at clinic. Although I missed four days, I thought I could just pick up

2. Fear

where I left off. As I unlocked the door to the ward, I began to feel slightly anxious. Thoughts—such as clients can change in a day's time, even more so in a week—are going through my mind. Attending a team meeting alleviated the anxiety to a small extent. In addition to running groups, evaluating a new client, and writing a discharge summary on an old client, I spent most of the next two days getting reacquainted with my clients.

My highest level of frustration is associated with the discharge of one of my clients. Since he was being transferred to a TDTP in this hospital, I was required to complete an evaluation of his baseline occupational performance. His discharge occurred the day I returned, allowing me only a few minutes to speak with him before he left the ward. Although I reviewed his chart and approached colleagues to obtain and update information, I still had a difficult time ascertaining his level of occupational performance at discharge.

There are some good moments also. Two of my clients improved significantly during my absence. It is exciting to see them well groomed and walking with more of a purpose and direction in their stride. It also means I have to spend more time than usual with them in order to know and understand fully their present functioning levels.

As if to spite me, two other clients decompensated after the progress notes were signed and returned to me. I contemplated rewriting their notes, but decided against it. The main reason for this decision is a lack of time. Other documentation and responsibilities need my immediate attention. Additionally, the contents of the progress notes were accurate at the time they were written. The new information just has to wait until next week's progress notes.

By the end of day two since my return to clinic, I felt I was back to normal. The only difference between the other colleagues and myself is that they are receiving their midterm evaluation this week while I am forced to wait another two weeks before receiving mine.

Log 16. 7/19–7/20

11. Anger about limitations and inadequacies of the system

17. Integrating theory and practice

Lately, I am feeling frustrated. Five classes in psychiatry are not enough preparation for this field, in my opinion. Many goals my colleagues and I are writing are not realistic, especially when setting goals for someone in a psychotic state. People who are delusional display poor insight and judgment. Without insight, awareness of problems, and ability to check reality, how are we supposed to motivate people to improve in their occupational performance? I think my colleagues and I lead group activity sessions extremely well. However, recreational therapists could just as easily lead the task groups and the verbal groups are led by psychologists.

Two weeks ago, a social worker approached me concerning a specific client. She wanted to know if I thought this client was ready to go on group walks and the reasoning behind my opinion.

While stating proofs for not allowing group walks, I mentioned the goals I set in the intervention plan with this person. The social worker was surprised that I was already working on increasing problem-solving skills besides improving social skills, in view of the fact the psychology department was still working on building a trusting relationship. What ensued was a 15-minute discussion with the social worker. She began the discussion by saying that new psychology interns make the same mistake, jumping from step one to two so quickly, because that is how it is taught in the textbooks. Also, it should be mentioned the goals I set with this person were based on a discussion with fellow colleagues, since I was at a loss as to how I should continue with a person who was still denying her illness and the facts that led up to her hospitalization (*). While the conversation with the social worker was very informative, I was left feeling frustrated.

This week I am finally hearing solutions to my questions and frustrations. The role of occupational therapy versus recreational, art, or dance therapy and psychology was addressed during intern seminar, a weekly seminar dedicated to open discussions of issues important to interns. Based on the seminar, I realized that, as an occupational therapist, I focus on a client's current occupational performance during group sessions, something a psychologist, art, or recreational therapist would not do. I, however, still feel I need a stronger background in psychiatry to be a more effective therapist when setting goals and meeting one on one with people in a psychotic state.

This issue was addressed a few days later during team meeting. Tom's symptoms were finally decreasing. Dr. M., when discussing Tom, mentioned that sometimes there is nothing a health professional can do until the medication takes full effect. He continued to say that, while in most situations it takes approximately three weeks for the medication to reach its full potency, it is not unheard of for the medication to take up to 60 days. Dr. M. could not have stated my sentiments any better.

Tom, who happens to be my client, was already in the hospital for over 40 days. Due to extreme agitation, denial of symptoms and illness, and lack of insight and judgment, it is impossible to write a contract with Tom or work on any goal besides behavior modification in the form of decreasing the number of times he uses profanity when expressing his anger during a discussion with staff members. The statements made by Dr. M. helped me realize that I know more than I am giving myself credit for, my expectations may be too high, and at times I will feel totally ineffective until the clients' medication takes full effect (*).

Log 17. 7/21–7/26

Sonia has been my client for the past three weeks. As I wrote the discharge summary today, I reflected on her hospitalization, including the client-therapist relationship.

17. Integrating theory and practice

11. Anger when limitations are not solvable

10. Becoming aware of the limitations of interventions

4. Inadequacy

I administered an evaluation on the third day of Sonia's hospitalization, two days later than the nursing and psychiatric evaluations. Sonia was cooperative during the evaluation, spontaneously supplying the necessary information. Prior to my evaluation, the staff had a sparse history on her.

Initially, I thought Sonia's compliance was due to the time difference between the first two interviews and mine. Sonia was disoriented on admission. Two days could have given her enough time to recuperate, enabling her to provide details of personal history and the event that led to the admission. Periodically, answers contradicted each other. However, Sonia clarified the mistakes once they were brought to her attention.

As her hospitalization progressed, I contemplated the possibility that my Jewishness may have contributed to her willingness to talk openly to me. Sonia referred to my Jewishness during a group session in her second week at the hospital, jokingly saying we were a team since we are Jewish. Until this point, I did not realize that Sonia knew I was Jewish. Religious Jews recognize one another based on the attire, since we follow a specific dress code. I was not aware that Sonia had prior exposure to the religious Jewish community.

Today, as Sonia waited for the discharge papers, she discussed a variety of Jewish topics with me. It was a "neighborly" type of conversation. Last week's comment during group session in combination with this conversation seem to confirm the possibility that initially she trusted me more than other staff members (*).

Log 18. 7/27–7/28

15. Recidivism

The first client to return since my internship began was admitted today. Only one week has passed from Ibrahim's discharge to readmission. The reason for readmission was the same as for the previous admission, noncompliance with medication. At the team meeting, staff members mentioned this was his sixth admission, all for the same reason. Apparently, Ibrahim was not ready to accept the fact he has psychosocial problems (*).

10. Becoming aware of the limitations of the intervention center

Another client of mine will be discharged in a few more days. Although Tom has complained continuously throughout the hospital stay, unconsciously he really likes the attention he receives. As proof, Tom's anxiety level escalates on hearing his discharge date. Instead of pacing the hallways, Tom remained in bed to prevent total decompensation. Additionally, his speech returned to being pressured. I am fearful he will decompensate once he returns home. Unfortunately, the health care system does not allow a transition from institutionalization to community living.

Insurance companies mandate client care, causing a significant decrease in clients' functional levels during the hospital stay. The clients enter the hospital on a sicker level and leave stabilized but not necessarily functional. While I do not perceive the

15.
Discouragement
around lack
of progress,
regression, or
recidivism

8. Empathy

"revolving door" client as a personal failure, the phenomenon definitely affects work satisfaction, contributing to a sense of helplessness.

In addition, on a certain level, I feel some intervention plans written by mental health professionals are unrealistic. Some people improve solely due to medication. These people deny their barriers, lack insight, or are too psychotic to benefit from any form of therapy. If I feel frustrated and helpless at times, one can only imagine what these people must feel like.

Log 19. 7/29–7/30

Today I interviewed Pamela. When assigned Pamela, I was warned to proceed with caution since she has a history of physical violence and verbal abuse. Sure enough, on day one, she started yelling at me as soon as I said my name. As Pamela pronounced each word, I heard the anger rise in her voice. I felt safe from her anger, since I maintained a considerable distance from her. Pamela was sitting on her bed while I stood 2 inches from the door. Also, I was not alone. Pamela's room is in full view of a nursing attendant.

By day two, I was able to say two complete sentences before she started screaming and yelling. By day three, Pamela was very friendly and amiable. We spoke for approximately five minutes before she expressed the need to end the conversation. By day four, I was already attached to her.

Once medicated, Pamela is an adorable lady. She has a long psychosocial history. Her son was in a correctional facility at the time of her hospitalization. Her son's absence exacerbated the psychosocial issues, since they shared an apartment. Pamela is in her forties and has been around. She has her stories to tell. The cutest part to her personality is that she has her ways for doing things. As the nurses said, "Pamela is Pamela." She sets her own rules. When assigned to special care, she roamed around the entire ward instead of staying within the limits of the special care wing. If she felt like attending a structured group activity, she went, even though group activities are off limits to the special care population. She needs to smoke. A nurse takes her out to smoke, a privilege usually reserved for the highest functioning clients on the ward, in return for accepting a certain amount of responsibility for themselves and their barriers.

Even with all her sweetness, Pamela is a challenge. She recognizes that she has problems. She knows her decompensation was associated with her son's absence, so much so that she expressed a wish to be transferred to a state hospital because she cannot live alone. However, she is ineligible for a state placement. She already refused home care, an option offered to her a few months ago, during the last hospitalization. Discharge planning for this hospitalization focused on finding a well-structured day treatment program with a tremendous amount of emotional support.

As for her intervention plan, I concentrated on her attending and participating in as many group activities as she can tolerate (*). Once in group, I spent energy on getting her to participate. My reasoning behind this is that most of the day in continuing day treatment programs is spent in group activities. If she does not start developing an interest in group activities in the inpatient unit, what are the chances she will participate in a day treatment program once discharged?

18. Consolidation

Log Summary

Even though students are constantly warned and reminded regarding countertransference, one is not always aware of its existence. I went into great length discussing Leah in Log 1; however, not until Log 3 did I acknowledge my thoughts and reactions as countertransference by stating, "my presence on the ward is . . . not an issue for Leah, but for me." Countertransference appears again in Log 7, when I mention the difficulty I experienced working with people who are depressed, since "Brian and Michael feel a tremendous amount of pain and sadness. . . . It is hard to watch them struggle with the illness. . . ." By now, I am more attuned to when my feelings affect my actions (*).

In Log 11, I discuss Sharon's presentation the day following her court appearance. I describe a feeling I share with Sharon, stating "it is hard for a mother to be separated from her child." The thoughts that crossed my mind during the actual court session on the previous day I did not record in the logs. Sharon's arguments in court were very persuasive. Her explanations for the behaviors that led to the hospitalization made the behaviors appear as normal and appropriate reactions to the situation. So much so, that if I had been the judge, I would have released her from the hospital. Overidentification, another problem common to interns working in the mental health field, may have affected my view of the situation. The only saving grace is that, when Dr. B. and I rehashed the court case in the taxi ride back to the hospital, Dr. B. told me that, if another judge had handling the case, Sharon would have been released. This particular judge has been biased toward doctors in the past.

6. Overidentification

As the internship progressed, I learned to become more assertive with the clients, challenging their behavior or distortions of reality. Rob went on and on with his monologue (Log 1). Instead of setting limits on the client's behavior, I made an excuse for leaving him. Felicia saw completing college as her panacea (Log 2). Instead of doing some reality testing with her, I chose to leave the discussion as is. Not until after I meet with Dr. B. (Log #5) did I start confronting clients directly. As stated in the log, "The next time I met with Leah I asked her why she uses Yiddish." In Log 13, I am already at the point where "I feel comfortable expressing ideas to clients, even when I know it might cause them to add my name to the black list of staff members."

Reading charts, questioning clients, and speaking with team members from all the disciplines helped in my growth. "Although fellow interns recommend not reading charts" (Log 3), I disagreed (*). The doctors and psychiatry interns at this site also read clients' charts before and after meeting with them. It helps one hone into the important issues when doing the initial evaluation. One can see which areas are weak or lacking information. It may also help the professional find a topic that is important to the client, a topic that may be used to help build an immediate rapport with the client at the time of the initial evaluation.

An interview I observed Dr. B. administer begins with a discussion of a particular client's child. Dr. B. asked the client if she had any children, knowing the client dotes on this child and her relationship with the child is one of the client's strengths. This information, gleaned from the chart, aids in the development of a good rapport.

It is not enough to read charts. It is also necessary to go directly to the clients. I approached Jean (Log 2) to discern the truth regarding her business. I could have read the diagnosis in her chart, but it was more beneficial to speak with Jean directly. Reading a chart is similar to working with the analysis of a case study, while speaking with the person allows one to learn by direct observation.

Meeting with those in other disciplines is also very important in one's growth as a professional. There is no better setting than mental health for this, since the field of mental health is very team oriented. In this affiliation, I am able to attend team meetings three times per week and staff meetings once a week.

16. Understanding symptomatology as it relates to diagnosis and functioning

Log 4 gives an example where the information supplied at a team meeting increased my understanding of the symptoms I observed in a client on the previous day (*). I often asked nurses or psychiatry interns for suggestions for handling particular situations. One reference is in Log 5, regarding factors used to determine a client's hygiene and grooming status. Throughout the logs, I also mentioned some of the more significant questions I posed to attending doctors.

As part of my experience, I also tried to clarify my perception of the role of occupational therapy in the mental health field. I first alluded to it in Log 14 and then discuss it in more detail in subsequent logs. It seems my initial reasons for needing to define the role is precipitated by feelings of frustration when clients do not show signs of improvement from one-on-one sessions with me. I go on to explain in Log 11 that "many clients are improving due to the benefits of medication." Even though I acknowledged that my role is "to provide clients with ample opportunities to learn new skills . . . that will enable them to return to their roles," I am still not satisfied with my function in this setting. I keep reverting to more psychosocial issues, such as helping clients gain insight and awareness into their barriers and facilitators. In Log 16, I finally question the difference in domains between recreational therapists, psychologists, and occupational therapists.

Several factors affect my ability to be more accepting of the role of occupational therapy in mental health (*). I became more comfortable in challenging and confronting clients' distortion of reality or inappropriate behavior "even when I know it might cause them to add my name to the black list of staff members." I tell myself "I cannot change people . . . just try to do the best I can" (Log 13). Additionally, Dr. M. said in a team meeting, "Sometimes there is nothing a health professional can do until the medication takes full effect." Medication cannot be removed from the picture, since it does play an important role in helping clients regain their ability to function. Finally, an intern seminar session provided a definitive answer. My job was to focus on a clients' current occupational performance. I needed to do an activity analysis, a common occupational therapy task in the physical disability setting. However, instead of looking at physical barriers, I needed to look at barriers due to psychosocial issues.

Until this point, I kept looking at a client's barriers and associated them to broad issues, such as lack of insight and awareness, denial, or psychosis. I was using a psychotherapy type of approach. Now I began to use a top-down approach, by listing a client's barriers and the actual performance components that impeded occupational performance. I still needed psychiatric knowledge to be able to discern symptoms, such as if a client is delusional or not, but I did not need to focus my therapy on eradicating the symptoms only. I will still provide psycho-education. The difference is that I am really looking at final outcomes based on daily function. Additionally, I will analyze peoples' occupational performance by their task performance while engaged in an activity, something psychologists and psychiatrists do not observe.

> 16. Understanding barriers as they relate to diagnosis
>
> 18. Consolidation

The final theme I would like to discuss is the attachments interns develop with clients in the mental health setting. Building a rapport with people is crucial in any setting to be able to build a good working client-therapist relationship. It, however, plays a more significant role in mental health. People with psychosocial issues tend to have a more difficult time building relationships, since many are paranoid or have learned to distrust people. This population, more so than others, has had many disappointments in life, specifically connected with close relatives or friends deserting them.

> 19. Feelings of loss around termination

I find myself often thinking about clients that were discharged weeks ago, wondering where they are now. Did they readmit themselves to a different hospital? Are they attending the outpatient programs? Are they managing their responsibilities at home? Since I am moving on to a new affiliation in a couple of weeks, I will never know the answers to these questions.

Analysis of Growth Throughout Marsha's Internship

Marsha begins her log by describing her preconceived ideas about clients (stage 1). Like many interns, she has had exposure to people with mental health issues, but unlike most interns, her preconceived ideas seem to be void of prejudice. Since she appears to be somewhat comfortable with this population, her apprehension (2. Fear) centers around procedural details such as meeting documentation deadlines and arriving to the unit on time. She expresses a feeling of confidence in being able to form trusting therapeutic relationships, a skill carried over from her level I affiliation, until she meets Leah, which put Marsha in somewhat of a shocked state (3). Her initial reaction to Leah is sympathy (7), followed immediately by overidentification (6).

Marsha elevated some of the pressure of working with Leah by switching to a funny moment in her narrative regarding a new client, Rob, who constantly moves his feet. Marsha grapples with understanding his "symptomatoloy" (16).

Concrete thinking appears in her second log, when she describes the procedure of the community meeting. She then becomes angry at the limitations of the context of the meeting (9), thinking that the staff is ignoring the clients' complaints.

Instead of taking what her clients say at face value, Marsha now can question the validity of Jean's wreath business and the feasibility of her return to work (16). Next, Marsha describes two instances on which she is able to focus (12): whether or not Leah may be able to gain insight into her illness and why the attendance is low for her movement group.

By Log 3, Marsha has moved from sympathizing (7) with Leah to empathizing (8) with her, demonstrating an ability to distance herself from Leah enough to observe her from "her [Leah's] standpoint" instead of through her own sympathetic reaction. Even though Marsha has been confident in the past, she becomes fearful (2) when she hears about two incidences of violence in the special care area, which she now avoids.

Marsha then learns from a meeting that Sharon's crying and refusal to speak with her are symptoms of depression instead of Marsha's previous notion that crying was a side effect of medication and unwillingness to speak was out of anger (16).

In Log 6, 13 days after the beginning of her internship, Marsha lost her confidence (4) and became discouraged over her clients' lack of progress (15). She then underestimated Brian's pathology (5) but, after initiating a meeting with his doctor, is able to assimilate the newly learned material to better understand Brian's symptoms of hypomania (16). Marsha then overidentified (6) with Brian's, Sharon's, and Michael's pain and sadness, followed by being afraid (2) of Sharon, which resulted in postponing her intervention session until after the weekend.

After more frustration (11) and discouragement around lack of progress (15), more rescue fantasies (11), and more underestimation of pathology (5), by Log 13, Marsha is able to start the consolidation process (18), where she experiences hope (14) and is better able to provide realistic interventions (13). Feelings of inadequacy (4) and fear (2) resurfaced to a certain degree, only to be followed by an integration of theory and practice (17) spurred on by her anger about limitations of the system (11). Recidivism (15) was mentioned and worked through.

Marsha ends with an insightful summary that includes more consolidation (18) and briefly mentions the termination process (19).

As you can see, the growth process is intricately woven throughout the internship. Phases are worked through only to reappear again, then worked through on a deeper level, ideally ending in some consolidation and productive treatment.

KATE HARRINGTON

In the following log by Kate Harrington, identify the stages of maturation through your own bubble writing as was done in the previous log by Marsha Eiserman.

Log 1. 6/1

Am I ready? This was all I could think about in the days before internship started. *Anxieties*, *nervous*, and *apprehensive* were the words that fluttered in my mind. I did not know what to expect on arrival to my site. Rather, the day finally arrived and the smiling faces of interns and staff pleasantly surprised me as I made my way into the office. For a moment I felt relieved; however, I knew I still had to face the unit. I had never been on an inpatient psychiatric unit. In the classroom, we had discussed common issues faced in an inpatient unit, and quite honestly, I did not know how I would fare. Only time would tell. Within an hour of my arrival, we, the other interns and I, were sent down to the unit.

Our orientation guide, another intern who was ending his 12 weeks, dropped us off near the nurses' station. We were to wait for "team rounds" to end, and then the rest of the interns would orient us further. On waiting for this to occur, a client approached us and asked who we were. Surprisingly, I responded calmly. My insides, of course, were doing something completely different. Why was I so nervous? Was I scared I would say the wrong thing? Was I scared of the client? These questions were foremost in my mind. I do not think, however, that it was apparent to the client. We introduced ourselves as interns. The client then responded by saying, "Why would you want to do that? You look too put together to do that." These statements threw me, as I did not know how to respond. I suppose this is where my nervousness kicked in and I just smiled. I did not know what to say. This frustrated me, as I wanted to reply with an insightful response.

Another significant component of the day was when I observed another intern perform an evaluation. The woman she evaluated was very confused and distracted. The client did not know why she was in the hospital, as her stories conflicted with each other. The intern, however, was able to gather some valuable information about the client by observing her mannerisms and listening "between the lines." I say "between the lines" because much of what the client was saying made no sense. It was that very observation that helped the intern identify problem areas and goals to work on.

The transition from classroom to clinic is not an easy one to make. You want everything to be "by the book" and it is difficult to accept that this is not the way it is. Although I know this to be true, it will still be a challenging transition. I did, however, walk away today feeling more confident than when I walked in.

Log 2. 6/3

As I stated before, I had felt somewhat more confident about being on the unit after yesterday's end. This feeling, however, changed slightly after the staff meeting today. The primary topic discussed at the meeting was the issue of violence on the unit. Recently, two clients had acted out toward staff members and had to be restrained for constant observation. Unfortunately, the restraints do not always adequately restrain the client, as there were situations where clients were able to free themselves. This information has instilled in me a heightened sense of anxiety. I do think, however, that this increase in my awareness will benefit me. For example, had these situations not occurred, then the topic of violence may not have been thoroughly discussed and I may have had more of a relaxed attitude. I am now aware of specific precautions and procedures to follow if a violent situation arises.

Prior to the staff meeting was a community meeting involving clients, staff, and interns. This is a forum where clients can vent their concerns, problems, and comments about the unit. This is an open forum; however, one client who compiles a list of the clients' complaints leads it. As of yet, I had not been to a community meeting, and it was interesting to see how it was run. The client was allowed to read the list of complaints, and then the staff commented on the complaints and concerns. All clients were allowed to voice their concerns. There were certain clients who dominated the forum, but everyone was given a chance, if they wanted to speak. I was able to gather valuable information about clients from observing them during the meeting. The various positions, mannerisms, and speaking patterns gave way to much interpretation. To be honest, I do not know if what I was thinking was correct, but the community meeting stimulated thought and observation.

Today was yet another day of eye-opening realizations. I am slightly overwhelmed, still anxious, and very excited. I am excited to see and experience evaluations, groups, and of course the daily issues faced on an inpatient psychiatric unit. I am excited to dip my feet into the water, so to speak. I know I have a lot to learn, but I have a feeling this experience will help pave the way for that knowledge.

Log 3. 6/6

Our team got three new admissions last night. It was time for me to perform my first evaluation. Again, the question remains, Am I ready? Well, there is no time like the present. In the moments that I had free during the day, I introduced myself to the new clients. Through the brief conversations I had with each, I made a decision regarding whom I would interview later that afternoon.

I had found the person I wanted to interview in the solarium reading the Bible. I asked if he would mind if I asked him a few questions. He did not seem to mind, so I proceeded with the interview. We sat down at a table, I gave him a copy of the unit's information packet, and we began talking. He would not look at me; in fact, his entire body was facing away from me. He was not completely turned around, but he definitely was facing a direction away from me. This made me slightly uncomfortable. Although he said he did not mind that we spoke, his body language alone stated he was not interested. I took out my list of questions pertaining to work, family, leisure, educational history, and activities of daily living; however, I soon realized I did not need it. The first questions I asked pertained to work history. He told me not even to go there, because he had not worked since 1994, and he would not because he was HIV positive. I got similar responses when I asked about his family and living situations. I realized I needed to ask my own questions, separate from the specific questions on my cheat sheet. When I made this transition, the forum opened a little, and he gave me more information. We discussed his diagnosis of HIV, and the impact it has had on various areas of his life (i.e., work and family).

Needless to say, this was a difficult interview for me. Not only did I have difficulty getting the information I needed, but I also had to be cognizant of his behaviors, mood, affect, and cognitive skills. When I have observed other colleagues and supervisors give interviews, it always seemed so easy. With practice, though, I am sure it will get easier—at least, I hope so.

Log 4. 6/8

Another day has passed and I have survived. It is definitely difficult to adjust to a 9–5 schedule. I have been used to the haphazard school schedule. I must admit, though, I enjoy working, or as I like to call it *pseudo-working*. I like having definitive hours and being able to leave work at work, or at least I try to leave work at work. I have taken some work home with me, as I read about certain diagnoses to refresh my memory of what I learned in the classroom. I also write these logs nightly, so in a sense it is taking work home. I also tend to think about the clients a lot. I think about their cases and wonder what I can do to be of service to them. I constantly think of how I am making, or not making, a difference.

A different kind of stress has been placed on me. I have not, at least yet, had to worry about deadlines or grades. I realize things have to be completed within a certain time limit, but I think I am capable of this aspect of the job. The kind of stress I feel comes from something internal, if that makes sense. As I stated before, I think, "How am I affecting these people?" I have also not had the luxury of leading a group. This will raise my stress level a little. One of my biggest fears to date is dealing with an unruly group. It is not that I am dwelling on this, but I do have a heightened sense of stress over it. As with everything in life, things will work themselves out, or at least I like to think they will. I hope I am able to rise to the occasion when it is my turn to step up to the plate. I think I will survive, as long as I believe in myself. Unfortunately, this is easier said than done.

Log 5. 6/9

Anxiety sets in. I am to lead my first group tomorrow, a grooming group. I am to lead this group in front of my cohorts, so that they may observe my techniques and provide constructive criticism. In a way, this almost makes me more nervous. Knowing that my colleagues will critique me adds a touch of pressure. In the past, however, when speaking in front of people, I feel the nervousness often helped. I only hope this is the case tomorrow. As stated in previous entries, a heightened sense of awareness can be beneficial. I just pray that the group runs smoothly.

Today was a moderately busy day. Another intern and I were to present the clients at team rounds. Unfortunately, I was not aware of this until 15 minutes prior to the start of the meeting. In a panic, I tried to gather my thoughts and observations about the clients. Why was this suddenly so difficult? Actually, I know why it was difficult. I did not want to look like an idiot. In trying to figure out and interpret my observations, I realized I needed a lot of work in one particular area. I can factually state what I see; however, I run into trouble when trying to interpret these observations. What does psychosis look like, constricted, guarded? I hear these and many more descriptors so often, but I have trouble identifying them. This is something I need to work on. The rest of the day, when walking around on the floor, I would observe clients and try to determine such things as their mood, affect, motor activity, and so on. I hope these observations will aid in my awareness of what these descriptors look like when exhibited by clients. I know that with time comes experience. Unfortunately, I want all the answers now.

Log 6. 6/11

Well, I successfully survived my first group today, a grooming group. I think it went really well. Approximately seven clients attended. Most people were concerned about their nails, clipping and filing them. Some people started grooming right away, while others needed a little more guidance and direction.

A few conflicts did arise during the session. For example, one client was very insistent about putting her nail polish on, and repeated the same question over and over, "Where is the nail polish?" Another client, looking at the various colors, was getting frustrated by the constant repetition of the question and stated to the client, "Stop asking me, you are annoying, and a nag." I thought this was the end. Was a fight going to break out? How was I to handle this situation? I took a deep breath and addressed the client asking the question first. I said, "The other client is looking at the colors, and she is aware that you are waiting for the polish." I then thought it would be appropriate to address the client who was looking at the colors. I said, "There are nicer ways to handle situations like this," and she responded, "I heard you and when I am finished I will give you the bin [of nail polish]." I do not think this was received well, as the client rolled her eyes at me. At this point I dropped it. I am not sure if I handled the situation appropriately, but I thought it needed to be addressed.

Toward the end of the group, many of the group members were socializing as they continued to groom their nails. Another intern and I tried to facilitate the conversation, and in doing so, the topic of families came up. Clients were talking mostly about their children. One client, however, began talking about all the abortions she'd had and began, what seemed to be, talking about her delusions. I was not sure how to address this scenario. As it ended up, another client said to her, "Do not go there, you are digging yourself deeper in a hole, just do not talk about that," and that was the end of it. The client ceased talking. I was surprised and relieved but wondered if I should have said anything. Sometimes, I tend to look too far into things, and this may have been one of those times. Regardless, the group went well. With an increased sense of confidence, I look forward to my next group.

Log 7. 6/13

Out with the old, in with the new. The interns who preceded us are leaving; today was their last day. It was fortunate to have them around, as they were of great assistance. This is not to say that, if they were not around, I would not have acclimated to the unit, but they did make it easier. They showed us the ropes, introduced us to groups, and provided us with feedback. On the flip side, however, it will be nice to do things myself. It has been a little difficult to get started, as I felt that I did not have a place yet; I was not sure where I fit in.

Aside from the intern issues just described, I am still trying to define my role on the unit. The interns and one certified occupational therapy assistant make up the occupational therapy direct care staff. We, the interns, have much autonomy and responsibility. From what I gather, it is not like this at many places. A few months ago, if I had heard it would be like this, I would have been very nervous. I have, however, adjusted somewhat to the format. If I had

had a slow, gradual introduction to the unit, the anxiety would have built up and I would be constantly worried about what lay ahead. There was no time for worry. We immediately had to take over client cases and begin groups. I should recommend this method to everyone. Of course, it may not be for everyone, but it has worked for me. I truly enjoy the atmosphere and the way the unit is run. I am asked for my opinion; in fact, on Tuesdays, I am required to present the clients at team rounds. This was nerve-racking at first but at the same time invigorating. I think, to myself, my opinion is respected and valued. This, in itself, provides a great source of confidence. This is turning out to be a great experience.

Log 8. 6/16

Slowly but surely, I am adjusting to the likes of the unit. I am becoming more comfortable with interviewing clients; however, I am still learning and developing my interviewing style. I realize, though, that my interview will change with every client. What works for one may not necessarily work with another. I had a challenging interview today, as the interviewee did not want to be interviewed. Her main concern was smoking a cigarette, followed by getting "the f—k off the unit." She did not think she needed to be here or in any other psychiatric setting for that matter. She has been using heroin for 18 years and had voluntarily admitted herself to the detoxification unit. It was determined that she may have an underlying depression and may benefit from an inpatient psychiatric stay, so was transferred. She says she is feeling better and wants to go home. I asked her if she felt she could keep herself off of drugs on her own, and she said, "This time I know I can do it." What was I supposed to say? Should I have mentioned the other times when this plan did not work? Given that this was our initial interview and I was not sure how to respond, I moved forward with the questioning. I did, however, suggest that options were available to aid her in the rehabilitation process.

Log 9. 6/21

Everyone was out today—well, not everyone but those who count. Our supervisor, the certified occupational therapy assistant, and the dance therapist were out. It was a little strange. The day had to continue on. I had two evaluations that needed to be signed. Luckily, I was able to contact an occupational therapist, in another unit, to review and sign my evaluation. I should have been more on top of the work; had I done the evaluations on Friday, I would not have been faced with so much work today. Enough said, the work got done, and that is all that matters.

On another note, let me talk about setting limits. This is something I need to work on. I have a difficult time setting limits with the clients, especially in a group format. It is relatively easy to set limits, at the beginning of the group, for all group members to adhere to; however, this becomes tricky when group members do not follow the guidelines. For example, the other interns and I led an exercise group today. Approximately nine clients attended. We told the clients, in the beginning, that if they wanted to leave, they could not return. We also told them that if they were not going to participate, they would have to leave. During the warm-up, a couple of clients became agitated. They were not following directions. They were talking and performing their own exercises. We instructed clients to do five jumping jacks in place. One client got very excited and performed approximately 20 jumping jacks at an extremely high intensity. It was as if he could not hear us tell him that he needed to stop and follow the directions of the leader. We simply could not get through to him. He remained difficult to redirect throughout the entire group. It was difficult to set limits with him because he was not listening to what we were saying. Should we be stricter? It is difficult to decide which approach to take. As with all issues I have faced, the answer still remains, only time will tell.

Log 10. 6/24

I do not have too many complaints thus far. I enjoy the people with whom I work, but more important, I really enjoy the population. The cases I encounter are fascinating, and I often find myself running to the textbook to look up diagnoses, symptoms, and pharmacology information. As I have said before, I have so much to learn, yet I am coming to terms with this. At first, I was anxious and disappointed, realizing there was so very much to be learned. I have, however, changed my school of thought. I am still an intern—in fact, I will always be an intern—in the sense that there is always more to learn. Slowly, the pieces will come together.

I led a goals group today, which, unfortunately, did not go as planned. The group started off well and limits were set; I had an outline; I knew where I wanted the group to go. About three quarters of the way through the group, when I asked clients to share their goals, the group went awry. One client stated, "I have no goals. What is the point anyway? The doctors decide everything." She went on to describe how she followed all the rules on the unit, went to all the groups, had her sheets signed, and still could not go on a group walk. Apparently, her doctor had told her that the team did not feel she was ready. Her question to the group and me was, "Why?" She was angry and frustrated and basically told everyone in the group that it does not make a difference whether they work on goals or not, because ultimately it was up to the doctors, who make the decisions. I was floored. In one sense, I saw her point; however, I also wanted the clients to understand that they set goals for themselves. True, the doctors and team members decide when clients are ready for level changes and, ultimately, discharge, but this was not the only reason we set goals for ourselves. The group was getting angry. They wanted answers, and I wanted to be able to give them the answers, but this was not so easy. I think I was able to bring the group full circle. I am not sure how everyone interpreted what I was saying, but I gave it my best attempt. Knowing what to say and what not to say is my greatest challenge thus far. Slowly but surely, I am getting there.

Log 11. 6/30

Starting today, four and a half weeks into this internship, I am starting to feel settled. I know what is expected of me during the day, and I am comfortable with this role. I know how long it takes to do an evaluation, relatively speaking, as in certain situations it can take longer or shorter. I know what is expected of me regarding groups (i.e., how they should be run and what my role is). I am beginning to figure out which clients require one-on-one intervention and which clients may not. I think I am balancing my time well, between getting documentation completed, visiting with clients, and running groups. Somehow, it is all coming together, and this makes me happy. Of course, there are difficult days, difficult clients, and difficult situations, but for the most part, this experience is going very well. These are generalized feelings, a midpoint perspective. I do not have much more to say today, other than what I have stated already; this is a great site, and a wonderful first internship.

Log 12. 7/2

Feelings of abandonment and autonomy run through me. Our supervisor is out, the certified occupational therapy assistants and creative art therapists are on vacation, and the attending doctors and residents are ending their rotations. This has left the nurses, social workers, and interns to pick up the pieces. I have been told that this is the hardest time of the year on the unit. Unfortunately, the staff are not the only people to have a difficult time adjusting. I have noticed clients acting differently toward staff members and interns. This was especially evident today at the community meeting. Many of the clients talked about wanting to have a priest or chaplain visit the floor more often. It was hypothesized that this could be related to the staff leaving, as the clients may see religion as a central source of comfort and solace. It could very well be that this is not the case; however, it is strange that the topic of religion has not come up until today.

Aside from feelings of abandonment, I have a strong feeling of autonomy and responsibility. I am in a situation where I can spread my wings without feeling as if others are watching me constantly. In a sense, I can test the waters, see what I really know and what I truly have difficulty with. For example, I have had some challenging clients that keep me guessing; that is to say, I have to ask myself, "What can I do for them that will help them?" Granted, this has given me a chance to problem solve and hypothesize various interventions, but it all leaves me with a sense of uncertainty. What if I am completely off-track? I know the only way to find this out is to try, but this is easier said than done.

Soon enough, our supervisor will be back, and until then life goes on. Luckily, there are people to turn to within the hospital, but they are just not as easily accessible. I do consider myself fortunate, though; I have been given the chance to be autonomous, while knowing that the autonomy is not indefinite.

Log 13. 7/4

I think, therefore I am, or shall I say, I speak, therefore I am. You must be wondering to yourself, why is this intern quoting philosophical statements? I have a client with a long history of schizophrenia, who has unfortunately been hospitalized yet again. He has very apparent positive symptoms, including delusions and paranoia. He does not, however, display problems with socialization often exhibited by persons with schizophrenia. In fact, this client constantly socializes and interacts with staff, clients, and anyone who will listen. He is always by the nurses' station or on the telephone, waiting to interact and talk with others. He is often intrusive and meddlesome and has very poor impulse control. The social worker on my team suggested that perhaps this client needs to validate his existence by constantly speaking aloud, that maybe when he is quiet he gets confused and lost, and he needs to hear his voice and receive feedback from others to feel present.

This was an interesting thought, and the social worker suggested that perhaps I could pursue this idea with the client. This suggestion actually fit into the intervention I had begun with the client. We, the client and I, had been working on communication skills, more specifically, how to improve interpersonal communication. Initially, the client was working on controlling the rate and volume of his speech, as he frequently spoke fast and loud. Today, after speaking with the social worker, I visited the client, and we discussed what it was like for him to not speak or to be quiet. He said in one word, "Helpless." He could not really provide me with further information regarding how he felt. Perhaps he meant that he felt as if he was not in control when he was not speaking. I plan on asking him more questions about this topic, specifically, what it may be like for others when they are talking to him, and how we can learn to manage our conversations with others.

Log 14. 7/10

"You have done good work." A social worker said this to me this morning in team rounds, and it made me feel great. I was acknowledged for the work I have done with one of the clients—actually, it was the client I have mentioned in the preceding log. The staff has seen this client as rather intrusive and meddlesome, as he constantly talks and interrupts many of the staff members. We, the client and I, have been working on his interpersonal skills, more specifically, how to interact with people in a controlled and concise manner. The staff reports that this patient has been less intrusive and calmer. It makes me proud to feel that I may have been part of this process.

We, the interns, are to be observed this week leading groups. I am to lead a goals group. To say the least, I am nervous. Sometimes, the group goes according to plan; and sometimes, it takes on a mind of its own. Last week, only two clients showed up to the group. I am not sure what I think is more challenging, a small, one-on-one type of group or a larger, dynamic group. I suppose it depends on the clients. Needless to say, I am slightly on edge about the experience to come.

It is hard to believe I am halfway through with this experience. Where did the time go? It feels like just yesterday that I was thinking how nervous I was to talk to clients. These feelings have subsided, as I am more confident in my approach and work with clients. Granted, not all feelings of nervousness have subsided, as there are moments, such as when I lead groups, when the anxious feelings surface. All in all, I feel as if I have acclimated well to this environment thus far.

Log 15. 7/15

I have come to a point where I am comfortable on the unit. I enjoy interacting with staff and clients and developing intervention plans to help my clients. I enjoy leading groups, albeit it has taken some time to get used to. At the moment, though, I continue to struggle with assisting those clients that seem to be resistant or noncompliant with treatment. There is a client who voluntarily admitted herself to this unit because she was having suicidal ideations. She is a MICA, mentally ill chemically addicted, client. She prostitutes for money to buy drugs and has not worked in the past six months. She does not think she has any problems or areas in which she feels she can improve. She does not want to attend groups and talks of being discharged. The social worker suggested at team rounds that this client appeared no longer to be a threat to herself and that she should be transitioned to a dual-diagnosis program for people suffering from both a mental illness and substance abuse. Some members on the team suggested that she probably would not attend, and the social worker sadly agreed. So my question is, Why send her? If she is not going to attend the program, then why send her there? Should my intervention shift to trying to convince her to attend the program? I am not sure what my role is, because she seems so resistant to wanting help.

It is frustrating when you want so much to help someone, when you have so many ideas and thoughts about what you can do to make a difference in someone's life, and unfortunately they want nothing to do with you or what you have to offer them. I remember a professor saying that you have to find your "in," a way in which you can reach the client and ultimately help. I have realized finding the "in" is often easier said than done. I will continue to try though, as maybe something I choose to say or do will open the door to helping this client.

Log 16. 7/20

I wish I could help everybody; I want to be able to help everybody. I have been thinking that, perhaps through some fault of my own, I am not capable of reaching everyone. This is a difficult concept to understand and define, as I feel there must be a way to intervene and make a difference.

In one of my classes, Mental Health Perspective II, a professor said, "You have to find your in." She described an "in" as some way for us to connect to the client and, therefore, a possible means to guide intervention. For example, when talking with a client, you discover you share a common interest; this could be an "in." The "in" in question is the common interest, something for the both of you to talk about. The "in" may act as a mechanism in helping you to develop a rapport with the client. This is often easier said than done, as I am currently having difficulty finding the "ins" with many of my clients.

Some of my clients have been in the hospital longer than I have. Their status has not changed; they are not decompensating, but they are not improving. I am constantly struggling with this concept. How can I find my "in" with these clients? What can I do to make the "in" more obvious? As I stated, the "in" is often difficult for me to see, or maybe it is so obvious that I often overlook it.

I do, however, think that I made a mini-breakthrough with one of my clients. Janna has been in the hospital since early May. She was not compliant with her medication regimen and had decompensated at her residence. She is noncompliant with the medication in the hospital, does not attend groups, isolates herself in her room, and rarely talks to me. I visit her daily, as I try to discover my "in." Yesterday, when I made my daily rounds, I found her doing a crossword puzzle. I casually asked her about it, and she told me she really enjoyed word puzzles. I then asked her if she would like me to bring her more crossword puzzles and word games. Her face brightened up, as she gladly accepted. One of my goals had been to increase Janna's interpersonal skills. As I mentioned, she usually talks to me for a limited amount of time, less than five minutes. Perhaps we could do a crossword puzzle together, at least part of one. Since I am not very good at crossword puzzles, I can ask if Janna would mind teaching me different strategies. This is a start, and I am not sure if I will be successful, but it is worth a try.

The funny thing is, I have seen Janna reading the paper and doing crossword puzzles before, but I never thought to utilize this as a possible treatment strategy. I think this may be my "in." The "in" in question (crossword puzzles) has been in plain sight all along; I was just looking too hard. I hope my idea works.

Log 17. 7/22

This week has gone very well. In thinking about the "ins" I was describing last week, I have made some progress with some of my clients. For example, Janna, the woman who enjoys crossword puzzles, loved the fact that I brought her in some puzzles. She explained how to start the puzzles, and how to come up with answers to the clues. We interacted for about 5 to 10 minutes, which was the goal I had set with her this week. When we were speaking she was not irritated or on edge; in fact, I actually think she enjoyed the conversation.

I have another client who has a very long history of schizophrenia. She has had multiple hospitalizations and is often non-compliant with her medication. She is in the hospital this time because she was not eating at her residence. Our plan was to increase her self-care skills, including eating meals during the day. When I ask her to do things with me (e.g., her laundry), she often says she does not feel well. Today, I was able to get her to do her laundry. Unfortunately, she still says she does not want to eat. I am not sure what is prompting this behavior, and I am not sure how to get her to eat. I think I need to start small, with snacks, and perhaps work toward a larger meal in the future. I have asked her why she does not want to eat, and she simply replies that she is not hungry. This could be a side effect of her medication, but again, I am not sure. I plan on bringing this problem up at the staff meeting to gain some insight into this issue.

Another client, who has a long history of major depression, recently tried to commit suicide. She continues to express passive suicidal ideations to the residents and nurses, but she has not expressed this to me. She actually said she is all right, a little down, but mostly fine. She is very well dressed, has a secure job, and secure housing. We discussed different types of coping mechanisms and stress management techniques; and although she is accepting, I feel as if she is just going along with me to please me. The information I have given her is simplistic in nature and may be too low functioning for her. When we do discuss stress-related issues, she turns the conversation around on me, and I end up being questioned. She is very good at this. I guess I feel as if I have hit a wall with her. I am still trying to figure her out, but she is making it very difficult. I am going to try and find her more sophisticated information on visual imagery and aromatherapy.

Log 18. 7/27

I want to be able to help all of them. I want to find the "ins" to all of them and help them get better. I thought I was making headway with Janna, but when I went to see her yesterday, she told me the crossword puzzle was no good because she did not have the newspaper to go with the puzzle, and she did not want to talk to me. I hope I am able to find another "in" with her.

Log 19. 7/29

I initially thought I would have no problems gathering information from clients regarding their drug or alcohol addictions. I have, however, encountered some difficulty. It has not been as easy as I thought it would be. When I first began this experience, I had one client who had been addicted to crack and heroin since her late teens. I have been able to gather some of her past history; however, it was not easy to come by. When I asked her questions about her drug use, she would initially become excited that we were discussing it; but as the conversations continued, she would ask me if we could change the subject, because it was making her want to use the drugs. She had never completed a rehabilitation program and was currently still using. She had stated that the programs simply did not work for her and she did not know why this was so.

I met one person who has been sober for over two years. He is able to freely discuss his past drug and alcohol use without necessarily feeling overwhelmed by the conversation.

On a completely different subject, I cannot believe this experience is nearing its end. Where did the time go? I have thoroughly enjoyed my experiences at this hospital. The staff was very friendly, and the clients were always interesting. I am going to be sad when my final days roll around. I had originally thought that I was destined for a physical disability setting as my initial job postgraduation. I have, however, begun to second-guess that thought. I am beginning to entertain new thoughts of becoming a mental health occupational therapist. The people with whom I have worked have been fascinating, exciting, and a pleasure. Of course, there have been extreme moments of frustration, but there have been several more occasions of satisfaction and joy. I think I will save the rest of this retrospective testimony for when I am closer to the end.

Log 20. 8/1

Some make it to discharge, others do not. Lois, a client who has been here about two weeks, was supposed to be discharged today. She resides at an adult home for women and was considered to be at baseline and therefore eligible for discharge. Over the weekend, Lois had begun to decompensate. It was reported that she stood in front of a sign near the nurses' station and talked to herself for approximately six hours. She was completely incoherent, and the nurses were unable to communicate with her. Lois has been destined to stay with us for a little while longer.

I went to see Lois today. She asked me if I could get her a newspaper and a soda. She loves the newspaper. She is always reading the paper, although I am not quite sure if she actually reads the paper or simply scans the headlines. After Lois asked me to get her these items, she asked what my name was. Mind you, I have been working with her for two weeks. This was a little disconcerting, but I attributed it to her gradual decline in mental status.

I think my "in" with Lois will be the newspaper. She seems to enjoy this so much, and perhaps I can find a way to integrate this into her intervention. Perhaps we can read a short article together and discuss it when we are finished. This is a purposeful activity that works on concentration, memory, organization, and interpersonal skills. I hope this identified "in" will be successful.

Log Summary. 8/15

It has been a short three months. The time has passed so fast it almost seems surreal. I have learned a lot during this three-month excursion, much more than I had thought possible. I learned much about myself, how I learn, my "style" as a future therapist, and what I need to do to succeed in a psychosocial setting. I also became aware of how much I have yet to learn.

I began this internship with feelings of anxiety, apprehension, and nervousness. I did not know what to expect, or more important, what would exactly be expected of me. To my surprise, the other interns and myself were thrown right in. We were immediately expected to evaluate clients, write progress notes, lead groups, and participate and work with a collaborative team of professionals. At first, I was taken aback by this approach. I thought, *I am definitely not ready for this.* I thought I would be given more time to adjust, to get acquainted with the environment, to be able to take in my surroundings before attempting to spread my wings. Right away, I was destined to sink or swim. Luckily, I swam. I was able to rise to the occasion and perform to the best of my ability. In retrospect, I would have it no other way. The feelings of anxiety and nervousness were short-lived. Had I had a slower introduction, the feelings of apprehension and anxiety would have only grown, not subsided. I was also given more time to practice evaluating, writing progress notes, and running groups. I actually felt as if I was part of the staff. Granted, I am an intern, but the services I provided on the unit and the feedback and perspective I was able to give the team made me feel more than an intern. It was a sense of responsibility and professionalism that I had been longing to feel. This has truly been a great experience, and I am sad to see it end.

As stated already, I learned a lot about myself through this experience. I became aware of the many differences that exist between the classroom setting and the clinical setting. For example, in the classroom, one receives grades and direct feedback regarding such work as intervention plans or knowledge of material. In the clinical setting, you must rely more on clinical judgment and reasoning as a basis for checking your work. You must integrate knowledge learned in the classroom with actual experiences and situations in the clinic. There are no cookbook answers to develop intervention plans for clients. Often times, you learn specific ways to treat different diagnoses in the classroom; but when you get to the clinic, it is a completely different scenario. You must integrate what you learned in the classroom with what you observe in the clinic and, more important, with each individual client. Everyone is unique, and you must take that perspective when thinking about how you want to intervene.

Another important aspect I learned was the importance of building rapport. Some clients wanted to open up and receive what I had to offer. I did, however, have difficulty establishing rapport with others. I had to work hard to find my "in." Regardless of how hard or easy it was establishing that rapport; it was something that had to be done. I found that, once I was able to build rapport and find my "in," I was able to develop and implement successful interventions.

Something I struggled with during this affiliation was defining my role on the unit. We were the ones who were going to help clients become functional and better able to deal with daily life skills. I was able, toward the second half of my stay, to engage myself more in conversations with the social workers and residents. I would ask in-depth questions, so I was able to gain a broader perspective. I would also explain what I was working on and why, so they would be aware of my perspective and the reasoning behind what I was doing.

I have come to realize that I cannot help everyone all the time. People who have just had their first break and are in denial may not be receptive to the services I have to offer. Oftentimes, people have been too psychotic to talk to me, much less attend groups. The changing health care system has also made it difficult to implement interventions, as the length of stay is becoming shorter and shorter. I know I can only do my best, no more and no less. This has been a hard concept for me to accept, but I have forced myself to do so. I did the best I could, in the time frame with which I had to work. More important, knowing that I put my best foot forward and that I learned a lot about my strengths, my weaknesses, and myself has made this experience one that I shall never forget. I have even decided to keep the idea of becoming a mental health occupational therapist in the forefront of my mind. As stated in previous logs, only time will tell.

Client-Centered Reasoning Activities

1. Identify Kate's types of clinical reasoning.
2. Return to Chapter 11 on substance abuse and trace Philip's stages of maturation.

14

Analysis of Logs II: Writing Between the Lines

The purpose of this chapter is to further the development of an ongoing dialogue in your head as you respond to written or spoken information about clients. The awareness of your dialogue's content is helpful in directing interviews, reading charts, and running groups. It helps you know what to focus on, what to ask more about, and how to direct the situation.

ANONYMOUS INTERN

Client-Centered Reasoning Activity

Write between the lines.

Log 1. 5/20

Today was the first day of my second internship. I had my first internship on a similar unit, which I attended two times per week for six weeks. This first experience consisted of mostly observing and running a few groups. I had seen locked doors, people under constant observation because of suicide ideations and possible attempts, and all different types of diagnoses before. Even though I had previous exposure, being on the unit and seeing the sick clients still affected me as I watched them wandering on the unit. Some clients were very disheveled, dressed in hospital clothing, roaming the halls, while others seemed just like the other staff members and me—like normal people.

It is so important to realize that, no matter what the clients look like or act like, they are people just like us. They have the same difficulties that we have and the same feelings but may not be able to control them as we can. Impulses, feelings, and moods are taken to the extreme and carried too far. For instance, almost all of us have been depressed at one time or another in life, but we have the coping skills to get ourselves back into life again. The clients need that extra push to do what comes naturally to us. That is why we are here. We can give that extra push. We can help them discover new ways to cope when things seem so bad that life is not worth living. We can help them to discover what they do have and to develop their self-esteem. We can listen and empathize.

Log 2. 5/24

On my way to my internship, I was looking at all of the people around me on the subway. I kept thinking that this person sitting beside me could end up in the hospital where I am doing my internship. The clients on the unit look and act like many people on the subway and many people I nonchalantly pass and deal with in everyday life. What makes these people end up in the hospital? I have seen that, many times, the people who care for the client bring them to the hospital. The outside person either cares for the well-being of that client or cares for the client's family and friends enough to try to make a difference. Other clients end up in the hospital because they do not have a strong support system. These clients may act out and do something drastic that may cause the police or emergency medical technicians to bring them into the hospital. Is the not-so-normal-looking person sitting at the end of the subway car going to end up in the hospital? Does this person have anybody to show any concern for his or her well-being? Or will it take something drastic to happen to this person? It seems so sad to me not to have somebody who cares enough to try to make a difference in the life of another human being. What a lonely life these people must live. Maybe this is why they do something drastic and eventually end up in the hospital with many staff members who seem to care.

Log 3. 5/27

I am frustrated. Not only is there tension among the team members but also tension among the interns. This is frustrating because we are supposed to be our own team. We are supposed to be able to count on each other as colleagues and confidants. There are differences of opinions, which are fine, but there is no discussion of these differences. This tension and the way in which it is handled are frustrating. If people have problems, I wish they would go to the source and work it out as adults.

I sat in on the team meeting without any of the other interns today. I was confident. I was nervous. I was intimidated. I was informed. I did fine when the time came for me to give my input. I now realize how much I retained from school. Not that I did not expect to, but it is scary to come into a setting that you have learned about from books and try to apply the information. It seems that, when you are learning the information in the classroom, you will never remember all of it. It amazes me how much has stuck with me through my program. I realize that I will be learning from now until the last day of my 12th week and everyday after when I am working, but I certainly have learned and retained the basic foundation of knowledge and clinical reasoning necessary for a practitioner.

Log 4. 5/28

Today, I had to write notes for the clients on my team. Writing progress notes that will actually be put into charts was a more difficult task than I thought. I have written notes and evaluations before but in class. When doing this for a real person, it made me think, *this is a person's life I am dealing with.* It would be put in the chart for other professionals to read. I had some difficulty at first with writing them, but by the end of the stack, I found it easier. I was able to pick out the important things to write about. Describing what I saw in group or on interaction was easier to record after completing a few progress notes and evaluations.

A client from the unit escaped yesterday. He was going with his doctor to the day treatment program that he was going to attend after discharge. When they got off the bus, the doctor went one way and the client went the other. The doctor let him go because he was ready to be discharged anyway; they were just waiting for the day treatment program plans to go through. This client was an English professor down South and decided to come up to New York with his partner. They felt that there were more opportunities up here. They were subletting an apartment and looking for jobs. They lost the sublet on the apartment soon after they arrived, which forced them to go into a shelter. Soon after, this client found out that his partner was HIV positive. His partner left him, and then he found out that he was HIV positive. Not long after this, he found out that he also had hepatitis. This client was in the hospital for depression. All I could think was, *Would not you be depressed, too?* This man had so many things happen in such a short period of time. He did not seem like he belonged in a hospital. It proved to me that there is a very fine line between mental stability and mental illness. Now I understand why the doctor did not chase after him.

Log 5. 6/2

Nancy was in a catatonic state when she came into the hospital, so I had been unable to interview or communicate with her. I was on the unit today when she came walking out of her room. The previous night, she ventured out to see the unit. I was so excited. She walked around the hall for a little while and then walked up to the schedule of groups. She looked at it for a few minutes. I walked up to her and introduced myself. She told me that she was interested in the activities on the unit. I explained the schedule to her and left it at that. I did not want to pressure her or force her into anything.

I told her when the next group would be, where it would take place, and that I would love to see her in there. The next group was the grooming group. This group would be very helpful for her. Since she had come in, she had not taken care of any of her activities of daily living. This was one of her goals while on the unit. I was so happy to see her. I was surprised to feel that way. I had not even talked with or communicated with her prior to this. However, I wanted to help her and so badly wanted to see her get well.

Log 6. 6/3

Nancy attended the grooming group on her own. She took the initiative and walked into the group to see what it was all about. She sat in the group and observed for a few minutes and said that she was going to watch for a little while because this was her first group and she was still feeling a little weak. After only a short time, she saw what was expected of her and figured out what she needed from us. When she felt more comfortable, she asked us for the necessary supplies to take care of her activities of daily living in her room. She even expressed a desire to take a shower. Before she left, she even painted her nails. This initiative of her activities of daily living, to me, was a huge step. She was on her way to recovery, and I was going to be there to support her. I was so happy for Nancy.

Log 7. 6/4

I really feel that I am getting to know the clients well. The clients will now approach me to talk or ask me questions. I feel as though I am creating a good rapport with most of them. They seem to trust me and feel comfortable with me. I, too, am feeling much more comfortable with them, not only because I know them better but also because I know the ways of the unit better. I know more of the processes (levels, discharges, and even medical terms) on the unit; therefore, I feel able to answer more questions and not have to look for support from others or redirect the clients to someone else if I do not know. My confidence in myself is obvious to the clients. Their trusting me and feeling comfortable with me coincide with my trusting myself and feeling comfortable with myself. They are very perceptive.

Log 8. 6/7

Today, some of my first clients were discharged from the hospital. I heard others say that you become attached to the clients and get used to seeing them around the unit. I felt so much for the ones that were leaving. I was excited for them, nervous, and worried all at once. They were moving on, but would they make it in the community? I was excited that they were getting back into life and would be able to see their families again, but I could feel their nervousness. One man was pacing the halls and biting his nails, anxiously waiting for his wife's arrival. Another man had his jacket on and bag packed waiting by the nurses' station for almost an hour before he was scheduled to leave. They were going back to their family members, some of whom brought them into the hospital, to try again. They were definitely nervous but had to move on and try to put their lives back together.

Log 9. 6/9

I led my first group on my own on Tuesday. It was the community task group. I felt as though it went very well. I did not know some of the clients very well because they were new to the unit, and I did not know the community tasks very well. I did not know every requirement of all of the jobs around the unit. Taking this into consideration, the group ran very smoothly. The group consists of having people volunteer for jobs to be done around the unit. These jobs include watering the plants, setting up snacks, and representing the community. After each of the jobs is assigned, each person in the group can voice any suggestions regarding the unit, complaints, comments, or compliments. The community representative makes a list of all of the comments and then presents them the following day at the community meeting to the entire staff and the rest of the clients. It is very interesting to hear the comments made by the clients. Sometimes, the client who seems the most disorganized will come up with a very important complaint. For instance, one client who did not speak much to the other clients, stayed in his room a lot, and seemed very preoccupied and distracted came up with the suggestion that people should not be wandering into other's rooms, especially at night. After he said this, other clients started to tell their own stories about waking up in the middle of the night to see another client standing in the dark, looking out the window. They spoke about how scary this can be. They are in an unfamiliar place, on a lot of medications, and in a psychiatric hospital that has scary and negative stereotypes associated with it. To wake up to find another client standing in your room would be a terrifying experience for anyone. The hospital is a place where the people should feel safe. Having others wander into your room would not give anyone this feeling of security. If people do not feel safe and trust the environment, their intervention could be compromised. It all goes back to creating rapport. Not only are rapport, trust, and security important, but clients need to determine that their needs will be met by the hospital itself, including all those that work on the unit. If they think that the staff is not keeping them safe, they will not trust them or rely on them for help.

At the end of the group I felt that we had all accomplished something. Each member gave his or her input and conversations were flowing. I feel that I facilitated conversations and expression of feelings well and also set limits when they needed to be set. I was comfortable with the clients and that, in turn, allowed them to feel comfortable with me.

Log 10. 6/11

In the staff meeting, we had an inservice on how to "take a client down" if he or she was becoming agitated. This was a follow-up from the meeting before where the staff spoke of violence on the unit, after a client became very agitated on the unit and hit a nurse. The attending doctor showed techniques on how to do this. I thought the inservice was a great idea, especially since most of the staff had not known how to do this. It just seems to me that this rehearsed technique would be very difficult to accomplish on the spur of the moment and very quickly. The inservice will be continued another time because there was not enough time to practice the technique and finish the instructions.

To be honest, the violence is scary but something that scares me more than the violence is the prevalence of HIV-positive clients on the unit. This is related to the violence, in that if someone is cut or hurt and begins to bleed, this could be very dangerous to those involved. I could not believe when I heard that 90% of the population on the unit was HIV positive. This may seem strange, but if I were to get hit in the face, I know that it would heal because broken bones are fixable, HIV is not. I realize that universal precautions are always to be taken, but what if something happens suddenly, without notice? During the grooming group, I had to go with someone to his room to watch while he shaved. Going in, I knew he was HIV positive and had hepatitis. I was scared. I wore gloves as I was supposed to, but what if an accident occurred? What if he cut himself and when I took the razor back from him, there was a slipup of some sort?

Log 11. 6/13

I walked into the day room to introduce myself to a new client. When I walked in, there were a few clients that I already knew and another person that looked like a visitor. I thought to myself, *it is not visiting hours, so why is that person in the day room now?* I went back to the nurses' station and asked if anyone had seen the new client, Gina. A nurse told me that she had just seen her in the day room. She told me that she was wearing a yellow shirt and blue pants and had her face all made up. I went back into the day room and, to my surprise, the person that I thought was the visitor was Gina.

I learned some information about Gina in the team rounds that morning. I found out that she is a social worker and a therapist and has been practicing for 17 years. She had some problems with alcohol in the past but had been treated for them. Gina was brought into the hospital because she was expressing suicidal thoughts after having drunk two bottles of wine by herself. A friend found her in her closet. Gina was very depressed. When I saw her, I thought, *How could this happen to someone with a background like hers? She is a social worker. She should be helping the clients that were sitting around her in the day room, not watching television with them, waiting for groups to start.*

When I approached her, she gave me a big smile and said, "Hi." I asked her if I could speak with her for a few minutes, and she agreed. I told her about the unit and gave her the orientation packet. I felt awkward giving it to her because I felt she could probably teach me about a unit like this one. She looked at the orientation packet and asked if she could take it with her when she leaves because she starts up and runs many programs and would like to use the ideas in the packet as a reference and a guide. She also told me that she came to this particular hospital, rather than going to a hospital closer to where she lived, because she was known in the field where she lived and wanted to maintain her confidentiality. We had a very pleasant conversation and she seemed more like a staff member.

Gina left the next day because her insurance would cover only three days in the hospital. She went into a rehabilitation center for her alcohol problems. She knew that this was what she needed and had already picked out a center for herself. I really wonder what it was like for her to stay in a hospital like this one. How did she feel being on the other side of the fence? Would she change the way she dealt with clients after being one herself?

Log 12. 6/16

During my second week of my internship, someone was admitted to the unit who had been there previously, not too long ago. The interns that were finishing up their internships and showing me the ropes had worked with her previously. The first thing they said was, "You are going to have your hands full with this patient." Sheila was a 17-year-old woman who had been diagnosed with schizophreniform disorder. She was getting into trouble because she had been smoking a lot of marijuana and cigarettes. Her grandmother was worried and had her admitted because her behavior was bizarre. The client told me she was here because her "grandmother thinks I smoke too much weed." But, she informed us that she was not going to give it up. There was nothing wrong with it. Unfortunately, she really believed this. Her mother is a drug addict, and her father abuses drugs and alcohol. Her grandmother raised Sheila, but both her mother and father lived close by, allowing the client to see them often. This drug use was somewhat normal to her. After having her on the unit for a few days, I realized what the other interns meant when they said that she was going to be a handful. She was caught smoking on the unit, was soliciting sex for cigarettes, and finally eloped during her first week here.

Sheila, I found out, was hospitalized because of her bizarre behavior and not just for smoking too much "weed," as she told us. We found out that Sheila has a 2-year-old daughter and was found putting her finger in her daughter's vagina and then in her own mouth. How could she think she was in here for smoking weed and cigarettes?

Not 10 days after she eloped from the unit, she was back. The police brought her in in handcuffs. She got right back to her old ways. She was caught smoking twice in one day, her second day here. No one on staff could figure out from where she got the cigarettes. We found out later that the last time she was here, she "stashed" a couple of cigarettes on the unit, and they were still there when she came back.

When talking to this girl, it seems as though everything goes right over her head. She does not have any insight into her illness and the things she does. You could tell her not to do something five times, but she will do it anyway. I just wonder what goes on in her head. All she wants to do is smoke and get out of the hospital. She wants this so badly that she attempted to elope again. This time a nurse who recognized her caught her in the elevator. As much as things seem to go right over her head, she is very manipulative and knows exactly what is going on. What can be done to help this girl? How do you help her gain insight into her illness when she will not even talk about it? What is this girl's future going to be like?

I find it very difficult and frustrating to work with Sheila. Nothing I say is heard. I believe this girl has more of a conduct problem. She is a teenage girl that has lived in the city all of her life. She hangs out on the streets with friends that have the same interests as she does. I have a tendency to avoid her. She is not allowed to participate in groups because of her inappropriate conduct, such as testing limits by trying to elope and stealing objects; she has little contact with others on the unit, unless she wants something. I try to check in on her daily, but all I get is an attitude from her. She has a very good way of making one feel that he or she is a bother to her or interrupting her when approached. I guess I avoid her because I do not know what to do with her. I do not know how to motivate her or even get her to listen to anything that I say. It makes me feel better that all of the other team members have the same difficulty and that it is not just my own lack of knowledge or expertise. I would really love to do something for

Sheila and help her in some way, but I do not know if it is possible. Is it something that she may grow out of when she becomes mature? Or is this who she is for life?

Log 13. 6/18

Denise was diagnosed with paranoid schizophrenia and has spent most of her time in her room. She stays in bed with the covers over her head and avoids contact with others as much as possible. Just recently, she has begun to emerge from her room every couple of days. I have approached her many times in her room and tried to encourage her to come to groups. At first, she would ignore me and keep the covers over her head. Now, she is more attentive and acknowledges my presence. I stopped her in the hallway one day to comment on her being showered and dressed and out on the unit. I said to her, "Denise, you look great all showered and dressed." She said, "Yeah? Well, I feel pretty good." We got into a long conversation about her showering and the problems she is having. She opened up and told me many things I could not find out from the chart. For instance, she spoke of her old boyfriend, who died of AIDS five years ago, and how it affected her. She spoke of her fear of AIDS and fear regarding the future. The conversation ended with our talking about the things she feels that she wants to work on for herself while in the hospital. It was amazing that she was much more motivated to help herself when she chose what it was that she wanted to work on. Even though I knew that these things needed to be worked on and knew that her intervention plan actually consisted of most of the same goals, it took her realizing and stating them herself to become motivated. One of the things she told me was that the shelter where she lived may not take her back because of her temper and anger and how she expresses them. She said that she really needs to learn how to control her anger so she can move back there and not be stuck without a place to live. We, together, came up with a plan for Monday. We would look at some of the information I have regarding stress and anger management techniques and come up with a way for her to express her anger in a more constructive manner. She seemed so happy that not only would we be working on something that could help her get her living arrangements back but also that she would be working on something that pertains directly to her. She stated that the groups are not helpful to her because she feels that they are not related to her and therefore a waste of time. We set up a time for me to come to her room and talk about our plan further. It was so great to see her smile and look interested in something. I also felt great that I was actually making progress with her. I felt that I was conducting effective intervention now and, I hope, making a difference in this one client's life. But we will see how receptive she is on Monday when I approach her about this. Was this just her mood or is she really interested in doing this for herself?

Log 14. 6/22

Well, I found out that Denise really does have an interest in working on her anger management but has a problem with motivation.

I went to her room on Monday to talk about how we would work on her anger management techniques. She was in bed, with the covers over her head, as usual. But this time, when I walked in her room and reminded her that we were going to talk about her anger, she actually sat up. I had picked out some anger and stress management worksheets to give to her. I showed them to her, and she thought they looked interesting. I gave her a time frame and asked if she would look at them that night since she stated that she was too tired to work on them at that time. She said she would try to work on them, and we decided that we would meet the following day to talk. I thought that giving her the worksheets to fill out on her own would give her some control as to how much time she wanted to put into it and when she wanted to work on them.

I went to see her the next day, and she had not looked at them. It is so difficult to judge her moods and motivation level. That afternoon, she attended groups and was very motivated. I always try to give her as much positive reinforcement as possible when she shows interest in groups, attends to activities of daily living, or even gets out of bed. I always tell her that she looks great when she showers and gets dressed, and I let her know when she does well in group. She always seems surprised but takes the compliment well. I have noticed a difference in her behavior, but her motivation level is always the deciding factor in how much she participates.

She has yet to fill out the worksheets. I have figured out that giving her complete control over the situation is not working. She is a person that may need more structure. Since she has shown a genuine interest in working on her anger management, she will complete the task but may need me there to work on it with her. I am going to try to sit down with her and help fill them out. I will let her set up the time that we meet. I feel that it is so important to give her some control because she has so little control in her life right now.

Log 15. 6/24

I saw Denise in the hall today, not doing anything. I asked her if we could sit down and work on anger management worksheets. We completed the worksheets. She did very well. She needed help identifying the signs of when she was becoming angry, but as we spoke, she began to recognize them. Later, she could describe them perfectly to me. As we proceeded, she identified things that make her angry and how she would normally deal with them. One thing that Denise loves to do is draw. She identified drawing as one way to express herself when she feels like doing something she may regret. Drawing helps her express other emotions such as sadness and anxiety. She came up with excellent, alternative ways of expressing her anger and many techniques on how to deal with her anger. She thought of counting to 10, taking deep breaths, and just turning and walking away from a situation before she does something. She knows how she is to deal with certain situations but has a lot of difficulty using these techniques. She seems to be a person who does not think before she acts. She has very little impulse control. The reasoning behind this intervention is so that she can begin to recognize that she is becoming angry and, I hope, remember that there are alternative ways of acting. She needs to act on her anger, not react to it.

Log 16. 7/1

The new residents, psychology interns, and attending doctors started today. I hope that this can be a new start. The team rounds used to be so tense because some members of the team did not like some other members who now have left. The team meeting seemed much more pleasant this morning. This could be a time for us to really make ourselves known to the team. We have already done that, but coming in new to a team that has been together for a while automatically put us at a disadvantage. We have to build a rapport with team members as well as clients, in order to feel confident and comfortable enough to work together. Now, the new team members are not familiar with the clients and we are the ones who know them very well. I spoke to the psychology interns on the team and let them know that we can help them out with getting to know the clients. I believe that the occupational therapy interns know the clients as well if not better than some of the other team members do, because we see them in so many different situations. We run so many different kinds of groups and see them using many different skills and thought processes.

Log 17. 7/7

Sheila continues to test limits and has little insight into her problems. I have tried to build rapport with her but to no avail. She does as she pleases and speaks only to those who she thinks can help her. She spoke to me one day regarding her hospitalization and then requested to have a copy of my keys for the doors on the unit so she could get out. It is very difficult to reach and influence her. Things had been fine between her and me, and we had a little bit of a therapeutic relationship. The other day I saw her coming out of another client's room. I asked her what she was doing in his room. She nonchalantly asked me if I had seen Victor. I told her that he was in a group, and that she should not be in another person's room. Clients are not allowed in each other's rooms. She said she understood and walked away. Not two minutes later, I walked past the same man's room to find her coming out of the room a second time after I reminded her that it was against the rules to do so. She looked as though she was hiding something in her hand. She denied being in the room as well as having something in her hand. I had to tell the nursing staff because this client was in special care and had a history of stealing from others as well as not abiding by the rules. The nursing staff approached her about the situation.

On the following day, I approached Sheila to check in with her to see how she was doing. She told me that she did not want to speak to me because I got her into trouble by telling on her. I told her that we all work as a team in the hospital, and I needed to tell the team about what I had seen. Thinking about it later, I think that I should have told her that she was the one who got herself into trouble by doing what she knew she was not supposed to do and that, no matter who catches her, the entire team will know. It bothered me that she said that she was not speaking to me because I got her into trouble, because having a good rapport with her is so important. It bothered me to think that one of my clients would not trust me or had a problem with me. I guess I have to realize that I am not there to be buddies with the clients; I am there to help them. If it means telling the nursing staff about what someone is doing, then I must do it. It seems that nobody has been able to get through to her, so I should not take it personally.

Log 18. 7/9

I set up a schedule of activities that Denise must attend. This is the person that has been in bed and not participating on the unit. Since I figured out that giving her structure usually helps her, I thought that this schedule would give her that extra push. I set up the schedule because the team informed Denise that if she participated in groups and was more visible on the unit, they would refer her to a rehabilitation setting, Denise enthusiastically told me. We set up the schedule together to ensure that she would be attending the groups that she needed. She required encouragement to attend the groups, but she went. Her medication was also changed. She felt that this medication adjustment helped her a lot. The new attending doctor who had worked with her in the past believed that her previous medication regime was more effective.

Denise did very well in the groups. She was now the client that led the conversations and initiated interaction most frequently. This is a change for her. I felt so proud of her, as a parent would for a child. Every time she progressed, I would boast about it to the other interns. Denise showed that she might do well in rehabilitation. She was allowed to participate in the outdoor group walks. I was so happy to be there when the nurse told her that she could go. She was so excited and jumped right out of bed. I was so happy for her. I hope that she continues to do well.

Log 19. 7/13

During school, there was always a debate about what people receiving intervention should be called. Do we call them *patients*, *clients*, or something else? There is a very vocal client on the unit that is close to discharge. He is now attending an outpatient program for a few days for a transition period. He will attend it full time when he is discharged. He came back to the unit after one of his intervention sessions and told me that the staff at the outpatient program referred to him as a *client*. He thought that *client* was a much more appropriate term for people than *patients*. He said that they are clients because they are involved in their intervention and they pay for what they receive. I thought that this was very insightful. I had thought about it before from the point of view of the patient but never had a patient actually say that he or she preferred to be called a *client*. Calling people *patients* automatically implies that they need to be taken care of and that they have debilitating problems. Many of the people on the unit will leave the hospital and be able to function independently and not need full-time help anymore, except for medications.

Log 20. 7/19

One of my clients that I had worked intensely with left today. This client had a lot of issues to deal with. She had been diagnosed with paranoid schizophrenia and had a long history of polysubstance abuse. She had improved on the unit and started to attend groups and interact much more. She was transferred to a rehabilitation program for a month and then was going back to her residence. I was so happy to see her improve so much on the unit. I am happy that she is going into rehabilitation, but I cannot help but think about what will become of her after she gets out of the rehabilitation program. I made an effort to work on things that were important to her in order to provide some motivation for her. We talked about what she could do after she returns to her residence to keep from coming back into the hospital, such as recognizing her signs and symptoms of her illness and what to do when she does recognize that these signs are emerging.

One thing in particular that worries me is that her boyfriend also lives in this residence, and he uses drugs with his friends. He will even use when she is around, knowing that she has a problem with them. We spoke about what she could do to avoid using and she came up with some very good answers, such as leaving her boyfriend or walking out of the room when he was using. When I asked her if she could follow through with any of these she said that she hoped she could but she did not know. I do not know if she could either. Will all the help she was receiving in the hospital and then in the rehabilitation program be for nothing? Will she end up back here the week she gets home from the rehabilitation program? I really feel that I worked on many things with her and spoke to her about many pertinent issues regarding her discharge, such as recognizing her signs and symptoms of her illness, medication management, and stress and anger management. I do not know if any of them sunk in for her. I hope that she remembers some of it, even if it is just one thing that will help her stay out of the hospital.

Log 21. 7/26

It is very frustrating when I feel that what I am saying in team rounds is important and others do not seem to feel that way. I was talking about a client in the meeting when some of the other team members started glancing at each other as if they were bored and one of them actually took out some photographs and began to look at them. I continued to speak and kept glancing in their direction, hoping that they would get the hint. The attending doctor even looked that way a few times. I try to give everyone the respect they deserve when they are speaking during the meeting. Each discipline brings something different to the table. Each discipline looks at different aspects of the clients and can help the clients in unique ways. I feel that I deserve respect from the other members.

I continued to speak to the rest of the team and got my point across. I want to give the two staff members who seemed bored the benefit of the doubt, that I was misinterpreting what I sensed from them, but if it happens again, I will have to bring it to their attention.

Log 22. 7/28

I was running the leisure group with the other interns. Dave wanted to draw. He began to draw a picture and was very intense and involved with this work. At one point, another person in the group asked him what he was drawing. Dave completely ignored his question. He asked a couple of times and then gave up. I was sitting next to Dave. I told him that Michael was speaking to him and that I did not know if he heard him. He said that he heard him but he did not know what he was drawing. He was just putting on paper what came to his head, and he did not know what the outcome was going to be. Dave is usually very pleasant and friendly. It was not like him to be so unapproachable and intense. He did not say anything the rest of the group and kept all of his attention on his drawing. After the group, I went in to talk with Dave to see how he was feeling. We sat down and he opened up so much to me. First he told me that he was exhausted from drawing that picture. He told me that he was drawing a flashback he has had about the house he grew up in. He continued to talk about all of the bad memories he had from that house and growing up. He explained that he is now claustrophobic because his parents used to keep him locked up in his room in the house and not let him out. He also spoke about how his parents always called him stupid and would compare him to his brother all the time. This intense and angry man suddenly seemed so vulnerable. He seemed like a little boy again.

Log Summary. 8/11

This 12-week internship has been one of extensive learning, finding out about myself, and learning to work with others. Keeping a journal has allowed me to follow what occurred during those 12 weeks and what I learned during that time. It displays the progression of clinical reasoning, ability to apply clinical knowledge, and confidence in my knowledge and myself.

It seems that, when I started, I was very concrete. I looked at the clients and thought about my textbooks from school. I tried to follow the "usual" procedure for intervention, how the client would present, and what the outcome should be. I soon learned otherwise. The knowledge learned in school is a foundation on which a new knowledge base will be built with experience. This new knowledge comes only from interacting with the clients and learning about them as individuals.

In looking through my logs, one recurring theme is empathy. In the beginning, it seems that I looked at the clients as clients that needed to be fixed. As time went on, I looked past the client and saw the person. I saw beyond my original fears and the stigmas. I found myself standing in his or her shoes. How does it feel to be going through something like this? What makes them tick? What do they like? What was their past like? This is all related to creating rapport. Sometimes, it is difficult to build rapport. With some clients, it happened very quickly and with others, it took some time to get to know them.

I began to take "bits and pieces" of what was learned in school and "fit" them to an individual. Not all people are textbook cases. Each person is an individual with his or her own symptomatology. More important, each person deems different things as important in life. These are the things that the therapist must focus on.

I found that it is easier to motivate an individual when the individual has a genuine interest in what the task is. I found this out by first deciding, on my own, what would be best to work on with a client. When the client was not responding to my pleas to participate in groups or individual sessions and would rather stay in bed all day, I knew something had to change. Somehow, I knew it was not going to be the client. She or he was not going to wake up and jump out of bed the next time I approached, ready to work on what I have been trying to work on for the past week. I had to adjust something. I thought I should find out what is most important to this person and then take it from there. More often than not, this worked. The client was finally given some control in what was very often a very out-of-control life.

In the beginning, decision making was a task that took a lot of thought and consideration. I would have to consider many different ways to intervene in order to achieve the best solution. After I did this in my head or even sometimes on paper in my logs, I would go to the other interns and ask what they thought about a situation. I questioned my own knowledge and did not trust my own thoughts and decisions. After deliberation, we would get all options out in the open and I would end up with my original decision. After doing this a few times, I realized that I was able to accomplish this decision-making task on my own.

It was not until later that I realized that my decision-making abilities were getting much quicker and that my fellow interns helped me to develop clinical reasoning. Expressing my thoughts and ideas to the others allowed me to hear them out loud and to also consider their opinions. The task of making decisions has become less thought out. I have the knowledge to consider both sides, make the decision, and be confident in my choice, in a timelier manner. This clinical reasoning and judgment have developed over the period of 12 weeks and will continue to develop with experience.

CLIENT-CENTERED REASONING ACTIVITIES FOR CHAPTER 14

1. Now that you have written between the lines, summarize what you wrote by identifying major themes in your writing. Break into groups and share your themes with your class-mates. Discuss how you would address these themes and problem solve around them.
2. Identify types of clinical reasoning.
3. Create your own futuristic log of your internship. Include a separate entry for each of the following issues. You may insert other entries, as you wish. When appropriate, you may wish to describe what happens, how you reacted to what happened, how you felt and what you thought about what happened, what problems arose, and how you circumvented the problems. Save your futuristic log and compare it to your real experience.

    Log 1. Describe your thoughts, feelings, and reactions to beginning your internship.

    Log 2. Describe the setting you are assigned to. Include the following: the funding, population served, mission statement, number of clients, number of staff members, number of students, location, type of facility, types of staff members and their educational backgrounds, hours that you will work there, hours of operation, and anything else you would like to describe.

    Log 3. Describe your first day.

    Log 4. Describe a supervisory session.

    Log 5. Describe your first interview with a client.

    Log 6. Write about your first team meeting.

    Log 7. Explain how you would work with others.

    Log 8. Describe your work with someone with whom you overempathize because you have an issue in common and you are still sensitive about this issue in your own life.

    Log 9. Describe how it is to treat a very sad, depressed person.

    Log 10. Describe the first team meeting where you had to present input.

    Log 11. Describe your first group.

    Log 12. Describe your typical day.

    Log 13. It is now midterm. Obtain a copy of your professor's evaluation and score yourself on the midterm. What areas do you think you would be good at? What areas do you think you might be having a problem with at this point in the internship? What help would you like to have to improve your skills in these areas?

Log 14. Describe what your student seminar would be like back at school. What would you talk about? What would your friends' experiences be like.

Log 14a. Describe an instance where you had to set limits with a client.

Log 14b. Describe an instance where you had to set limits with a staff member.

Log 15. Describe your work with a client in denial.

Log 16. Describe how you handled a sexually inappropriate client.

Log 17. Describe how you got a resistant client to participate in your treatment.

Log 18. Describe how you dealt with an angry client.

Log 19. Describe how the presentation of your student project would go. To whom would you be speaking? What would you be speaking about?

Log 20. You just received your final evaluation. Are you going out to celebrate or are you staying for an extra week to finish honing those hard-to-achieve skills? List your areas of strength at this time. What areas of difficulty may affect your next internship?

Log 21. Describe your last day.

Log 22. Write a log summary of your internship experience.

4. Throughout this book many client-centered reasoning activities have required you to identify the types of clinical reasoning you used in various situations (assessments, occupational performance analyses, intervention plans, discharge plans, referrals, and group protocols). Which type of clinical reasoning did you use the most frequently? The least frequently? How did your use of clinical reasoning types change over the course of this book? Did you use more of a variety of clinical reasoning types as you progressed through the book? Did you change from using predominantly one type to a different type? Which types of clinical reasoning would you like to improve on in the future? For each type, list skills that you would like to cultivate to improve your clinical reasoning in this area.

Index